ZACCAGNINI & WHITE'S

Core Competencies for Advanced Practice Nursing

A Guide for DNPs

Diane M. Schadewald

DNP, MSN, RN, WHNP-BC, FNP-BC, CNE

Clinical Professor Emeritus
University of Wisconsin-Milwaukee
School of Nursing

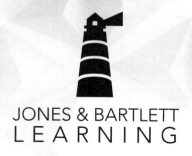

JONES & BARTLETT
LEARNING

World Headquarters
Jones & Bartlett Learning
25 Mall Road
Burlington, MA 01803
978-443-5000
info@jblearning.com
www.jblearning.com

Jones & Bartlett Learning books and products are available through most bookstores and online booksellers. To contact Jones & Bartlett Learning directly, call 800-832-0034, fax 978-443-8000, or visit our website, www.jblearning.com.

28842-1

Production Credits

Vice President, Product Management: Marisa R. Urbano
Vice President, Content Strategy and Implementation: Christine Emerton
Director, Product Management: Matthew Kane
Product Manager: Tina Chen
Director, Content Management: Donna Gridley
Manager, Content Strategy: Orsolya Gall
Content Strategist: Christina Freitas
Content Coordinator: Samantha Gillespie
Director, Project Management and Content Services: Karen Scott
Manager, Project Management: Jackie Reynen
Project Manager: Roberta Sherman
Program Manager: Dan Stone
Senior Digital Project Specialist: Angela Dooley
Senior Product Marketing Manager: Lindsay White
Content Services Manager: Colleen Lamy
Senior Director of Supply Chain: Ed Schneider
Procurement Manager: Wendy Kilborn
Composition: S4Carlisle Publishing Services
Project Management: S4Carlisle Publishing Services
Cover & Text Design: Briana Yates
Senior Media Development Editor: Troy Liston
Rights & Permissions Manager: John Rusk
Rights Specialist: Liz Kincaid
Cover & Title Page Image: © Comaniciu Dan/Shutterstock
Printing and Binding: CJK Group

Library of Congress Cataloging-in-Publication Data

Names: Schadewald, Diane Marie, editor.
Title: Zaccagnini & White's core competencies for advanced practice nursing
  : a guide for DNPs / [edited by] Diane M. Schadewald.
Other titles: Doctor of nursing practice essentials | Core competencies
  for advanced practice nursing
Description: Fifth edition. | Burlington, MA : Jones & Bartlett Learning,
  [2024] | Preceded by The doctor of nursing practice essentials / [edited
  by] Mary Zaccagnini, Judith M. Pechacek. Fourth edition. 2021. |
  Includes bibliographical references and index.
Identifiers: LCCN 2023020123 | ISBN 9781284288391 (paperback)
Subjects: MESH: Education, Nursing, Graduate | Advanced Practice
  Nursing--education | Clinical Competence | Nurse Clinicians | Nurse
  Practitioners | United States | BISAC: MEDICAL / Nursing / General
Classification: LCC RT75 | NLM WY 18.5 | DDC 610.73071/1--dc23/eng/20230714
LC record available at https://lccn.loc.gov/2023020123

6048

Printed in the United States of America
27 26 25 24 23   10 9 8 7 6 5 4 3 2 1

This book is dedicated to my colleague, Mary Zaccagnini, and in memory of Kathryn Waud White who together envisioned the value of and need for a text to describe how the 2006 AACN *Essentials* of Doctoral Education were actualized in practice. I had the privilege to contribute to the first four editions of this book and am honored to be able to serve as an author/editor of this fifth edition. I hope this edition will be found to be as useful for Doctor of Nursing Practice students and faculty as the previous editions.

This book is also dedicated to all of my current and future DNP colleagues, especially those who so graciously gave of their time and volunteered to author chapters for this book.

—Diane

Brief Contents

Contents

PART 1 The Essentials   1

CHAPTER 1 Knowledge for Nursing Practice 3
Adrienne M. Markiewicz, DNP, RN, AGACNP-BC, CHSE

CHAPTER 2 Person-Centered Care 27
Jeana M. Holt, PhD, DNP, MSN, RN, FNP-BC, APNP

Carol Flaten, DNP, RN, PHN, Clinical Associate Professor
Stephanie Gingerich, DNP, RN, CPN, Clinical Assistant Professor

Catherine Tymkow, DNP, MS, APN, WHNP-BC

CHAPTER 5 Quality and Safety. 151

Carol G. Klingbeil, DNP, RN, APNP, CPNP-PC, CNE
Carolyn Ziebert, DNP, RN, PCNS-BC

CHAPTER 6 Interprofessional Partnerships 181

Cheri Friedrich, DNP, RN, CPNP-PC, IBCLC, FNAP, FAAN
Diane M. Schadewald, DNP, MSN, RN, WHNP-BC, FNP-BC, CNE

CHAPTER 7 Systems-Based Practice. .207

Sandra Petersen, DNP, APRN, FNP-BC, GNP-BC,
PMHNP-BE, FAANP
Amy Roberts, PhD, APRN, FNP, FAANP
Diane M. Schadewald, DNP, MSN, RN, WHNP-BC, FNP-BC, CNE

CHAPTER 12 DNP Project Types and Abstracts 353
Diane M. Schadewald, DNP, MSN, RN, WHNP-BC, FNP-BC, CNE

Foreword

The demand for nurses capable of delivering care at an advanced nursing practice level to meet society's needs for health care has fueled the expansion of DNP education. While regional practice differences exist, the need for standardization of a comprehensive and robust curriculum is necessary to ensure that every student can receive the same educational foundation and all employers can anticipate the same competencies in the nurses they hire to work at an advanced level. That standardization has now been provided by the American Association of Colleges of Nursing through their publication of *The Essentials: Core Competencies for Professional Nursing Education* (2021).

The *Essentials* are the result of collaboration between both practice and academic experts to identify meaningful competence at both the beginning level of nursing practice (level I) and the advanced level of nursing practice (level II). Ten domains for nursing practice are identified, reflecting long-standing expectations of nursing education that include incorporating knowledge of the physical and social sciences as well as professionalism and leadership expectations. Additionally, the domains represent requirements for all healthcare professionals identified by the Institute of Medicine's competencies (IOM, 2003) that were later described through the lens of nursing practice with the Quality and Safety Education for Nurses Competencies (Cronenwett et al., 2007, 2009).

The 10 domains of the *Essentials* are further defined by actual nursing practice expectations identified as competencies. Each competency contains subcompetencies specific to level I, which applies to those beginning nursing practice, and level II, which applies to those broadening their nursing career in one of the four advanced practice registered nurse (APRN) roles or in an advanced nursing practice specialty such as informatics, leadership, or population health. Additional enhancements to the structure provided by the *Essentials* includes eight concepts to be threaded across the curriculum and spheres of care that are a requirement of undergraduate nursing.

Zaccagnini & White's Core Competencies for Advanced Practice Nursing: A Guide for DNPs provides a comprehensive and detailed overview of the competencies that nurses practicing at an advanced level need to meet the demands of today's constantly changing, technology-driven, and culturally diverse world. Healthcare organizations expect competent practitioners with the ability to understand quality metrics and interpret and analyze data to drive change that improves care and processes and ensures safe, high-quality, consistent patient outcomes. Faculty, students, and clinicians will find that this text is an excellent resource to support their work in today's complex healthcare system. Each chapter carefully addresses the AACN *Essentials* domains at the competency and subcompetency levels, describing expectations and providing evidence-based strategies learners can employ as they gain knowledge, skills, and attitudes on the continuum of competence toward mastery.

Throughout the text, the role of the DNP in the translation of evidence into practice, the initiation of process improvement projects, and the evaluation of outcomes is emphasized through alignment with the national organizations that represent each role specialty as well as the standards set by the *Essentials*.

The textbook is written by nationally recognized nurse educators, nurse researchers, and thought leaders representing all the advanced practice nursing roles of the consensus model as well as the advanced nursing practice specialties. Contributors to this text come from all over the United States representing a diverse and broad view of DNP practice and education. Each chapter explores principles that guide readers to professional growth to build expertise at the graduate level as effective leaders, expert caregivers, proficient communicators, collaborative team members, and staunch patient advocates capable of improving care for individuals and populations as well as improving the systems in which they work. This textbook provides the resources needed for students to frame their professional nursing identity and build a strong foundation for their current and future nursing practice.

Gerry Altmiller, EdD, APRN, ACNS-BC, ANEF, FAAN
Professor, The College of New Jersey
Director, Quality and Safety Innovation Center at The College of New Jersey

References

American Association of Colleges of Nursing. (2021). *The essentials: Core competencies for professional nursing education.* Author.

Cronenwett, L., Sherwood, G., Barnsteiner, J., Disch, J., Johnson, J., Mitchell, P., Sullivan, D., & Warren, J. (2007). Quality and safety education for nurses. *Nursing Outlook, 55*(3), 122–131.

Cronenwett, L., Sherwood, G., Pohl, J., Barnsteiner, J., Moore, S., Sullivan, D., Ward, D., & Warren, J. (2009). Quality and safety education for advanced nursing practice. *Nursing Outlook, 57*(6), 338–348.

Institute of Medicine (IOM). (2003). *Health professions education: A bridge to quality.* National Academies Press.

Preface

With the development of the 2021 American Association of Colleges of Nursing's (AACN's) *The Essentials: Core Competencies for Professional Nursing Education*, a new edition of this time-honored text was vital. To provide continuity of the role this text has had in doctor of nursing practice (DNP) education and to honor the previous author/editors, the fifth edition of this text is titled *Zaccagnini & White's Core Competencies for Advanced Practice Nursing: A Guide for DNPs.*

The new AACN *Essentials* (2021) include eight concepts central to nursing, four spheres of care, and ten domains with competencies and subcompetencies associated with the domains for entry to practice (Level I competencies) and advanced-level nursing (Level II competencies). This text focuses on the AACN Level II competencies that advanced-level nursing education prepares graduates to meet and can serve as a guide for DNP students, graduates, educators, and policy makers. These AACN competencies are reflective of the quality and safety in nursing education (QSEN) competency domains of patient-centered care, teamwork and collaboration, evidence-based practice, quality improvement, safety, and informatics (Wang et al., 2022), and also correlate well with educational competencies for other healthcare professional roles (Jenkins-Weintaub et al., 2023).

It is understood that students in advanced-level nursing educational programs need to be competent at Level I in order to demonstrate Level II competencies. Therefore, any student in an advanced-level program having difficulty demonstrating Level II competencies may need evaluation of competency at Level I and remediation. In addition, because the four spheres of care identified by the new AACN *Essentials* are focused on the undergraduate level and Level I competencies there isn't an elaboration on the spheres of care in this text.

In this edition, all chapters are new and updated. Chapters cover all 10 domains as well as associated competencies and Level II subcompetencies essential for advanced practice nursing and advanced nursing practice specialties. Chapters 1 through 10 also include a description of concepts for nursing practice which were selected as highlighted in the domain of the particular chapter. Chapter 11 outlines a step-by-step template for the development of a DNP project. Chapter 12 includes more information on DNP project types as well as abstracts authored by DNP graduates practicing in advanced practice nursing roles and/or advanced nursing practice specialties.

Advanced nursing practice specialties include informatics, administration practice leadership, public health, population health, and health policy according to the AACN (2021). Students pursuing a degree in one of the advanced practice nursing specialties are most often being prepared at the DNP level. There is not a recognized abbreviation or titling for these specialties similar to abbreviation(s) and titling for those in advanced practice nursing roles. The AACN identifies advanced practice nursing (APN) roles as certified nurse practitioner, certified nurse midwife, certified clinical nurse specialist, and certified registered nurse anesthetist (AACN, 2021).

These are roles consistent with those identified by the 2008 Consensus Model (APRN Consensus Work Group, & NCSBN, 2008) which uses and promotes the title advanced practice registered nurse (APRN) as the overarching title and abbreviation for such roles. However, not all states are using APRN as the abbreviation to identify nurses in APN roles. To be inclusive, in this text, the abbreviation APN/DNP is used as appropriate for advanced-level nursing roles as well as specialties in regard to Level II competencies.

This text is authored by nurses who practice at an advanced level. Many of the authors have educationally achieved a DNP degree. The author for Chapter 2 also has a PhD as this degree combination (PhD, DNP) has been found to be complementary. One of the coauthors for Chapter 7 is an APN who obtained her PhD before the DNP degree was widely available.

For this edition, all of the chapter contributors, in addition to their APN role or advanced nursing practice specialty, are nurse educators who are implementing the new AACN *Essentials* as part of their academic role. I am grateful for each of these contributors who took hours of their already busy lives to author these materials. The abstract contributors are currently in clinical practice.

Purpose of the Text

This text is intended to serve as a core text for DNP students and faculty to use to achieve mastery of the AACN *Essentials* as well as a "shelf reference" for DNP-prepared nurses as they practice in their chosen field, advancing innovation and policy change in healthcare transformation. The AACN *Essentials* are all covered herein; each essential and associated competencies are covered in adequate detail to frame the foundation of the DNP educational program. This text provides the infrastructure for students, faculty, and those practicing with a DNP degree to achieve and sustain the highest level of practice. This text gives students the foundation necessary to enter into the highest level of practice in APN roles or advanced nursing practice specialties and develop that practice to the highest level possible for the benefit of patients and the health of the population. For faculty, this text provides a framework that they can partner with their creativity to make their own unique programs, different from each other but all coming to the same endpoint: graduates who practice at the clinical doctorate level. This text will support all DNP-prepared nurses to engage in advocacy, show leadership, and demonstrate the skills of clinical competency to ultimately impact and improve the health of the nation.

References

American Association of Colleges of Nursing. (2021). *The essentials: Core competencies for professional nursing education*. Author.

APRN Consensus Work Group & NCSBN. (2008). *Consensus model for APRN regulation: Licensure, accreditation, certification & education*. https://www.ncsbn.org/public-files/Consensus_Model _Report.pdf

Jenkins-Weintaub, E., Goodwin, M., & Fingerhood, M. (2023). Competency-based evaluation: Collaboration and consistency from academia to practice. *Journal of the American Association of Nurse Practitioners, 35*(2), 142–149.

Wang, T., Nelson, Y. M., Alexander, F., & Dolansky, M. A. (2022). Future direction of quality and safety competency-based education: Quality and safety education for nurses teaching strategies. Guest editorial, *Journal of Nursing Education, 61*(6), 287–288.

Contributors

Gerry Altmiller, EdD, APRN, ACNS-BC, ANEF, FAAN
Professor
Director, Quality and Safety
  Innovation Center
School of Nursing, Health, and
  Exercise Science
The College of New Jersey
Ewing, New Jersey

Emily Bartel, DNP, RN, FNP-BC, APNP
Family Nurse Practitioner
Froedtert Menominee Falls Hospital
Menominee Falls, Wisconsin

Joy Elwell, DNP, FNP-BC, APRN, CNE, FAAN, FAANP
Professor & Director DNP Program
University of Connecticut
School of Nursing
Storrs, Connecticut

Carol Flaten, DNP, RN, PHN
Clinical Associate Professor & Director
  of Pre-Licensure Nursing Programs
University of Minnesota
School of Nursing
Minneapolis, Minnesota

Cheri Friedrich, DNP, RN, CPNP-PC, IBCLC, FNAP, FAAN
Clinical Professor & Katherine R. &
  C. Walton Lillehei Chair
Coordinator of Pediatric Nurse
  Practitioner-Primary Care Specialty
Co-Director, Center for
  Interprofessional Health
University of Minnesota
School of Nursing
Minneapolis, Minnesota

Ashley D. Fry, DNP, AGACNP-BC, ACHPN
Palliative Medicine Nurse Practitioner
UCHealth
Colorado Springs, Colorado

Megan Galske, DNP, RN, AGPCNP-BC, APNP
Nurse Practitioner
SSM Health
Madison, Wisconsin

Stephanie Gingerich, DNP, RN, CPN
Clinical Assistant Professor
University of Minnesota
School of Nursing
Minneapolis, Minnesota

Suelhem A. Grochowski, DNP, RN, FNP-BC, APNP
Family Nurse Practitioner
Sixteenth Street Community Health
  Clinic
Milwaukee, Wisconsin

Amy Heidenreich, DNP, RN, AGCNS-BC, PMHNP-BC, APNP
Behavioral Health Advanced Practice
  Nurse
Psychiatry and Behavioral Medicine
Froedtert Hospital and the Medical
  College of Wisconsin
Milwaukee, Wisconsin

Jeana Marie Holt, PhD, DNP, MSN, RN, FNP-BC, APNP
Assistant Professor
University of Wisconsin-Milwaukee
School of Nursing
Milwaukee, Wisconsin

Carol Klingbeil, DNP, RN, CPNP-PC, CNE, APNP
Clinical Associate Professor & DNP
    Program Director
University of Wisconsin-Milwaukee
School of Nursing
Milwaukee, Wisconsin

Adrienne Marire Markiewicz, DNP, RN, AGACNP-BC, CHSE
Clinical Assistant Professor
University of Wisconsin-Milwaukee
School of Nursing
Milwaukee, Wisconsin

Lauren Petersen, DNP, MPH, APRN, CPNP-PC
Clinical Assistant Professor
University of Minnesota
School of Nursing
Minneapolis, Minnesota

Sandra Petersen, DNP, APRN, FNP-BC, GNP-BC, PMHNP-BE, FAANP
Professor & PMHNP Coordinator
University of Texas
College of Nursing and Health
    Sciences
Tyler, Texas

Amy Roberts, PhD, APRN, FNP-BC, FAANP
Professor
University of Texas
College of Nursing and Health
    Sciences
Tyler, Texas

Diane Schadewald, DNP, MSN, RN, WHNP-BC, FNP-BC, CNE
Clinical Professor Emeritus
University of Wisconsin-Milwaukee
School of Nursing
Milwaukee, Wisconsin

Catherine Tymkow, EdD, DNP, APN, WHNP-BC
Professor of Nursing
Governors State University
College of Health and Human Services
Department of Nursing
University Park, Illinois

Michelle Ullery, DNP, APRN, CNP
Faculty & DNP/FNP Program Director
Augsburg University
Department of Nursing
Minneapolis, Minnesota

Carolyn Ziebert, DNP, RN, PCNS-BC
Clinical Assistant Professor
University of Wisconsin-Milwaukee
School of Nursing
Milwaukee, Wisconsin

Contributors to Fourth Edition

A special thank you and recognition goes to those who contributed to the fourth edition of this book and whose work, in part, informed sections of the current text.

Laurel Ash, DNP, APRN, FNP-BC and Catherine Miller, DNP, RN, CNP
Interprofessional Collaboration for
    Improving Patient and Population
    Health

Robin R. Austin, PhD, DNP, DC, RN-BC and Anne E. LaFlamme, DNP, RN
Information Systems/Technology
    and Patient Care Technology for
    Improvement and Transformation of
    Health Care

Carol R. Eldridge, DNP, RN, CNE, NEA-BC

Nursing Science and Theory: Scientific Underpinnings for Practice

Angela Mund, DNP, CRNA

Healthcare Policy for Advocacy in Health Care

Jeanne Pfeiffer, DNP, MPH, RN, CIC, FAAN

Clinical Prevention and Population Health for Improving the Nation's Health

Mary E. Zaccagnini, DNP, APRN, ACNS-BC and Judith M. Pechacek, DNP, RN, CENP

A Template for the DNP Project

PART 1

The Essentials

CHAPTER 1

Knowledge for Nursing Practice

Adrienne M. Markiewicz, DNP, RN, AGACNP-BC, CHSE

> *"Our dilemma has not been what is known and how we come to know it (our epistemology)—rather our problem (or dilemma) has been how to express what we know in living/being nursing (our ontology) . . . the focus of our discipline— our epistemology—is not a "thing"—it is experience and process—or more accurately many particular manifestations of particular kinds of experiences or processes."*
>
> —**Peggy Chinn** (Chinn, 2019, pp. 3–4)

Introduction

Practice of nursing at the doctoral level is a highly complex, rich, multileveled experience that demands deeper insights if we are to effectively help our clients and represent our profession. Nursing knowledge is built on relevant science and theory. Understanding that foundation is central to effective advanced nursing practice. The reason we use science and theory in nursing is to improve practice and to positively impact the health of our patients (Parker & Smith, 2010).

Advanced practice nurses (APNs) provide care to patients across the entire continuum of health and illness. This practice may be directly patient-facing or may be related to systems management, informatics, public health, health policy, or executive leadership as performed by those with a doctor of nursing practice (DNP) in one of these advanced nursing practice specialties. Regardless of setting, nursing knowledge is a formative part of practice for APNs/DNPs. Despite this, APNs/DNPs struggle at times to articulate exactly "what" nursing knowledge is and to distinguish the science of caring from knowledge found in other disciplines. In the current model of health care, this distinction can be further devalued in favor of processes which favor and emphasize positivist, empiric knowing to the detriment of other ways of knowing. This struggle becomes more poignant in advanced practice as one performs tasks historically reserved for other disciplines. APNs look for actions and their consequences, believing that every effect has a discernible and, it is hoped, treatable cause, understanding that science is essential to clinical practice. However, clinical practitioners are often inclined to discard theory as too abstract for practical purposes and too broad to have meaningful application to daily nursing practice. DNP-prepared APNs bring specific expertise to their work, based on a very particular grounding in the scholarship of application and translational science. The APN/DNP must therefore be intimately familiar with the ways in which nursing knowledge is defined, formed, shaped, and integrated into the care of individuals and systems. This chapter will explore the formation of nursing knowledge and how the APN/DNP uses knowledge to impact the care of individuals, communities, and populations.

Nursing Knowledge Defined

If the APN/DNP is to create change by translating the body of nursing knowledge to practice, that translation must begin with a mastery understanding of nursing's beginnings and its disciplinary and scientific transformations. This process starts with the knowledge that the definition of nursing itself is continually becoming. As the actions entrusted to the nurse have expanded and the experience of health and illness have evolved over time, so has its definition, often dependent on the philosophical or professional paradigm of those responsible for shaping its trajectory. Parse (1997) wrote that nursing is a discipline organized around nursing knowledge and that the practice of nursing is a performing art. Rogers (1994) wrote that it is not the practice of nursing that defines nursing; rather, it is the use of nursing knowledge to improve the human condition. Reed (1997) proposed that, just as archaeology is the study of ancient things and biology is the study of living things, nursing is the study of promoting well-being. In a notable shift from the medical model, Reed's definition was independent of the presence or absence of disease. Perhaps, Newman, Sime, and Corcoran-Perry (1991) most sweepingly capture the concept as they write, "Nursing is the study of caring in the human health experience" (p. 3). While eloquent and aspirational, these definitions can be difficult to operationalize in the context of "real-world" constraints of clinical practice. Additionally confusing is the fact that despite a relatively well accepted metaparadigm, no one theorist has created an operational definition of nursing that has been universally accepted. Recently a growing coalition has attempted to create consensus around the term "nursology" in place of "nursing" as a descriptor for the science and the discipline, building upon the work of Paterson and Zderad (1988) and reinforced by Fawcett and colleagues (2015). This term, they argue, would be more consistent with other disciplines whose names describe the study of a phenomenon rather than the action that surrounds it.

If a universally accepted definition of nursing can't be found, how can nursing knowledge be defined? Nurses utilize several means or "ways" of obtaining knowledge; however, it first must be accepted that "knowing" is not a concrete destination, rather a continuing process of enlightenment. As nursing continues to seek academic and professional credibility among the healthcare disciplines, nurses must be cautious not to abandon more abstract ways of knowing in favor of those more concrete while understanding that scientific knowledge indispensably underpins everything nurses do. This is a paradox of advanced nursing practice. Several great minds have contributed to the body of literature describing how nurses know what they know, perhaps none more well known than Barbara Carper and Patricia

Benner. Carper's (1978) seminal work describes ways of knowing in nursing: empirics (science of nursing), aesthetics (art of nursing), personal knowledge in nursing and ethics (moral knowledge). These descriptions ultimately legitimized the idea that knowledge outside empirics was valid to inform and guide nursing practice. Importantly, Carper made clear in her description of these ways of knowing that all are essential for the development of the professional nurse; however, none alone are sufficient for nursing practice. Benner's novice to expert model (1984) further solidified that the nurse gains knowledge through experiential learning and reflection, a process that progresses to expertise, though not always in a directly linear fashion.

The American Association of Colleges of Nursing (AACN) renders a portrait of the DNP-prepared nurse through its newest essentials for advanced practice education (AACN, 2021). These competencies and subcompetencies scope the role, responsibilities, and core functions of advanced nursing practice. Knowledge for nursing practice is a foundational domain to this rendering and its realization is dependent on continual evolution of what is possible rather than a fixed destination of mastery. As said by Peggy Chinn in a keynote address at Case Western Reserve University to commemorate 50 years of nursing theory (2019),

> Consider for a moment the difference between what it means to "doctor a drink" and to "nurse a drink." We hardly need to go into the potential explanations of the differences—I have yet to encounter a person (at least a native English speaker) who does not immediately already understand this difference, and who also immediately knows the actions associated with each of these phrases. But notice that "doctoring" involves a "thing"—an action to change the character or effect of a drink. "Nursing" on the other hand is a process that requires many different actions and that can take many forms, depending on who is doing the "nursing" and where! Nursing the drink probably involves an action (sipping the liquid) but what happens to fill the spaces between sips is the real key to understanding what this phrase means—it involves a process that makes it acceptable, in the context of drinking the liquid, to keep the same drink going over a period of time—implicitly understood to be a social context. Note that the "in-between" actions cannot be anticipated in advance; these actions that fill in the time/space between sips depend entirely on what is called for and what is possible in the social space where the person is sipping on the drink. (pp. 4–5)

Nursing knowledge cannot be simplified to theory, nor completely captured in experience. Instead, theory and careful reflection through experience must guide the DNP-prepared nurse to engage with patients, communities, and populations.

Selected Concepts for Nursing Practice Represented in the Domain

Clinical Judgment

Clinical judgment, or the ability to make sound decisions about patient care, is an essential aspect of APN/DNP practice. Nursing knowledge forms the basis for clinical judgment. The decisions made by the APN/DNP must therefore be systematic and defendable, grounded in theory, informed by experience and reflection. APNs/DNPs must bring analysis and critical thinking to bear on a variety of patient problems, drawing from a broad base of knowledge in multiple scientific disciplines to synthesize the data and make creative inferences to help the client. They are prepared to do so by advanced education and training in their area of specialization. Furthermore, APNs/DNPs are guided in this complex reasoning process by nursing theories that shape and inform reflections and provide the foundation for clinical practice (Kenney, 2006).

Communication

Communication is an exchange of information and ideas through various modalities, including verbal and nonverbal mechanisms. Health and illness provide ample situations in which productive and effective communication is not only the ideal, but crucial to a good outcome or recovery of an outcome that is not optimal. Nursing knowledge in all its forms must underpin communication with patients, families, communities, and populations. It must also be the hallmark of communication with other healthcare disciplines to accomplish the goal of forward movement on the health continuum. APNs/DNPs are able to communicate with physicians, other nurses and the multidisciplinary team in a clear and concise manner, providing them with all necessary information about the patient's care and displaying leadership to manage the complex aspects of each case. The DNP-prepared APN must incorporate and synthesize facets of nursing knowledge into communication to be fully effective.

Ethics

Ethics is a fundamental aspect of the discipline of nursing and nursing knowledge plays a crucial role in informing the ethical decision making of APNs/DNPs. All nurses operate under the American Nurses Association Code of Ethics. The principles of autonomy, beneficence, nonmaleficence, and justice are foundational to the practice of APNs regardless of context. APNs/DNPs demonstrate mastery knowledge of the application of these principles in clinical practice. Even in complex and ethically nebulous situations, nursing's knowledge of the "whole" patient drives partnered decision making with the patient or surrogate decision maker. The APN/DNP is also able to seamlessly integrate medico-legal aspects of care into ethical care of patients. Ethical principles are also inextricably linked with the generation of new knowledge and its implementation into clinical practice through translational research. For example, an APN may care for a patient who is seeking access to assisted suicide. The APN's holistic care of the patient includes knowledge of the applicable federal and state laws governing this process and synthesis of legal procedures with the ethical implications of assisted suicide. This is inclusive of position statements from professional bodies and key stakeholders. Through this process, the patient receives care compatible with their beliefs and wishes via joint decision making within the established ethical and legal boundaries of health care.

Evidence-Based Practice

Nursing knowledge provides the foundation for the use of research and data to inform clinical decision making. Multiple studies indicate that an average of 17 years is required for evidence-based practices to be integrated fully into clinical care (Green et al., 2009). APNs/DNPs can reduce this gap by critically appraising new findings and acting as change agents in their practice areas. The holistic and systems-based thinking that guides the nursing discipline uniquely equips APNs/DNPs to lead change, guide implementation, and perform process evaluation in a wide variety of practice settings.

Level II Competencies of the Domain

Demonstrate an Understanding of the Discipline of Nursing's Distinct Perspective and Where Shared Perspectives Exist With Other Disciplines

Much of the controversy about nursing's disciplinary perspective centers on the distinctiveness of nursing's body of knowledge, particularly its differentiation from medical science. The study and practice of medicine focuses on the diagnosis and treatment of disease. Nursing focuses on the human response to illness and its treatment. Yet, medicine and nursing overlap at many points, and seemingly even more so in advanced practice nursing. Do medicine and nursing truly differ in anything besides mere scope of practice.

Newman and colleagues (2008) explored this very question by examining the evolution of the disciplinary focus over time. They describe a receptive phase in which nursing knowledge was primarily a composition of pieces of knowledge obtained from other disciplines. This led to a self-generative phase in which nurse theorists began to concentrate on disciplinary nursing knowledge. Finally, nursing knowledge underwent a transformative phase, wherein nursing knowledge not only impacted nursing practice but informed the perspective of other disciplines. Much of early nursing knowledge followed a positivist perspective by controlling and testing reliable variables and emphasizing control and predictability. This reflected the dominance of the biomedical model of care. They argue that the advent of Rogers's *The Science of Unitary Human Beings* (Rogers, 1994) shifted the disciplinary perspective to one of "relationship," giving rise to other theories integrating the whole person as a unitary concept of health, where "pathology is relevant but not separate and dominant" (p. E17). As the focus becomes relationship, health, caring, consciousness, mutual process, and patterning, presence, and meaning emerge as central concepts to the disciplinary perspective. This is not to the detriment of biomedical knowledge; rather, the APN/DNP must unify biomedical knowledge with the insight of their personal worldview and must do so without devaluing either perspective. The future of advanced practice nursing is not absorption into the biomedical model to the exclusion of relationship nor is it rejection of empiric data in favor of intuition. In writing about an expanded view of health, Jean Watson said, "The evolved future becomes large enough to hold the paradox of both side by side" (Watson, 2007, p. 14). It is indeed the nurse–patient relationship that must unite the discipline through all roles and practice settings.

As APNs/DNPs articulate this disciplinary perspective, common ground with other disciplines can and should be achieved. Nursing shares many central concepts with other disciplines. A wonderful example of this is the presence of Orem's

Self-Care Deficit Theory (1971) in the multidisciplinary literature. Orem describes the phenomena in which a patient's capacity to self-manage their condition is overwhelmed, which can be due to a variety of factors. The patient is viewed not as a dependent or othered into the "sick" role, but rather as reliable, responsible, and capable of seeing to their own health needs if equipped with the correct tools. The nurse–patient relationship is pivotal for the acquisition of education and skills needed by the patient to self-manage their condition and promote their own health. These requisite actions are known as "activities of daily living" (ADLs). Orem's theory continues to be central to the nursing care of many populations (Mohammadpur et al., 2015; Isik & Freland, 2021; Drevenhorn et al., 2015); however, many components of Orem's work are on display as common ground in other disciplines, including physical therapy (Kongsted et al., 2021) and pharmacy (Van Eikenhorst et al., 2017; Cani et al., 2015; Dokbua et al., 2018), even if the theory itself is not explicitly referenced. Physical and occupational therapists seek to empower patients to regain mobility and the ability to perform ADLs, moving the patient to an improved state of health. This enables self-management of illness and ultimately, it is hoped, a return to health for the patient. Pharmacists provide medication teaching and consultation to patients to assist them in managing medication regimens. For many patients, these regimens can be incredibly complex, with a wide range of adverse effects and drug interactions. The pharmacist can intervene to empower the patient to self-manage their condition. As each discipline approaches patient care from a unique disciplinary perspective, mutual understanding of shared aims and connected purpose can drive a new healthcare team fueled by this multidisciplinary approach to patient care based on a shared perspective. Use of a multidisciplinary approach results in better outcomes for patients and populations (Clarke & Forster, 2015; Jo et al., 2017). The disciplinary perspective is key to a functional multidisciplinary team. This multidisciplinary approach will be further delineated in subsequent chapters.

APNs/DNPs are the keepers of the nursing disciplinary perspective in clinical practice, in the creation of systems of care, and in administrative decision making. The nurse–patient relationship centers the disciplinary perspective and should be at the forefront of shared ground with other disciplines. As Newman and colleagues conclude on the power of nursing's perspective in health care:

> Nurses are thirsting for a meaningful practice, one that is based on nursing values and knowledge, one that is relationship-centered, enabling the expression of the depth of our mission, and one that brings a much needed, missing dimension to current health care. What is missing in health care is what nursing can provide when practiced from the heart of our disciplinary perspective. (Newman et al., 2008, p. E25)

Translate Evidence From Nursing Science as Well as Other Sciences Into Practice

Knowledge translation is the process through which research is created, circulated, and adopted into clinical practice. This process is dynamic and involves a complex system of interactions between investigator, existing knowledge, and the audience to which knowledge is disseminated. An iterative approach is necessary but rarely results in a linear process (Curtis et al., 2017). For these reasons, the gap between existing science and the actions that occur individually and systemically in clinical practice can be incredibly wide. Furthermore, not all evidence generated is translatable. Evidence may lack generalizability, or the studied phenomena may be difficult to measure with rigorous methods. Distillation of the current literature on a particular topic into systematic reviews or clinical practice guidelines is one way to combat these issues; however, these findings or guidelines still require interpretation when held up to specific patient populations in a particular practice setting. In short, the question becomes one of operationalization.

Several models and frameworks exist for evidence translation. One particularly salient approach is described by Graham and colleagues (2006) as the knowledge to action cycle. This process is guided by two major phases: knowledge creation and the action cycle. DNP-prepared APNs have prominent roles in both of these phases, though this role is distinct from that of nurse scientists or researchers. Though DNP-prepared APNs do not generally create new knowledge in the form of primary research, they are very qualified to synthesize new knowledge created through research into relevant clinical practice guidelines, formal statements, or systematic reviews. This is a critical part of ensuring that available evidence is rigorous and well suited to address clinical problems. The action cycle follows knowledge generation and is comprises seven steps.

1. Identify the problem and relevant research.
2. Adapt research to the local context.
3. Assess barriers to using that knowledge.
4. Select, tailor, and implement interventions.
5. Monitor knowledge use.
6. Evaluate outcomes.
7. Sustain knowledge use.

DNP-prepared APNs first actualize the translation of evidence into practice by identifying clinical problems or gaps between available evidence and current patient-facing practice. Every practice setting has unique challenges in workflow, patient population, and resources. APNs are well positioned to identify and scope problems in real time, using organizational knowledge to identify and connect key stakeholders. While narrowing a clinical problem, the APN can utilize evidence-based practice (EBP) models to inform the approach. Several important EBP models can guide practice change. These models are further elaborated on in Chapter 4.

Knowledge must be adapted to the local context to be effective. Every institution has individual needs, resource limitations and patient-specific factors that influence how evidence can and should be applied. The DNP-prepared APN provides nursing perspectives on these factors as a primary source, not removed from practice but inextricably connected to it.

Change management requires a proactive approach to common barriers. APN/DNP-related barriers include limitations in understanding of terminology or evidence-based frameworks, lack of confidence, time constraints, and lack of support from colleagues or leadership. Organizational barriers include financial considerations, time constraints, and competing alternative priorities. While these are significant barriers, the largest barrier is the acceptance of established practice simply for its being "established practice" rather than practice informed by evidence. The challenge to the status quo is often the most intimidating part of translating evidence to practice, particularly for novice APNs.

The next step is to select, tailor, and implement interventions. The evidence should guide the options for available interventions and the local context should inform the decision of which option to choose. Often, new interventions require some upskilling of staff, new education, or re-education to be successfully implemented. Careful consideration of current state processes and the "ask" of change is needed. Does the intervention pose additional steps in a known process or involve a foundational change to workflow? How many staff may be affected? These questions and more should be assessed in detail prior to implementation and addressed within the implementation plan. The APN/DNP should expect that despite careful planning, unforeseen issues may arise during implementation. Should this happen, the APN/DNP should remain calm, flexible, and open to different approaches so long as the purpose of the project is not compromised. On occasion, even projects with the best intentions and well-laid plans are unsuccessful. This can be due to a variety of factors and should be carefully debriefed with the project team. Evaluation of efforts should be comprehensive with a focus on sustainability of the change.

Every project plan should include a plan for sustainability of the change. Teams can usually be easily engaged in solving short-term problems; however, the question of sustainability can pose a serious challenge to even the most experienced group of multidisciplinary professionals. Sustaining a process or practice change, even when evidence is strong and initial morale is high, can be incredibly taxing. Falling back on old knowledge, practices, and processes is human nature. APN/DNPs can mitigate this risk. Armstrong and Sables-Baus (2019) outline two focus points for sustainability in DNP-led team projects. First, the APN/DNP must ensure that the project aligns with the organization's mission, vision, values, and philosophy. This ensures greater stakeholder support beyond the initial push of a project, especially if further resources become needed. Second, the APN/DNP must ensure that resources exist to sustain the change and, if warranted, to spread it. Transparency with stakeholders and planning with sustainability in mind is crucial. Specific interventions to ensure continuance of the change will vary by project.

Demonstrate the Application of Nursing Science Into Practice

The APN/DNP first demonstrates the application of evidence to practice through the DNP project, the details of which are discussed elsewhere in this text. Beyond the initial DNP project, APN/DNPs must continue to forge new collaborations and find innovative ways to bring nursing science to bear in practice. One of the most important and effective ways this can be accomplished is through strategic DNP–PhD partnerships.

The APN/DNP must effectively apply nursing science into practice. As growth of DNP programs has exploded over the past decade, academic nursing has grappled with the role of a practice doctorate in scholarly inquiry, knowledge generation, and dissemination—roles traditionally held by nursing colleagues with a PhD. Role confusion and overlap, as well as competition for similar positions in organizations that do not fully realize the unique skillset of each can stagnate opportunities for uninhibited collaboration (Cowan et al., 2019). Though academic preparation is different, the common disciplinary perspective of nursing provides a common focus and opportunity for transcendent collaboration, with the PhD-prepared nurse as a research scientist and the APN/DNP as an expert in translation and implementation science (Falkenberg-Olson, 2019). DNP-prepared APNs are uniquely positioned not only to apply science from the nursing disciplinary perspective but to partner with PhD-prepared nurses to create and disseminate nursing science, each within their own role. This is one of the most effective strategies DNPs can use to ensure nursing science is applied and translated to practice.

PhD-prepared nursing colleagues offer a wide breadth and depth of skills in clinical inquiry, methods, data management, and analysis that complement the DNP-prepared nurse and can enhance the application of nursing science. **Table 1-1** highlights effective strategies for promoting DNP–PhD synergy.

Table 1-1 How to Promote DNP and PhD Collaboration

Goals or Impetus	Persons or Groups to Engage
Organization and Culture	
Create a supportive colearning environment based on mutual respect, trust, and credibility to enable DNP and PhD collaboration.	Facility leadership Nurse leadership Facility DNPs and PhDs
Employ an office or nursing leadership position to centralize resource utilization in facility and/or to coordinate unit projects and staff expertise.	Chief nurse of education Chief nurse of research Hospital-shared governance committee
Identify DNP- and PhD-prepared staff within facility.	Facility DNPs and PhDs
Identify DNP expertise such as using the electronic health record for retrospective chart reviews and PhD expertise such as conducting qualitative analysis.	Academic DNPs and PhDs Nursing education/research Shared governance council Unit practice management
Create academic practice partnerships (APPs) as research and scholarship teams to address facility issues.	Facility DNPs and PhDs
Through collaboration of facility, academic, and student DNPs and PhDs, identify quality improvement, EBP, or research projects.	Academic DNPs and PhDs
Project Specific	
Create brainstorming group of PhD and DNP nurses to address a topic or clinical problem and form a project team. Challenge team to focus on research that:	Shared governance members
■ Aligns with facility goals.	Facility leadership
■ Is translatable to clinical practice.	Designated nursing educators
■ Solves an existing problem.	Quality improvement

(continues)

Table 1-1 How to Promote DNP and PhD Collaboration   (*continued*)

Goals or Impetus	Persons or Groups to Engage
■ Demonstrates sustainability.	Research office
■ Advances the science of nursing.	Academic DNPs and PhDs DNP and PhD students
Focus projects on outcomes. Design a research study or quality improvement project that is:	DNP and PhD in partnership
■ Clinically relevant.	Project team members
■ Timely. ■ Useful to the population served.	Other key stakeholders (such as unit leadership)
Agree on roles, responsibilities, and time line.	Collaborating DNPs and PhDs
In collaborating, DNPs and PhDs should be flexible in working together and open to developments that make the end result meaningful to each other.	Project team members Other key stakeholders
Communicate on a regular basis such as at weekly meetings.	Facility DNPs and PhDs
Acknowledge strengths and unique contributions of each. Revise plans as appropriate.	Collaborating DNPs and PhDs
Build relationships with other disciplines to assist with PhD–DNP collaboration projects or teams.	Interprofessional stakeholders
Publications and presentations. ■ Before starting, determine the order of authorship.	Collaborating DNPs and PhDs
■ Determine which author will coordinate and serve as corresponding author.	Other project team members
Professional Development	
Encourage motivated colleagues to pursue advanced degrees early in their careers.	Collaborating DNPs and PhDs Academic DNPs and PhDs
Lay a foundation for mentoring and retaining doctoral students.	Facility DNPs and PhDs Facility leadership Interprofessional stakeholders

Note: APP = academic practice partnership; DNP = Doctor of Nursing Practice; EBP = evidence-based practice; PhD = Doctor of Philosophy.
Data from Cowan, L., Hartjes, T., & Munro, S. (2019). A model of successful DNP and PhD collaboration. *Journal of the American Association of Nurse Practitioners, 31*(2), 116–123. https://doi.org/10.1097/JXX.0000000000000105

Integrate an Understanding of Nursing History in Advancing Nursing's Influence in Health Care

Nursing has a long and rich history, dating back to ancient civilizations. In most societies, caregivers were female, though notable exceptions existed in male shamans or medicine men. These caregivers were mostly unpaid and learned through oral tradition, providing care in the home of the sick individual. Nursing began to organize around religious ideals in the early Christian era and this marked the beginning of the influence of Christianity on caregiving in the Western world of the time. Through the Middle Ages, nursing continued to be heavily influenced by religious orders. Hospitals existed of a form; however, care was largely provided in family homes, with hospitals reserved for individuals who had no living family members. Nursing in these times did not require formal education and often, women were conscripted to unpaid caregiving. The first secular nursing schools were established in the 19th century with the advent of modern nursing in the West.

Florence Nightingale is considered the founder of modern nursing in the West. Her distinct legacy paved the way for the beginning of nursing science and scholarly inquiry, which would fuel an explosion of nursing as a distinct discipline separate from the biomedical model. For the first time, nurses were taught theory along with psychomotor skills and nursing's body of distinct knowledge began to develop beyond the scope of passed-down oral tradition. In the United States, the outbreak of the Civil War further cemented nursing as a distinct discipline, not only in the eyes of the healthcare model at the time but also in the court of public perception. Nursing helped to fundamentally change the perception of acceptable "women's work" outside the home environment at a time when society mandates were quite the opposite. Dorothea Dix, Clara Barton, Harriet Tubman, Louisa May Alcott, and others established the value of formal education in the "caring" of the sick, paving the way for schools of nursing to be formed in the late 19th century (Egenes, 2017).

With the advent of the Industrial Age came advents in established healthcare models. With so many sick in clustered city areas, hospitals began to form and nursing's influence continued to grow both inside and outside these structures. Despite general lack of support from physician colleagues, schools of nursing grew in number and quality of nursing education continued to improve. Community and public health nursing as well as midwifery care saw huge gains due to the rampant need and the work of pioneers like Lillian Wald (Egenes, 2017). Advanced practice nursing saw its advent in the Industrial Age as nurses began to administer anesthesia, a precursor to the nurse-anesthetist role of today (Murphy-Ende, 2002).

It was also during this time that nursing professional identity continued to emancipate itself in more concrete ways, separate from the idea of "handmaiden" to the work of the physician. In 1903, North Carolina became the first state to pass a licensure act and by 1941, 48 states had followed suit. Title protection of the term "registered nurse" occurred at this time, but in a permissive capacity rather than a mandatory one, allowing individuals to call themselves "nurses" and be compensated for nursing work so long as the term "registered nurse" was not used. Mandatory laws requiring licensure as a registered nurse to perform nursing tasks were not passed until the later 1940s. The World Wars provided ample opportunity for nurses to work more autonomously in a battlefield setting due to lack of human resources, further demonstrating the ability of nursing as a discipline to contribute to health care independent of complete subservience to the traditional medical model (Egenes, 2017).

Following the World Wars, a massive shortage of qualified nurses led to the formation of Associate Degree Programs as an addition to the model of hospital-based diploma training programs. It should be noted that during this time and until the 1960s a nurse was expected to resign from the role upon becoming pregnant. In 1965, the American Nurses Association published a position paper encouraging a baccalaureate degree as the standard for entry to practice; however, this did not significantly alter the growth rate of these programs (American Nurses Association, 1965). Still, this position statement and later federal funding from the Nurse Training Act of 1964 did increase the depth and breadth of graduate nursing programs, particularly programs dedicated to the development of nursing faculty (Egenes, 2017). The role of the APN within the context of the nurse practitioner and clinical nurse specialist specialties also became more concrete and legitimized in the pediatric and community-based care settings.

The shortage of physician healthcare providers in the 1970s–1990s further fueled the establishment of hospital-based APN practice for adult and pediatric populations. The Information Age also propelled growth in informatics in the nursing discipline. As APN/DNPs became more and more integrated into health care, the influence of nursing on the whole grew. Hanson and Hamric (2003) describe this phenomenon in three stages:

1. Specialty develops in practice settings.
2. Organized training for specialty begins.
3. Knowledge base grows and pressure mounts for standardization and graduate educational programs emerge.

As APNs/DNPs communicate and create value within the current healthcare system, it is the knowledge of nursing's collective history that must inform and guide new frontiers. While challenging to communicate value within a system that prioritizes monetary and hard, empiric outcomes, it has never been more apparent that nursing's value is transcendent of these simple aims. In the post–COVID-19 world, healthcare consumers are amplifying the cries for systemic change that adds value to care and prioritizes person-centered and population-focused interventions. These arenas are ripe for APNs/DNPs to meaningfully advance nursing's influence from the heart of its own disciplinary perspective.

Apply Theory and Research-Based Knowledge From Nursing, the Arts, Humanities and Other Sciences

APNs/DNPs must apply, synthesize, and translate a wide variety of knowledge to patient- and population-specific contexts. This requires a broad awareness of the knowledge base of other disciplines in addition to mastery level knowledge of nursing's unique disciplinary perspective. We will discuss specific examples of the synthesis of multidisciplinary knowledge, ethical decision making, socially responsible leadership, and the utilization of theory in advanced nursing practice.

Synthesize Knowledge From Nursing and Other Disciplines to Inform Education, Practice, and Research

We have already discussed that knowledge can be obtained in nursing through several mechanisms. Knowledge from nursing informs and directs the care that APN/DNP provide; however, the disciplinary knowledge of nursing is not the limit of knowledge. On the contrary, many disciplines offer evidence-based knowledge from which the nurse can synthesize parts to form the whole of a patient's care. For example, the APN/DNP may use biomedical evidence to inform the diagnosis of the patient with an acute stroke and evidence from the social sciences to inform the rehabilitation of speech, activities of daily living, and communication. Furthermore, the APN/DNP may utilize knowledge from the arts, such as thanatology, to aid in healing. This knowledge may include theories, conceptual models, diagnostic and treatment algorithms, epidemiological data, music, art, and much more.

Apply a Systematic and Defendable Approach to Nursing Practice Decisions

Nursing practice decisions can be made across all points of care, in both patient-facing and non–patient-facing roles. Regardless of context, the APN/DNP must be systematic in the approach to the problem to create an easily defendable framework for nursing practice decisions. First, the APN/DNP should assess the scope of the problem and identify stakeholders, if applicable. Depending on context, this could look like a patient interview and physical assessment, a learning needs assessment, a SWOT analysis, a focus group, and many others. The APN/DNP must have a keen awareness of those problems which necessitate focused assessment and which may require a more comprehensive approach. This sense is honed through experiential knowledge, professional development, and active mentorship by more experienced colleagues. Once the problem has been identified and scoped, the APN/DNP should consider solutions. Depending on the problem, this may include one or more, sometimes many, members of the multidisciplinary team. The APN/DNP should display effective and collegial communication and should communicate back with any stakeholders or the patient if the problem is one in the sphere of patient care. The APN/DNP should have a clear rationale informed by evidence for any practice decisions and should bear in mind the ethical principles discussed in this chapter for communication with patients, families, and the larger multidisciplinary team. Every intervention requires evaluation and adjustment. In this way, the decisions made by the APN/DNP will be systematic and defendable, with appropriate context to the domain of care.

Employ Ethical Decision Making to Assess, Intervene, and Evaluate Nursing Care

Ethical decision making is the process by which the APN/DNP chooses among alternatives in a manner consistent with the ethical principles of autonomy, beneficence, non-maleficence, and justice. Health care abounds with ethical questions and dilemmas unique to each practice setting. It is important to note that APNs/DNPs practicing in non–patient-facing roles often encounter ethical issues as well. The nursing discipline brings clear consensus on these principles through the American Nurses Association *Code of Ethics* (2015), which is the standard for nursing education and practice, providing both normative and idealistic statements about how nurses, including APNs/DNPs, should employ ethics in practice. This code has nine provisions with accompanying interpretive statements for each. The general provisions are found in **Table 1-2**. The APN/DNP should bear in mind that the first duty is always to the patient. At times, situations arise in patient care or in systems management that challenge ethical provisions or give the illusion that one ethical principle is exclusionary to another. This chapter will discuss ethical decision making within the context of informed consent for care and for participation in human subjects research.

Table 1-2 ANA Code of Ethics Provisions

Provision	Description
Provision 1	The nurse practices with compassion and respect for the inherent dignity, worth, and unique attributes of every person.
Provision 2	The nurse's primary commitment is to the patient, whether an individual, family, group, community, or population.
Provision 3	The nurse promotes, advocates for, and protects the rights, health, and safety of the patient.
Provision 4	The nurse has authority, accountability, and responsibility for nursing practice; makes decisions; and takes action consistent with the obligation to promote health and to provide optimal care.
Provision 5	The nurse owes the same duties to self as to others, including the responsibility to promote health and safety, preserve wholeness of character and integrity, maintain competence, and continue personal and professional growth.
Provision 6	The nurse participates in establishing, maintaining, and improving healthcare environments and conditions of employment conducive to the provision of quality health care and consistent with the values of the profession through individual and collective action.
Provision 7	The nurse participates in the advancement of the profession through contributions to practice, education, administration, and knowledge development.
Provision 8	The nurse collaborates with other health professionals and the public to protect human rights, promote health diplomacy, and reduce health disparities.
Provision 9	The profession of nursing, collectively through its professional organizations, must articulate nursing values, maintain the integrity of the profession, and integrate principles of social justice into nursing and health policy.

Reproduced from American Nurses Association. (2015). *Code of ethics for nurses with interpretive statements*. Silver Spring, MD.

Informed consent is a process of bidirectional conversation between a healthcare provider and a patient wherein the provider gives information about the risks, benefits, alternatives, and potential complications of a medical or nursing care intervention. The patient has the opportunity to ask questions about said intervention and retains the autonomy to decline the intervention without threat or coercion. This can sound straightforward; however, APNs/DNPs in patient-facing roles are often faced with ethical dilemmas surrounding informed consent. Bidirectional communication can be inhibited by language, cultural, and socioeconomic barriers. Patients may not feel heard or may feel judged for the information they provide or the concerns they bring forward to the care team. Even experienced APNs/DNPs may have difficulty elucidating the true risk of complications for high-risk procedures and articulating value. Omission of treatment alternatives is a common violation of the principles of informed consent. The availability bias of the provider may create an ethical dilemma wherein a patient provides consent for an intervention while unaware that another option exists.

Significant moral distress can occur for the APN/DNP and the other multidisciplinary providers if the patient or surrogate decision maker decides against the recommendations of the care team. One example of this is the well-known inability of Jehovah's Witness patients to accept blood transfusions on the basis of religion. Management of the acutely bleeding patient, invasive surgical procedures, and cardiopulmonary bypass is very complex in this population, yet the first duty of the APN/DNP is to that patient and to the preservation of their autonomy to make medical decisions free of coercion. This scenario becomes even more complex when it involves the pediatric patient. How should the APN/DNP apply ethical decision making in an incredibly vulnerable population who does not have full agency? In this case, the U.S. Constitution and courts have set precedent through several key legal cases that while parents retain the right to provide consent and to refuse medical treatments for a child, they do not have the right to withhold lifesaving treatment for a child in this context. This doctrine is referred to as *parens patriae* and describes the power the government retains to act in the best interest of the child when the treatment is deemed reasonable and necessary (Stevenson et al., 2023; Stern, 2019). The APN/DNP should consult with hospital risk management administrators and involve the ethics committee in such a case. If the blood loss is not immediately life threatening or time allows, mitigation strategies like erythropoietin-stimulating agents, cellsavers, and hemodilution are appropriate strategies. The APN/DNP must also carefully maintain open lines of communication with the patient and family members, being careful not to exercise implicit or explicit bias against deeply held beliefs, which could compromise the therapeutic relationship (Stevenson et al., 2023).

Nursing knowledge is continually becoming. The principles of beneficence and non-maleficence demand that the APN/DNP continually seek to translate new knowledge into practice through implementation science and to seek partnership with those qualified to operationalize primary scholarly inquiry to reduce the gap between knowledge and practice. Ethical decision making mandates that the APN/DNP base decisions on the best available evidence; therefore, the legacy of scholarship and scholarly inquiry belongs to all APNs/DNPs.

Within the endeavors of scholarship are embedded some specific ethical requirements for the protection of any entity whose participation would generate new knowledge. The APN/DNP must recognize that nursing has a dark and consistent history of complicity in egregious misuse of human subjects for research, leaving an understandably lasting and profound impact on those communities and populations. One poignant example is the Tuskegee syphilis study, in which the precursor to the modern-day Centers for Disease Control and Prevention intentionally withheld lifesaving treatment for a common sexually transmitted infection from 400 African-American men (Tobin, 2022). This is hardly the only example of the atrocities committed against minorities, women, and other vulnerable groups in the name of science. Formal protection of human subjects in research was not fully realized until the 1970s (Rice, 2008). Federal regulations require that research involving human subjects be subjected to an institutional review process. The review of such research is conducted by a research review board (RRB) or institutional review board (IRB), a committee responsible for ensuring that human rights and safety are protected, and that research is carried out ethically and in compliance with federal guidelines. Although the composition and processes of specific IRBs vary, federal law requires that members have adequate expertise to review research. Members must not have conflicts of interest pertaining to the research they review (Gray & Grove, 2020).

An IRB can decide that research submitted to the committee is either exempt from review, appropriate for expedited review, or required to undergo a complete review. The decision about the level of review is based on the risk to human subjects inherent in the proposed research. A proposed nursing study that posed nothing more than a small cost of time or inconvenience to subjects, such as a survey about working conditions, would probably be considered exempt from review. That decision cannot be made by the researcher, however. The researcher must submit information about the proposed study to the IRB. Usually, the chair of the IRB will decide whether the research proposal is exempt or should be presented to the full committee for review. No nurse researcher should conduct even the smallest human study in any institution without first obtaining approval from the IRB (Gray & Grove, 2020). APN/DNPs must always uphold the highest standards of ethical integrity when collecting or disseminating knowledge gained from clinical practice. Protection of human subjects in the generation or dissemination of knowledge is paramount. The DNP-prepared APN should be fully informed of all rules and regulations pertaining to the protection of human subjects.

Demonstrate Socially Responsible Leadership

Socially responsible leadership is inclusive of the areas of environmental responsibility, ethical responsibility, philanthropic responsibility, and economic responsibility. Social responsibility is defined as advocacy for the needs of others and program implementation that emanates a focus on social issues affecting contemporary individuals, groups, and populations. As a human caring and applied science, nursing has the expertise to advance society by creating change agents who consider socially responsible solutions to complex problems. APNs/DNPs can advocate for social change to enhance the well-being of a society. Because nurses represent the largest number of healthcare providers, it follows logically that the profession of nursing can and should assume the responsibility for acting in a manner that benefits all people (Tyer-Viola et al., 2009). APNs/DNPs have a unique presence to bear in leadership that is cognizant of social determinants of health as components of person-centered care, community and population health, and in the design imple-mentation and evaluation of quality improvement and research. These concepts will be further discussed in subsequent chapters.

Translate Theories From Nursing and Other Disciplines Into Practice

The explosion of nursing theory beginning in the 1940s forced nursing to truly reckon with its role as a distinct discipline with its own knowledge base. Giants of nursing theory like Dorothy Orem, Hildegard Peplau, Imogene King, and others developed grand and middle-range theories that conceptualized "caring" as science. However, with this Golden Age of nursing theory came deeper questions about the contributions of nursing to the larger healthcare enterprise and the value of theo-retical models in a positivism-dominated paradigm. While theorists envisioned a distinct and separate theory-based practice for nursing that transcended the medical model, the realities of the larger healthcare system often kept nursing subservient to the priorities of other disciplines. This complex dichotomy is perhaps most evident in advanced practice, as APNs/DNPs practicing in patient-facing roles use a signifi-cant amount of biomedical knowledge to inform and guide practice decisions.

In advanced nursing practice, nurses know and use knowledge and theories from many other disciplines. McEwen and Wills (2021) urged nurses to reframe shared concepts according to nursing's framework. Applying a theory from the field of psychology to assist patients in changing unhealthy behaviors transforms a shared theory into a nursing theory. Shared theories can and should augment and support nursing theory and practice. Concepts from behavioral, sociological, educational, biological, and medical sciences are commonly utilized as shared the-ories in the practice of nursing. In addition to these, leadership theories can be par-ticularly valuable to the DNP-prepared APN leading organizational, political, and system-wide change. By applying leadership science to nursing challenges, APNs enhance the ability to improve the health of patients, families, and communities.

Demonstrate Clinical Judgment Founded on a Broad Knowledge Base

Clinical judgment has taken many definitions within the discipline of nursing and, until recently, had been used colloquially as an equivalent to the terms "critical thinking" and "clinical reasoning." Development of critical thinking has long been a mainstay of traditional nursing education. Critical thinking is the process of actively and skillfully conceptualizing, analyzing, synthesizing, evaluating, and applying in-formation to guide beliefs and actions. It involves using evidence-based knowledge and information to make decisions and solve problems (Zuriguel et al., 2015). Critical thinking is a cognitive process that can be applied to any area of knowledge.

More recently, consensus has developed around the idea that clinical judgment is a distinct type of critical thinking and is the process used by the members of the healthcare team, including APNs/DNPs, to evaluate and synthesize patient informa-tion for the purpose of making decisions about the appropriate course of action to take in a particular clinical situation. Clinical judgment involves the ability to rec-ognize and interpret data, make accurate diagnoses, and develop effective treatment plans based on evidence-based practice and clinical experience (Tanner, 2006). This is essential for providing safe, effective, and patient-centered care, and it is a critical component of competency for APNs/DNPs. Several sources of knowledge inform clinical judgment.

1. Scientific evidence: Clinical practice should be based on the best available scientific evidence. The APN/DNP must synthesize this information in consideration of the other factors.
2. Patient preferences and values: Clinical judgment must prioritize and account for the unique needs, values, and preferences of each patient.
3. Clinical experience: The clinician's experience and expertise, including past successes and failures, can inform clinical judgment.
4. Contextual factors: Clinical judgment must consider the broader context in which care is being delivered, including environmental and organizational factors. This can include considerations of triage and availability of resources.
5. Ethical considerations: Ethical principles and considerations should guide clinical judgment, particularly in complex cases where there may be competing interests or values.
6. Interprofessional collaboration: Collaborating with other healthcare professionals can provide valuable perspectives and information, enhancing clinical judgment.

Challenges to effective clinical judgment abound. Patient complexity, cognitive biases, time pressure, resource limitations, lack of experience, and system level factors like work environment can all hinder effective clinical judgment (Goudreau et al., 2015). Clearly, the accumulation of knowledge alone is not sufficient for the development of clinical judgment. An APN can know about a particular disease or problem but may still not be effective in decision making at the patient or systems level. Evaluating clinical judgment is therefore a challenge in advanced practice nursing education.

Integrate Foundational and Advanced Specialty Knowledge Into Clinical Reasoning

Foundational knowledge refers not only to nursing's distinct disciplinary knowledge but also to the broader biomedical sciences and includes nursing theory, physiology, pharmacology, and pathophysiology. APNs/DNPs use foundational knowledge to understand the complex interplay of biological, social, and environmental factors that contribute to the patient's health status. APNs/DNPs apply foundational knowledge in the process of clinical judgment to identify risk factors, develop a differential diagnosis, and recommend appropriate diagnostic tests to confirm or rule out the diagnosis. This level of knowledge is essential to develop a treatment plan, including medication management, referral to specialists, or patient education.

Specialty level knowledge refers to the specific knowledge and skills required to provide care in a particular clinical area. APNs/DNPs with specialized training in anesthesia, oncology, cardiology, or midwifery care have acquired advanced knowledge in these areas, enabling them to provide expert care to patients with complex conditions. Specialty-level knowledge enables the APN/DNP to recognize subtle changes in the patient's condition, anticipate potential complications, and implement preventive measures. For instance, an APN/DNP with specialty-level knowledge in oncology can identify the common side effects of chemotherapy, provide or prescribe appropriate interventions, and monitor for potential adverse reactions. Similarly, an APN/DNP with specialty-level knowledge in cardiology can diagnose and manage complex cardiac conditions and provide appropriate patient education.

APNs/DNPs in non–patient-facing roles also exercise clinical reasoning in practice. For example, an APN/DNP informaticist may use clinical reasoning in the integration and evaluation of a clinical decision support tool into an organization's current electronic health record. These tools are frequently used to guide patient-facing clinicians and to recognize early signs of patient deterioration (Darvish et al., 2014). Foundational and specialty-level knowledge could be used in this case to enhance the tool's functionality and to evaluate its effectiveness.

Synthesize Current and Emerging Evidence to Influence Practice

The ability to synthesize evidence is a key competency for APNs/DNPs. This is not simply passive absorption. Synthesis requires systematically reviewing and analyzing research studies, expert opinions, and other sources of information to generate new insights or knowledge. It involves integrating and interpreting multiple sources of evidence to produce a coherent and comprehensive understanding of a particular problem (Melnyk & Fineout-Overholt, 2019). APNs/DNPs can synthesize evidence in several key ways.

One way in which APNs/DNPs synthesize evidence is through the use of clinical guidelines. These are evidence-based recommendations that guide clinical decision making in a particular area of practice. Clinical guidelines are developed by expert panels, who systematically review the existing evidence and make recommendations based on the strength and quality of the evidence. APNs/DNPs can use clinical guidelines to guide their clinical practice, ensuring that they are providing the best possible care based on the most up-to-date evidence. They are also qualified to write clinical practice guidelines within large interdisciplinary teams, professional organizations, and at the level of individual organizations.

APNs/DNPs can also synthesize evidence by using clinical decision support tools. As mentioned previously, these computerized tools provide clinicians with evidence-based recommendations for the diagnosis and treatment of various conditions or they can provide a warning of patient deterioration. Clinical decision support tools can be integrated into electronic health records, enabling APNs to access the latest evidence-based recommendations at the point of care. These tools do not replace clinical judgment on the part of the APN/DNP; however, they can be an effective adjunct, especially if the clinical picture is unclear.

Another way in which APN/DNPs synthesize evidence is through the use of quality improvement initiatives designed to improve the quality of care by identifying areas for improvement and implementing evidence-based interventions to address these areas. APN/DNPs can lead quality improvement initiatives in their practice settings, using evidence to guide the development and implementation of interventions. By using evidence to inform quality improvement initiatives, APN/DNPs can ensure that they are making evidence-based changes that will improve patient outcomes.

APNs can also synthesize evidence by using clinical decision-making models. These are structured approaches to clinical decision making that enable clinicians to systematically consider the available evidence and make evidence-based decisions. Clinical decision-making frameworks and models can help APNs to integrate the available evidence into clinical practice, ensuring decisions based on the best available evidence. This is discussed further in the following section.

Analyze Decision Models From Nursing and Other Knowledge Domains to Improve Clinical Judgment

APNs/DNPs can analyze decision models to improve their clinical judgment by examining the assumptions and principles underlying each model, assessing their own personal and professional values and beliefs, and considering the context in which decisions will be made. Though models exist using nursing disciplinary knowledge, models involving other domains may be used as well. This analytical process involves critical evaluation of the strengths and weaknesses of each model, and a determination of which model is most appropriate for a given situation. To analyze decision models effectively, the APN/DNP must have a solid understanding of the different types of models and their components and have the ability to apply these models to real-world scenarios. By analyzing decision models, advanced practice nurses can improve clinical judgment and make more informed decisions. While the decision models discussed here are by no means exhaustive to all existing possibilities, those discussed here are highly utilized in clinical practice and advanced practice education.

One example of a decision model that can be used to improve clinical judgment is the Ottawa Decision Support Framework (ODSF), which was developed to help clinicians make informed and effective decisions when faced with complex health problems. The ODSF consists of five components: problem identification, decision support, patient engagement, outcome evaluation, and feedback (Stacey et al., 2014). While this model is widely used, its applicability outside of direct patient care is quite limited and this should be a consideration for the APN/DNP seeking a model for process or operations decisions.

Another decision model that can be used to improve clinical judgment is the Six-Step Model of Clinical Decision Making, which involves identifying the problem, gathering information, formulating hypotheses, testing hypotheses, interpreting results, and evaluating the decision. This model has several advantages, including a systematic approach, use of evidence-based practice, a strong emphasis on patient-centered care, and a process for continuous evaluation (Banning, 2008).

Lasater's Clinical Judgment Rubric is a tool that can help nurse practitioners improve clinical judgment by providing a framework for evaluating the decision-making process. The rubric includes five categories: noticing, interpreting, responding, reflecting, and reasoning. Each category includes specific indicators that can help nurse practitioners identify areas where they may need to improve their clinical judgment. Noticing involves recognizing relevant clinical data. The rubric includes indicators such as recognizing patterns, identifying abnormal findings, and identifying changes in the patient's condition. Interpreting makes sense of the data that has been noticed. Indicators for this category include recognizing the significance of the data, identifying possible causes of the patient's condition, and considering the patient's history and context. Responding requires taking action based on the data and interpretation. The rubric includes indicators such as selecting appropriate interventions, prioritizing actions based on the patient's needs, and collaborating with the healthcare team. Reflecting evaluates the outcomes of the actions taken and making adjustments if necessary. Indicators for this category include evaluating the effectiveness of the interventions, considering the patient's response to the interventions, and modifying the plan of care if necessary. Reasoning analyzes the thought process used to make clinical judgments. Indicators for this category include considering evidence-based practice, using a systematic approach to problem solving, and considering the ethical implications of the decisions made (Lasatar, 2007). This approach provides a standardized method of evaluating clinical judgment and can be useful in the training and education of APNs/DNPs and also in clinical practice.

Summary

When APNs/DNPs fully embody nursing's disciplinary perspective by applying theory and knowledge as well as demonstrating clinical judgment, patients, communities, and populations receive the full scope of the value that nursing brings to modern health care. It is not just what the APN/DNP knows that matters. What matters is how APNs/DNPs apply and synthesize what they know through a perspective of continual improvement that brings about lasting practice change and ultimately improved health for the patients they serve.

References

American Association of Colleges of Nursing. (2021). *The Essentials: Core Competencies for Professional Nursing Education*. Washington, DC: AACN.

American Nurses Association. (1965). American Nurses Association's first position paper on education for nursing. *American Journal of Nursing, 65*(12), 106–111.

American Nurses Association. (2015). *Code of ethics for nurses with interpretive statements*. ANA.

Armstrong, N., & Sables-Baus, S. (2019). The DNP project deliverables: Sustainability and spread. In L. P. Williard & D. L. Edwards (Eds.), *Leadership and systems improvement for the DNP* (pp. 309–322). Springer Publishing.

Banning, M. (2008). A review of clinical decision making: Models and current research. *Journal of Clinical Nursing, 17*(2), 187–195. https://doi.org/10.1111/j.1365-2702.2006.01791.x

Benner, P. (1984). From novice to expert. Excellence and power in clinical nursing practice. Addison-Wesley Publishing.

Cani, C. G., Lopes, L. D. S. G., Queiroz, M., & Nery, M. (2015). Improvement in medication adherence and self-management of diabetes with a clinical pharmacy program: A randomized controlled trial in patients with type 2 diabetes undergoing insulin therapy at a teaching hospital. *Clinics, 70*, 102–106. https://doi.org/10.6061/clinics/2015(02)06

Carper, B. A. (1978). Fundamental patterns of knowing in nursing. *Advances in Nursing Science, 1*(1), 13–24.

Chinn, P. L. (2019, March). Keynote Address: The Discipline of Nursing: Moving Forward Boldly. Presented at "Nursing Theory: A 50 Year Perspective, Past and Future," Case Western Reserve University Frances Payne Bolton School of Nursing. https://nursology.net/2019-03-21-case-keynote/

Clarke, D. J., & Forster, A. (2015). Improving post-stroke recovery: The role of the multidisciplinary health care team. *Journal of Multidisciplinary Healthcare, 8*, 433–442. https://doi.org/10.2147/JMDH.S68764

Cowan, L., Hartjes, T., & Munro, S. (2019). A model of successful DNP and PhD collaboration. *Journal of the American Association of Nurse Practitioners, 31*(2), 116–123. https://doi.org/10.1097/JXX.0000000000000105

Curtis, K., Fry, M., Shaban, R., & Considine, J. (2017). Translating research findings to clinical nursing practice. *Journal of Clinical Nursing, 26*(5-6), 862–872. https://doi.org/10.1111/jocn.13586

Darvish, A., Bahramnezhad, F., Keyhanian, S., Navidhamidi, M. (2014). The role of nursing informatics on promoting quality of health care and the need for appropriate education. *Global Journal of Health Sciences, 6*(6), 11–18. https://doi.org/10.5539/gjhs.v6n6p11

Dokbua, S., Dilokthornsakul, P., Chaiyakunapruk, N., Saini, B., Krass, I., & Dhippayom, T. (2018). Effects of an asthma self-management support service provided by community pharmacists: A systematic review and meta-analysis. *Journal of Managed Care & Specialty Pharmacy, 24*(11), 1184–1196. https://doi.org/10.18553/jmcp.2018.24.11.1184

Drevenhorn, E., Bengtson, A., Nyberg, P., & Kjellgren, K. I. (2015). Assessment of hypertensive patients' self-care agency after counseling training of nurses. *Journal of the American Association of Nurse Practitioners, 27*(11), 624–630. https://doi.org/10.1002/2327-6924.12249

Egenes, K. J. (2017). History of nursing. In J. W. Kenney & D. L. Gregoire (Eds.), *Issues and trends in nursing: Essential knowledge for today and tomorrow* (pp. 1–26). Jones & Bartlett Learning.

Falkenberg-Olson A. (2019). Research translation and the evolving PhD and DNP practice roles: A collaborative call for nurse practitioners. *Journal of the American Association of Nurse Practitioners, 31*(8), 447–453. https://doi.org/10.1097/JXX.0000000000000266

Fawcett J, Aronowitz T., AbuFannouneh A., et al. (2015). Thoughts about the name of our discipline. *Nursing Science Quarterly, 28*(4), 330–333. https://doi.org/10.1177/0894318415599224

Goudreau, J., Pepin, J., Larue, C., Dubois, S., Descôteaux, R., Lavoie, P., & Dumont, K. (2015). A competency-based approach to nurses' continuing education for clinical reasoning and leadership through reflective practice in a care situation. *Nurse Education in Practice, 15*(6), e572–e578. https://pubmed.ncbi.nlm.nih.gov/26559351

Graham, I., Logan, J., Harrison, M., Straus, S., Tetroe, J., Caswell, W., & Robinson, N. (2006). Lost in knowledge translation: time for a map?. *The Journal of Continuing Education in the Health Professions, 26*(1), 13–24. https://doi.org/10.1002/chp.47

Gray, J., & Grove, S. (2020). *Burns and Grove's the practice of nursing research: appraisal, synthesis, and generation of evidence* (9th ed.). Elsevier.

Green, L., Ottoson, J., García, C., & Hiatt, R. (2009). Diffusion theory and knowledge dissemination, utilization, and integration in public health. *Annual Review of Public Health, 30*, 151–174. https://doi.org/10.1146/annurev.publhealth.031308.100049

Hanson, C. M., & Hamric, A. B. (2003). Reflections on the continuing evolution of advanced practice nursing. *Nursing Outlook, 51*(5), 203–211. https://doi.org/10.1016/S0029-6554(03)00158-1

Isik, E., & Freland, N. M. (2021). Orem's self-care deficit nursing theory to improve children's self-care: An integrative review. *The Journal of School Nursing*. Advance online publication. https://doi.org/10.1177/10598405211050062

Jo, H. J., Shin, D. B., Koo, B. K., Ko, E. S., Yeo, H. J., & Cho, W. H. (2017). The impact of multidisciplinary nutritional team involvement on nutritional care and outcomes in a medical intensive care unit. *European Journal of Clinical Nutrition, 71*(11), 1360–1362. https://doi.org/10.1038/ejcn.2017.108

Johnstone, M. J. (2015). Decolonizing nursing ethics. *International Nursing Review, 62*(2), 141–142. https://doi.org/10.1111/inr.12197

Kenney, J. W. (2006). Theory-based advanced nursing practice. In W. K. Cody (Ed.), *Philosophical and theoretical perspectives for advanced nursing practice* (pp. 295–310). Jones and Bartlett.

Kongsted, A., Ris, I., Kjaer, P., & Hartvigsen, J. (2021). Self-management at the core of back pain care: 10 key points for clinicians. *Brazilian Journal of Physical Therapy, 25*(4), 396–406. https://doi.org/10.1016/j.bjpt.2021.05.002

Lasatar, K. (2007). Clinical judgment development: Using simulation to create an assessment rubric. *Journal of Nursing Education, 46*(11), 496–503. https://doi.org/10.3928/01484834-20071101-04

McEwen, M., & Wills, E. M. (2021). *Theoretical basis for nursing*. Lippincott Williams & Wilkins.

Melnyk, B., & Fineout-Overholt, E. (2019). *Evidence-based practice in nursing and healthcare: A guide to best practice* (4th ed.). Wolters Kluwer.

Mohammadpur, A., Rahmati Sharghi, N., Khosravan, S., Alami, A., & Akhond, M. (2015). The effect of a supportive educational intervention developed based on the Orem's self-care theory on the self-care ability of patients with myocardial infarction: A randomised controlled trial. *Journal of Clinical Nursing, 24*(11–12), 1686–1692. https://doi.org/10.1111/jocn.12775

Murphy-Ende, K. (2002, January). Advanced practice nursing: Reflections on the past, issues for the future. *Oncology Nursing Forum, 29*(1), 33–38. https://doi.org/10.1188/02.ONF.106-112

Newman, M. A., Sime, A. M., & Corcoran-Perry, S. A. (1991). The focus of the discipline of nursing. *Advances in Nursing Science, 14*(1), 1–6.

Newman, M. A., Smith, M. C., Pharris, M. D., & Jones, D. (2008). The focus of the discipline revisited. *Advances in Nursing Science, 31*(1), E16–E27.

Orem, D. (1971). *Nursing: Concepts and practice*. McGraw-Hill.

Parker, M. E., & Smith, M. C. (2010). Nursing theory and the discipline of nursing. In M. E. Parker & M. C. Smith (Eds.), *Nursing theories and nursing practice* (3rd ed., pp. 3–12). F. A. Davis.

Parse, R. R. (1997). The language of nursing knowledge: Saying what we mean. In I. M. King & J. Fawcett (Eds.), *The language of nursing theory and metatheory* (pp. 73–77). Center Nursing Press.

Paterson, J., & Zderad, L. (1988). *Humanistic nursing*. Wiley.

Reed, P. (1997). Nursing: The ontology of the discipline. *Nursing Science Quarterly, 10*(2), 76–79. https://doi.org/10.1177/089431849701000207

Rice, T. (2008). The historical, ethical, and legal background of human-subjects research. *Respiratory Care, 53*(10), 1325–1329. https://rc.rcjournal.com/content/respcare/53/10/1325.full.pdf

Rogers, M. E. (1994). The science of unitary human beings. *Nursing Science Quarterly, 7*(1), 33–35. https://doi.org/10.1177/089431849400700111

Stacey, D., Legare, F., Col, N., Bennett, C., Barry, M., Eden, K. . . . & Wu, J. (2014). Decision aids for people facing health treatment or screening decisions. *Cochrane Database of Systematic Reviews, (1)*.

Stern, E. G. (2019). Parens Patriae and parental rights: When should the state override parental medical decisions. *Journal of Law and Health, 33*(1):79–106. https://pubmed.ncbi.nlm.nih.gov/31841618

Stevenson, J., DeGroote, N. P., Keller, F., Brock, K. E., Bergsagel, D. J., Miller, T. P., . . . & Castellino, S. M. (2023). Characteristics and outcomes of pediatric oncology patients at risk for guardians declining transfusion of blood components. *Cancer Reports, 6*(1), e1665. https://doi.org/10.1002/cnr2.1665

Tanner, C. (2006). Thinking like a nurse: A research-based model of clinical judgment in nursing. *Journal of Nursing Education, 45*(6), 204–211. https://doi.org/10.3928/01484834-20060601-04

Tobin, M. J. (2022). Fiftieth anniversary of uncovering the Tuskegee syphilis study: The story and timeless lessons. *American Journal of Respiratory and Critical Care Medicine, 205*(10), 1145–1158. https://doi.org/10.1164/rccm.202201-0136SO

Tyer-Viola, L., Nicholas, P. K., Corless, I. B., Barry, D. M., Hoyt, P., Fitzpatrick, J. J., & Davis, S. M. (2009). Social responsibility of nursing: A global perspective. *Policy, Politics, & Nursing Practice, 10*(2), 110–118. https://doi.org/10.1177/1527154409339528

Van Eikenhorst, L., Taxis, K., Van Dijk, L., & De Gier, H. (2017). Pharmacist-led self-management interventions to improve diabetes outcomes: A systematic literature review and meta-analysis. *Frontiers in Pharmacology, 8*, 891. https://doi.org/10.3389/fphar.2017.00891

Watson, J. (2007). Theoretical questions and concerns: Response from a caring science framework. *Nursing Science Quarterly, 20*(1), 13–15. https://doi.org/10.1177/0894318406296785

Zuriguel Pérez, E., Lluch Canut, M., Falcó Pegueroles, A., Puig Llobet, M., Moreno Arroyo, C., & Roldán Merino, J. (2015). Critical thinking in nursing: Scoping review of the literature. *International Journal of Nursing Practice, 21*(6), 820–830. https://doi.org/10.1111/ijn.12347

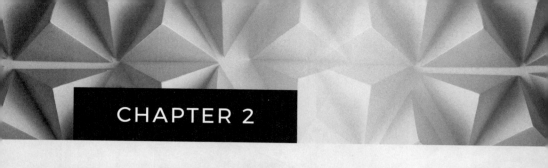

CHAPTER 2

Person-Centered Care

Jeana M. Holt, PhD, DNP, MSN, RN, FNP-BC, APNP

Introduction

What Matters to You?/What Is the Matter With You?

What emotions, feelings, or thoughts do these similarly worded phrases prompt? The first question, *What Matters to You?*, is an initiative that began in Scotland in 2016 to shift health conversations to listening and prioritizing what people want and need to achieve their best health. The second question, *What Is the Matter With You?*, still predominates health conversations in the United States. This chapter will explore the history of Person-Centered Care (PCC), its foundational concepts, applications, implications, and competencies. As you read the chapter, remember the image of a person surrounded by family, friends, and loved ones; surrounded by their neighborhood, work, and environment; surrounded by policies, government, and dominant cultural norms (see **Figure 2-1**). This chapter focuses on PCC, but advanced practice nurses (APNs) and those in advanced nursing practice specialties (especially those with a doctor of nursing practice [DNP] degree) must always understand that a person lives within a context that directly and indirectly affects their choices, opportunities, and health outcomes.

The National Academies of Medicine (NAM, 2001) (formally the Institute of Medicine) wrote a seminal book, *Crossing the Quality Chasm: A New Health System for the 21st Century*, that defined healthcare quality as effective, timely, efficient, safe, equitable, and patient-centered. However, there is a difference between patient-centered and person-centered care. Person-centered care is respectful and responsive to individual preferences, needs, and values, all pillars of nursing practice (Lauver et al., 2002). Emancipatory knowing is the human capacity to be aware of and critically reflect on the social, cultural, and political status quo and determine how and why it came to be that way (Chinn & Kramer, 2014). Emancipatory knowing calls for action to reduce or eliminate inequity and injustice. It validates that a person's context is central to a person-centered approach. The epistemology recognizes that social, political, economic, and gender injustices and professional forces support health and healing inequalities (Chinn, 2018). Current oppressive structures that exist in health care impede an individual's ability to engage in health-seeking and healthful

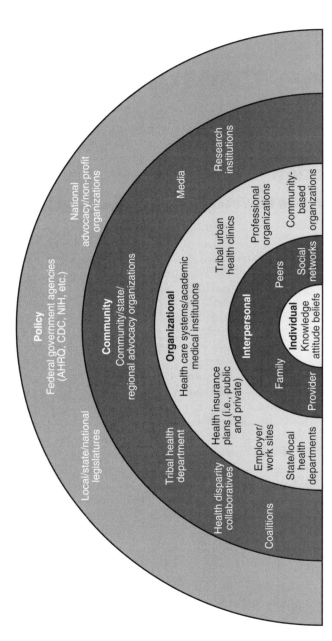

Figure 2-1 Socioeconomical Model of Health

behaviors. Emancipatory knowing intends to uncover and resolve social, political, economic, and gender injustices to empower people to seek and obtain their authentic well-being (Chinn, 2018). Nursing research and practice involve discovering and ameliorating inequities and injustices (Chinn & Kramer, 2014).

Person-centered care is increasingly central in nursing research, practice, and health and social policy (Bolster & Manias, 2010; McCance et al., 2009; B. McCormack et al., 2020, 2021). Conceptually, person-centered care is receptive and tailored to the person's needs, based on developing respectful and dignified therapeutic relationships (NAM, 2001). Person-centered care upholds the person's desires, needs, and principles to guide care decisions, thereby improving the power imbalances inherent in the current healthcare system. Person-centeredness advocates that all individuals are on a journey of health and healing. Person-centered care must be discernible and received as caring by the recipient (Bolster & Manias, 2010; Sharp et al., 2016). Often, clinicians respect the person, but they do not recognize the need to acknowledge and ameliorate discriminatory influences on health as part of the person-centered care approach (Chinn, 2018). It is, therefore, necessary to integrate the theory of emancipatory knowing to critically reflect on the multidimensional influences that affect health equity (Chinn, 2018).

Background of Person-Centered Care (PCC)

Historical Perspectives of Person-Centered Care in Medicine, Health Policy, and Nursing

In Nightingale's (1859) *Notes on Nursing*, she instructs nurses to "always sit down when a sick person is talking business with you, show no signs of hurry, give complete attention and full consideration if your advice is wanted, and go away the moment the subject is ended" (pp. 23–24). These simple instructions laid the foundation for the next 150 years of discourse on the professional interactions between nurses and patients. Other professions joined the epistemology much later. Medicine's PCC roots began when Engel (1977) called into question the centuries-old practice of dualism, the separation of mind and body in physician practice. Health policy makers came to the conversation still decades later, as they acknowledged the disparity in health outcomes and cited PCC as a potential solution (NAM, 2001). During this evolutionary process, scholars used different terms (*individualized care*; *patient-, client-, and resident-centered care*; and *patient-, client-,* and *person-focused care*) with subtle contextual variances to describe the phenomenon (Hobbs, 2009; Kitson et al., 2012; Morgan & Yoder, 2012; Zhao et al., 2016). Some authors proposed that the discordant language and definitions stymied the understanding of the phenomenon (Hobbs, 2009; Mead & Bower, 2001; Robinson et al., 2008). The following brief history of PCC in medicine, health policy, and nursing highlights sentinel texts from each discipline and their influence on the philosophical posits of PCC.

History of Person-Centered Care in Medicine

The origins of medicine's Biomedical Model can be traced to the early 1500s. Two paradigms were active: Descartes' analytical philosophy, where the whole body may be understood by examining its parts, and the Christian Church which supported that the mind held the soul in its domain. The mind-body dualism prevailed until Engel (1977) disputed the separation of biological-psychological-social influences of health. Engel (1977) denounced, "The biomedical model ignores both the rigor required to achieve reliability in the interview process and the necessity to analyze the meaning of the patient's report in the psychological, social, and cultural as well as the anatomical, physiological, or biochemical terms" (p. 132). This call to rebuke the Biomedical Model laid the groundwork for PCC in medicine.

Stewart (1995) authored the foundational PCC reference in medicine. The systematic review of the literature reported six domains of patient-centered care: (a) exploring the experience and expectation of the disease; (b) understanding the entire patient; (c) the physician and the patient finding common ground regarding management; (d) incorporating health promotion and self-management in the consultation; (e) attending to the quality of the physician–patient relationship; and (f) setting realistic expectations of outcomes. In a later text, Stewart et al. (2000) clarified that within patient-centered care, a physician does not relinquish control to the patient; instead, the patient and physician come to a mutual understanding of the patient's needs and respond accordingly. Although the element of "control" retained by the physician appears contradictory to the ontology of PCC, Stewart and collaborators (2000) were among the first to associate improved health status and efficacy of care with patient-centered practice.

A decade later, a team of physicians published a definition of patient-centered care much closer to that of the nursing discipline. Levinson, Lesser, and Epstein's (2010) definition of patient-centered care is from the perspective of physician communication skills. Patient-centered care is "characterized by continuous healing relationships, shared understanding, emotional support, trust, patient enablement, activation, and informed choices" (p. 1311).

History of Person-Centered Care in Health Policy

The seminal work in promoting change in health policy is attributed to the National Academy of Medicine's (2001) book *Closing the Quality Chasm*. In this publication, patient-centered care "encompasses qualities of compassion, empathy, and responsiveness to the needs, values, and expressed preferences of the individual patient" (p. 48). The World Health Organization's (WHO, 2007) policy framework affirmed the NAM's definition and provided an antecedent perspective to patient-centered care. A person-centered approach recognizes the imperative to educate and empower people to foster and safeguard their health before they become patients (WHO, 2007). The WHO's (2007) policy framework outlines four domains to promote person-centered health care: (a) individuals, families, and communities; (b) health practitioners; (c) healthcare organizations; and (d) healthcare systems. Each domain includes a strategic plan to promote the ideals.

History of Person-Centered Care in Nursing

PCC's ontology originates in nursing. Florence Nightingale (1859) described the work of medicine as removing obstructions, and nature does the work of healing. The work of nursing "is to put the patient in the best condition for nature to act upon [them]" (Nightingale, 1859, p. 82). This premise underpins PCC. To know the best condition for each patient is to know the person, understanding their perspectives, values, beliefs, and experiences and honoring how the collective influences health and behaviors.

Person. In the PCC literature, authors rarely define *person*, but scholars may glean characteristics of personhood in nursing and health policy works. A person is a relational, multidimensional human being with the potential to change and develop through and with others at all stages of life (McCormack, 2003a; Peplau, 1997; World Health Organization [WHO], 2007). This composite definition respects personhood in the young and old when traditional societal views may negate a person at these life stages as an autonomous individual. It also affirms that humans are communal beings who develop as social exchanges occur.

Environment. The environment concerning PCC is the healthcare system. The location may be community based, in a primary care clinic, in a school, and/or an acute care setting. Ideally, the values, mission, and actors in a person-centered healthcare system regard and respond to individual preferences, needs, and beliefs in humane and holistic ways that are in harmony and balance with people and the environment (IOM, 2001; WHO, 2007).

Nursing. The nursing profession's definitions in the context of PCC have advanced over the last 150 years. Florence Nightingale (1859) laid the foundation when she adeptly defined nursing as "the proper use of fresh air, light, warmth, cleanliness, quiet and the proper selection and administration of diet—all at the least expense of vital power to the patient" (preface). Peplau added the dimension of bonding between the nurse and the patient. According to Peplau (1997), nursing is a practice-based science founded on an interpersonal relationship between nurse and patient to promote the individual's well-being. Lauver and colleagues (2002) expanded beyond the nurse–patient dyad. They wrote that "nursing recognizes the uniqueness of individuals and the multidimensionality of human experience" (p. 246). Nursing is a profession that respects and works with persons, families, and communities through services and interactions that support persons, families, and communities "in regaining, maintaining, and attaining the fullest health possible in biopsychosocial-spiritual dimensions" (Lauver et al., 2002, p. 247).

Health. The PCC literature is nearly silent on the construct of health. Nursing authors speak to health with the other metaparadigm concepts of nursing, person, and care environment. Drawing from these paradigms, Lauver and team (2002) provide a comprehensive definition of the nursing profession that embeds health. Health is the fullest possible biopsychosocial and spiritual dimensions one may achieve (Lauver et al., 2002). McCormack (2003a & 2003b) contributed to the nursing discipline and PCC when he identified gaps in nursing theory, research, and practice in the epistemology of PCC. McCormack's (2003a & 2003b) sentinel works astutely recognize *that context in which the person-centered exchange* has the greatest potential to enrich or constrain the relationship. The context includes the professional's practice, which transpires within the confines of norms, values, milieu, power differentials, and organizational structure tolerance for innovation.

Person-Centered Nursing Framework. In subsequent years, McCormack and McCance (2006) published a middle-range theory, a person-centered nursing framework, which is the first to evaluate outcomes of person-centered nursing. Morgan and Yoder (2012), similar to McCormack and McCance's (2006) four constructs of person-centered nursing, delineate three domains of person-centered care, identified as antecedents, attributes, and consequences. Morgan and Yoder's (2012) contribution to epistemology includes empirical referents used in international acute care settings that aim to measure the "phenomena that demonstrate the occurrence of the concept" (p. 11). They urge U.S.-based researchers and practitioners to test the utility of the instruments across healthcare settings to develop and refine the implementation and practice of PCC.

Kitson and colleagues (2012) narrative review of the core elements of PCC synthesized 60 texts from nursing, medicine, and health policy. Contrary to other reports, the recognized seminal PCC texts had similar epistemology across disciplines. Health policy makers, nursing, and medicine included foundational themes of (a) patient participation and involvement, (b) the relationship between the patient and health professional, and (c) the context where PCC is delivered. Differentiation between professions developed with an emphasis on broader systems-level and contextual aspects of provider–patient relationships in nursing and health policy literature and circumscribed physician–patient therapeutic relationships in medicine articles. More discreetly described in the nursing literature was adhering to patient beliefs and values, where medicine devoted more exploration to understanding informed decision making (Kitson et al., 2002).

Contemporary Definitions of PCC

Building on the historical perspectives of PCC, several tenets guide current conceptualizations of person-centeredness: treating patients as individuals; respecting personhood; creating mutual trust and knowledge; and developing therapeutic relationships (McCance et al., 2021). Person-centered practice begins with humanistic caring and empathic listening to understand and facilitate care that aligns with an individual's context, roles, experiences, concerns, values, and aspirations (Morris et al., 2022).

Selected Concepts for Nursing Practice Represented in the Domain

Communication

The AACN *Essentials* concept of communication is most clearly present in the PCC domain through the subcompetencies included for engagement to establish a caring relationship and communicating effectively with individuals. In their sentinel paper, Street and colleagues (2009) ask, *How does communication heal?* They describe the communication functions and pathways that lead to proximal, intermediate, and health outcomes. They identified six communication functions: information sharing, acknowledging emotions, managing uncertainty, nurturing therapeutic relationships, decision making, and fostering self-management. Although not stated in the paper, information sharing goes beyond facts about the individual in person-centered communication. It must include the sharing of individualized information, such as genetic/genomic, environmental exposure information, social and fiscal resources, values, goals, and beliefs. One study invited individuals to identify preferences, values, goals, and barriers to care before their primary care visit using a digital tool linked to their electronic health record (Holt et al., 2020). They found that the digital tool users indicated notable increases in specific Communication Assessment Tool (Makoul et al., 2007) items rated as excellent: treated me with respect, showed interest in my ideas, showed care and concern, and spent about the right amount of time with me (Holt et al., 2020) versus nondigital tool users. These findings align with the proximal outcomes Street and colleagues (2009) identified.

Intermediate outcomes of person-centered communication may include trust in the healthcare system, consistent engagement in self-management activities, emotional regulation, and commitment to the co-designed care plan (Street et al., 2009). Notably, mistrust of healthcare providers and healthcare systems stems from egregious historical trauma and research misconduct (Bowen et al., 2022). In a nationally representative sample of 1,003 U.S. Black and Hispanic households, over one-third of households who received health care within the last year reported experiencing racism in care. Underscoring the importance of person-centered communication, only one-third of Black and Hispanic individuals who experienced racism reported satisfaction with care and care quality.

Health outcomes of person-centered communication patterns may lead to health equity and justice. Street and colleagues (2009) propose that health, well-being, functional capacity, and vitality restoration stem from person-centered communication. The therapeutic relationship must support culturally affirming agency and self-efficacy to manage health and access resources, leading to enhanced capability and motivation to solve health-related problems, manage complications, and consistently engage with treatment.

Social Determinants of Health

Social determinants of health (SDOH) are the conditions in which "people are born, live, learn, work, play, worship, and age that affect a wide range of health, functioning, and quality-of-life outcomes and risks" (Healthy People 2030, 2020). There is growing evidence that supports the remarkable sensitivity of health to the social and physical environment and political structures (WHO: Europe, 2003). Dagher and Linares (2022) recognize that the foundations of health begin before conception and are attenuated by early childhood experiences (Felitti et al., 1998), socioeconomic status, discrimination, working conditions, educational attainment, food access, and housing security (WHO: Europe, 2003). The environment and structures shape behavior, such as self-management practices, nutrition, physical activity, and substance use. Indeed, there is tremendous evidence that indicates that susceptibility to risk, healthcare choices, and health outcomes must be viewed with a systems-level lens and conditions within which people live, work, pray, and play (Prather et al., 2016). Furthermore, clinicians must acknowledge and reframe health inequities from race-based to racism-based disparities (Hardeman et al., 2020). For example, moving from a race-based statement, *Black pregnant people are at higher risk of preterm birth*, to a racism-based statement, the *lived experience of being Black in the United States puts Black pregnant people at higher risk of preterm birth* (Hardeman et al., 2020).

The healthcare system can prolong life and improve health in some conditions; however, the most impactful drivers of health stem from social and economic factors that make people ill in the first place (WHO: Europe, 2003). As nurses, we need to be cognizant of how people are affected by the context of their lived experiences. How is a person's living, working, and social conditions affecting their choices, behaviors, and health? Further, within the lived (and healthcare) experience, does the person feel heard, valued, and appreciated? How are we assessing them, and from whose perspective?

The AACN *Essentials* subcompetencies surrounding effective communication with individuals are imperative competencies in evaluating SDOH. Bourgois and colleagues (2017) challenge medicine to expand their assessment of social history beyond risk behaviors to acknowledge the impact of poverty, discrimination, and inequality on health. They highlight the overlapping and reinforcing power hierarchies (e.g., race, class, and gender), and institutional and political factors that inhibit healthcare access and the pursuit of healthy lifestyles (Bourgois et al., 2017). They developed a structural vulnerability assessment tool that assesses an individual's or a population's susceptibility to negative health outcomes by identifying eight domains of structural vulnerability, that is, financial security, residence, risk environments, food access, social network, legal status, education, and discrimination. In the healthcare environment, the structural vulnerability tool may lead to identifying susceptibilities and referring to mitigating resources. Although not explicit in their publication, personal agency must be included in a person-centered care environment to identify the desired intervention.

Risk Assessment Framework (2.9i)

The WHO's (2021) risk assessment framework defines *Risk* as the complex function of the probability of suffering harm or loss (adverse outcome) from exposure and susceptibility to some hazard. Applying this framework to the high rate of infant mortality in Milwaukee, WI (Capp, 2022), the risk is the scientific process of estimating the threat that hazards pose to adverse infant outcomes.

APNs/DNPs can use risk assessment to engage in risk management. First, identify what factors can be mitigated or managed. Second, focus on identifying predictors to address in the clinical and community settings. Third, share the assessment with community members and listen to their lived experiences. How do the patterns detected and health and risk factors identified align with their experience and goals for realigning or sustaining resources? See **Figure 2-2** regarding the complexity of

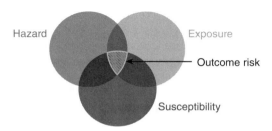

Figure 2-2 Risk = Complex Function of p[hazard] * p[exposure] * p[susceptibility]

Data from World Health Organization. (2021). Strategic toolkit for assessing risks: a comprehensive toolkit for all-hazards health emergency risk assessment. https://www.who.int/publications/i /item/9789240036086; Saulnier, D. D., Dixit, A. M., Nunes, A. R., & Murray, V. (n.d.). 3.2 Disaster risk factors – hazards, exposure and vulnerability. Retrieved March 20, 2023, from https://extranet.who.int /kobe_centre/sites/default/files/pdf/WHO%20Guidance_Research%20Methods_Health-EDRM_3.2.pdf

risk assessment. The community-engaged participatory research method can build consensus for community-identified health and risk factor prioritization for intervention development (McFarlane et al., 2022; Parker et al., 2020).

The AACN *Essentials* concept of SDOH is also prominent in the competencies surrounding development of a plan of care and evaluation of care outcomes. How the SDOH concept impacts subcompetencies within these competencies is described with more detail in the following paragraphs.

Strengths-Based Person-Centered Care

Person-centered health approaches, including explicitly naming how social, environmental, and political structures impact the community's health (Bowen et al., 2022) and resilience, are needed to enable a holistic picture of health. A holistic perspective may advance health equity by focusing on how individuals and communities thrive despite historical and contemporary health challenges (Chae et al., 2021). A person's strengths and resilience must be a part of a person-centered health approach. Strengths include individual, family, and community assets, talents, and capabilities (L. N. Gottlieb, 2014; L. N. Gottlieb & Gottlieb, 2017). Resilience is a learned and adaptable skill that can reduce an individual, family, or community's susceptibility to risk experiences and achieve a relatively good outcome despite adversities, traumas, challenges, or setbacks (Rashid et al., 2014). Person-reported strengths and clinician support promote resilience and prepare individuals to encounter challenges adaptively (Rashid et al., 2014). However, surveys and research rarely gather these data (Chae et al., 2021).

We can draw on the tenets of the Person-centered Practice Framework (B. McCormack & McCance, 2006) when screening for the SDOH. To begin, ask permission to complete the screening using culturally affirming communication, (i.e., communicating in the most respectful and effective ways to the individual). Also, ensure the healthcare system completes universal screening using a validated instrument to avoid bias in practice (NAM, 2020). If the person discloses a need, discuss potential and desired interventions, including resource and referral options. The discourse should be held within a compassionate, caring, and honest therapeutic relationship (Johnson et al., 2022). Steeves-Reece and colleagues (2022) systematically reviewed the literature to identify facilitators and barriers to resource connections. The facilitators included relevancy of the referral to social needs and context, simple to navigate and prompt connection, and inclusive of multiple social needs. Barriers to resource connections were referrals that were inaccessible, irrelevant, or restrictive; fears surrounding stigma, discrimination, and immigration status; impersonal or disrespectful interactions; inadequate knowledge about or capacity to connect to the resource; and language, culture, or literacy barriers (Steeves-Reece et al., 2022).

Driven by the critical need to advance health equity, researchers are rapidly developing instruments to survey health influences and connect people to needed resources. In 2016, the University of California–San Francisco (UCSF) established the Social Interventions Research and Evaluation Network (SIREN) to curate, mobilize, and disseminate rigorous research and inform the use of SDOH instruments (L. Gottlieb et al., 2017). Clinicians and researchers can submit a SDOH instrument for consideration of inclusion on the SIREN website. SIREN displays the instruments' number of social and nonsocial needs items, language availability, readability level, time to complete, and cost information. Further, they identify if an instrument contains the item(s) that assess any SIREN-identified 32 SDOH domains (e.g., discrimination, financial strain, and interpersonal violence). These instruments enable the various collections of SDOH; however, they are not standardized and are rarely harmonized to provide comparable and shareable data across information systems (Freij et al., 2019). The EHR needs better methods to incorporate whole-person health, including SDOH and strengths.

A strengths-based assessment tool option is MyStrengths+MyHealth (MSMH), a person-centered HIPAA-compliant web-based health assessment application designed for individuals to self-identify health and healthcare strengths, challenges, and needs. It includes Simplified Omaha System Terms (SOST), which are community-validated plain language versions of the Omaha System (Austin et al., 2022). MSMH aligns with national initiatives prioritizing social determinants measures for EHRs as it is mapped within SNOMED-CT and LOINC to enable interoperability within existing electronic health system platforms (Dzau et al., 2021; Rasanathan, 2018). MSMH was developed by employing user-centered design principles and validated among a diverse population (Austin et al., 2021). Participants or their proxy complete the MSMH app on their devices such as smartphones, iPad, or tablets.

Participants answer health assessment questions to identify strengths, challenges, and needs based on 42 health concepts in the Omaha System (Martin, 2005). Within MSMH, Strengths are defined as a rating of 4 or 5 on a 5-point Likert-type scale for each concept (e.g., "how would you describe your income"). Challenges are defined as binary signs/symptoms for each concept (yes if selected, no if not selected). Needs are defined as binary interventions for each concept (e.g., hard to buy the things I need; yes, if selected, no if not selected). MSMH app can be tailored to the health concepts relevant to a population (Austin et al., 2021). Participants receive a unique identifier when they complete the application to facilitate the retrieval and revision of their data. Participants can print or save their responses as a PDF at the end of the survey.

Some healthcare systems have been challenged by the implementation of SDOH screening (Imran et al., 2022). Chagin and colleagues (2021) developed a sequential six-step process to screen for SDOH and referral to a service organization when necessary. Developed for the primary care setting, all individuals are screened, it is determined if they have social needs, and they are asked for consent for a referral to a service organization. The healthcare team places the referral, monitors if the service organization accepts the referral, and documents the outcomes of the referral (e.g., did the individual accept the referral?).

Health Policy

The AACN *Essentials* concept of health policy is most clearly present in the competencies associated with communicating effectively, evaluating outcomes of care, and provision of care coordination. Each of these competencies has subcompetencies closely related to creation and/or development of policy.

When Does Policy Inhibit or Create Barriers to PCC?

Inequities experienced by non-White and non-heteronormative populations are largely due to systematic and structural racism in policy (Nickitas et al., 2022; Prather et al., 2016; Williams & Collins, 2001; Williams & Mohammed, 2013;

Yearby et al., 2022). Systematic and structural racism are "forms of racism that are pervasively and deeply embedded in systems, laws, written or unwritten policies, and entrenched practices and beliefs that produce, condone, and perpetuate widespread unfair treatment and oppression of people of color, with adverse health consequences" (Braveman et al., 2022, p. 171). Racially based socioeconomic and health inequities persist due to well-entrenched, unequal systems that uphold the legacy of overtly discriminatory practices, policies, laws, and beliefs (Yearby et al., 2022). These discriminatory legacies deny certain groups access to living wage jobs with benefits; safe neighborhoods; home ownership; high-quality education; accessible and acceptable health care; and fair treatment by the criminal justice system (Bailey et al., 2017; Gee & Ford, 2011; Williams et al., 2019; Yearby et al., 2022). There are many examples. Gee and Ford (2011) and Yearby and colleagues (2022) discuss over 30 racial and ethnic policies and actions, beginning in the 1700s, whose legacies maintain health inequities.

The path forward requires interventions at the individual, systems, and societal levels. The social ecological model (Bronfenbrenner, 1977) indicates that multilevel interventions yield greater and more sustainable benefits than interventions aimed at one level of influence (L. McCormack et al., 2017). Devine and colleagues (2012) reported on the success of a multifaceted program designed to decrease individual implicit biases by introducing multiple strategies to increase awareness of individual and societal biases. Results indicated that non-Black undergraduate student program participants sustained a reduction in implicit biases for at least three months after the program started (Devine et al., 2012). Additional implicit bias tests and training for healthcare providers are discussed later in this chapter.

Healthcare systems can review their policies and procedures to evaluate if they disenfranchise certain groups. Consider RC, who uses public transportation to travel to their clinic appointment from their place of employment. How could a late policy that states a person needs to reschedule if they are 15 minutes late to an appointment disadvantage people who use public transportation? Another example is the use of clear language principles across written and digital materials (Baur & Prue, 2014; L. McCormack et al., 2017). One principle is to prepare written materials at a seventh-grade reading level or less (National Institutes of Health, 2015). A 20-year review of patient education materials published in high-impact journals found the mean range of materials was approximately 11th to 14th grade (Rooney et al., 2021). The inability to understand written health materials has been linked with decreased self-management, reduced health engagement activities, and increased health disparities (Landis, 2021; Monsen et al., 2015; Rush et al., 2021).

Health policies at the state and national level also impact health outcomes. The Kaiser Family Foundation maintains a postpartum Medicaid extension coverage website (Medicaid Postpartum Coverage Extension Tracker, 2022) that illustrates states' postpartum Medicaid coverage. Twenty-seven states (as of 12/06/2022) have extended Medicaid coverage, and seven plan to implement extended coverage to one year postpartum. Wisconsin's Medicaid policy extends postpartum coverage to 60 days after birth, with an extension to 90 days under review in the legislature.

National organizations (e.g., American Association of Colleges of Nursing, 2021; NAM, 2021) call upon nurses to lead and advocate for policy changes. To do so, APNs/DNPs can review policies with a critical lens to evaluate how they impact the health of the people within their practice and organization (e.g., housing policies, and institutional policies). DNP-prepared nurses can also advocate for change by assuming leadership positions on boards at the local, state, and national levels (Ellenbecker et al., 2017). Nurses must take an ecological and holistic perspective toward policy change, including advocating for improving the quality of housing, food access, and neighborhood environments, access to financial opportunities, quality education, and accessible health care (Yearby et al., 2022). Remember that multilevel policy changes make the most impact on improving health outcomes (L. McCormack et al., 2017). Refer to Nethers and Milstead (2022) for a comprehensive review of the political process for nurses.

Level II Competencies of the Domain

Engage With the Individual in Establishing a Caring Relationship

Promote and Foster a Caring Relationship Through Empathy and Compassion and Facilitate Difficult Conversations

Empathy is a requisite of person-centered care and communication (Levett-Jones & Cant, 2020). It is a multidimensional construct that includes cognitive, affective, and behavioral elements (Everson et al., 2015). Levett-Jones and Cant (2020) describe a three-stage process of the empathy continuum used to establish a caring relationship. In the perceiving stage, the nurse senses the individual's emotional state. Then, using past and current reflections of personal biases, prejudices, and judgments, they must suspend these thoughts to be present unconditionally. During the processing stage, the nurse is respectfully curious about the person's experience and how the experience shapes the person's story. Finally, the responding phase is an altruistic expression of concern and offer of assistance to ameliorate suffering. The expression of concern includes active listening, being present, reflective listening, summarizing what was heard, and engaging in actions supporting the alleviation of suffering and promoting health and well-being. In other models, the responding stage is defined as compassionate care (Sinclair et al., 2017). Also, during the responding phase, the nurse engages in self-reflection to learn and improve empathetic skills going forward (Levett-Jones & Cant, 2020).

Sinclair and colleagues (2017) interviewed 53 individuals in advanced stages of cancer. The study compared and contrasted individuals' palliative care experiences of sympathy, empathy, and compassion. Participants described sympathy as receiving pity about regrettable circumstances and a shallow and superficial emotional response by the observer. Sympathy was always viewed as a negative care experience. Examples of sympathetic responses included, "I am so sorry" and "That must be so awful for you." Palliative care recipients positively viewed empathetic conversation, characterized by an affective response that recognizes and tries to comprehend an individual's experience through emotional resonance (Sinclair et al., 2017). Examples of empathetic responses included, "Help me understand your experience" and "I get the feeling that you are frustrated with your situation." Compassionate care builds on an empathetic response in an attempt to relieve suffering through actions (see **Figure 2-3**). Individuals receiving palliative care lauded compassionate care as

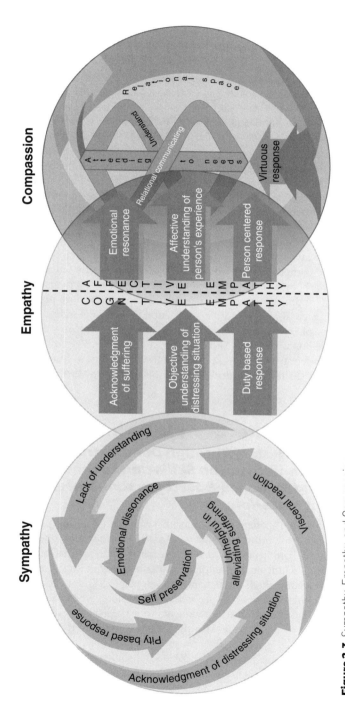

Figure 2-3 Sympathy, Empathy, and Compassion

the highest level of care. Examples of compassionate statements included, "I hear you saying . . . Would you be open to . . . ?" "I see that you are uncomfortable. How can I help you to feel more at ease?" (Sinclair et al., 2017).

To gain competency in establishing caring relationships with individuals, consider how you feel, engage, and react with interacting with others. A sympathetic reaction may be a coping mechanism used when the clinician feels inadequately prepared to address situational suffering (Sinclair et al., 2017). Empathy and compassion are a continuum of care valued by most individuals. In an empathic relationship, the clinician can share feelings of joy or suffering with an individual without losing perspective between self and individual (Singer & Klimecki, 2014). Singer and Klimecki (2014) propose that compassion is a protective action when a clinician feels concerned for another and is motivated to help. Clinicians can also practice being compassionate through meditation and other wellness activities.

In Fredrickson and colleagues' (2008) sentinel randomized control trial, they trained adults to become more compassionate using loving-kindness meditation. The one-hour per week for seven-week intervention consisted of 15 minutes of group meditation, 20 minutes of group sharing, and 20 minutes of education on how to apply mediation principles in daily life. The group meditation is built from directing love and compassion toward oneself to loved ones, acquaintances, strangers, and all living beings. The researchers predicted that as participants became skilled in loving-kindness meditation, they would experience more positive emotions, improving mental health and life satisfaction. The results indicated that the one-hour a week of loving-kindness meditation improved various positive emotions and interactions with others (Fredrickson et al., 2008). Refer to the Greater Good Science Center at the University of California Berkeley website to listen to the audio and read the loving-kindness meditation script (University of California Berkeley, 2022).

Communicate Effectively With Individuals
Create Cultural Safety Through Demonstration of Advanced Communication Skills and Techniques and Designing Evidence-Based, Person-Centered Engagement Materials

Recall when you were a "patient" in the healthcare system. Did the provider give you time to explain your priorities, values, or goals? Did they ask you about your agenda for the visit? Unfortunately, research results inform us that only 36% of clinical encounters include elicitation of the patient's agenda (Singh Ospina et al., 2019). When clinicians asked, the patient was interrupted 70% of the time, with a median time to interruption of 11 seconds. Furthermore, when the patient was uninterrupted, they completed their statements in a median of 6 seconds (Singh Ospina et al., 2019). Remember these startling statistics the next time you communicate with a person who is sharing their priorities, values, or experiences with you.

Actively listening to people is one step in establishing cultural safety. Cultural safety is when a person enters a health service, developed by someone of a different age, culture, race, ethnicity, gender, sexual orientation, (dis)ability, and/or belief structure, without the person losing their self in the process (Papps & Ramsden, 1996; Ramsden, n.d.). The person feels safe to authentically and fully engage in the therapeutic relationship to promote or restore their health. An outcome of cultural safety is clinician recognition and valuing of an individual's historical and personal narratives (Mukerjee et al., 2021).

Consider this clinical scenario adapted from The Fenway Institute (2015). Oscar is a 22-year-old Salvadorian female-to-male transgender person. Oscar has not had gender-affirming surgery or hormone therapy. Since arriving in the United States about 4 years ago, he has been a bartender in a nightclub. He has been with the same sexual partner for the past 6 months. Today he is visiting the clinic after taking a home pregnancy test, which was positive. Oscar is uninsured and an undocumented immigrant.

Take a moment to reflect on your assumptions or thoughts when you read this scenario. What mental imagines come to mind? How would you introduce yourself to Oscar? How would you ask Oscar to introduce himself? How can your (re)actions and words establish a culturally safe encounter? Clinician language and communication can support or hinder cultural safety. At the beginning of an encounter, a clinician may introduce themself using the following model: "Hi, my name is Dr. Jeana Holt; I am a family nurse practitioner. I use she/her pronouns. Please call me Jeana. What name and pronouns would you like me to use today?" (Mukerjee et al., 2021; Roe & Galvin, 2021).

Use Person-First Language by Applying Individualized Information in Delivery of Personalized Health Care

Creating a safety culture through language extends to using people-first language. Compare these descriptors:

- Diabetic vs. A person with diabetes
- Schizophrenic vs. A person with schizophrenia or a person with a mental health illness
- Nonadherent/Noncompliant vs. acknowledging the social and structural barriers to health
- Disabled vs. A person with dwarfism

Person-first language is founded on the principle that people are more than a condition, disease, (dis)ability, social class, race/ethnicity, or other characteristic (Dawkins & Daum, 2022). Acknowledging the holism of a person is critical for building and maintaining a culturally safe and therapeutic relationship. Using identify-first language has resulted in medical mistrust, decreased patient satisfaction, decreased engagement in care, and increased healthcare costs (Dawkins & Daum, 2022). Therefore, the words APNs/DNPs use must convey respect, cultural safety, and inclusion. Person-first language also aligns with the recommendations of trauma-informed care (Ravi & Little, 2017; Schimmels & Cunningham, 2021; Substance Abuse and Mental Health Services Administration, 2014).

Trauma-Informed Care as Part of Demonstration of Advanced Communication Skills and Techniques

Substance Abuse and Mental Health Services Administration (SAMHSA) provides healthcare organizations and clinicians with a trauma-informed approach to care that can be applied to all clinical encounters (SAMHSA, 2014). The framework consists of four pillars and six key principles. A trauma-informed organization *realizes* the insidious impact of trauma and various paths for recovery; *recognizes* the diverse signs and symptoms of trauma in individuals, families, clinicians, and others involved with the system; and *responds* by developing policies, procedures, and practices that acknowledge the widespread impact of trauma and *resists* retraumatizing those involved in the system (SAMHSA, 2014). Six key principles are fundamental to a trauma-informed approach, including establishing and maintaining safety, trustworthiness, and transparency; peer support; collaboration and mutuality; empowerment of voice and choice; and recognizing and validating cultural, historical, and gender experiences. In this context, establishing and maintaining safety and trustworthiness is the sense of physiological and psychological security (SAMHSA, 2014).

In a trauma-informed and culturally safe healthcare system, the organization and clinicians are transparent in building and maintaining trust with the person. Using a trauma-informed approach, clinicians validate past and current cultural, historical, and gender experiences and avoid retraumatizing the individual (Ravi & Little, 2017; Schimmels & Cunningham, 2021; SAMHSA, 2014). Empathizing and validating a person's experience with the healthcare system can also build trust. If someone discloses a negative healthcare experience, a clinician may respond, *I hear that you are angry and frustrated with how the clinicians treated you during your recent hospital stay*.

Clinicians recognize that trauma and chronic stress may present as alterations in sleep, appetite, libido, mood, and energy. Somatic symptoms may also occur such as nausea, headaches, and chest tightness. People may self-manage their symptoms by overexercising, restricting food or types of foods, or using alcohol, tobacco, or other substances (Ravi & Little, 2017).

A trauma-informed approach also recognizes the power relationships among the individual and clinician, the individual and health system, and the clinician and the health system. Please see **Figure 2-4** for principles of a trauma-informed approach. Clinician's actions can minimize the power differential, for example, sitting down, maintaining eye contact, and actively listening to the individual. Clinicians can also offer options during the interview and exam. For example, being alone or with a support person, using an interpreter, and ensuring that the individual knows their agency to decline to answer questions or decline portions of the exam (Ravi & Little, 2017). Clinicians can also be transparent about why they ask certain questions during the interview process. Mukerjee et al. (2021) offer the following phrasing when taking a sexual health history, "I ask all of my patients about their sexual activity so that I can make better recommendations about each person's sexual health" (p. 76).

Healthcare systems can offer peer support from trauma survivors to assist with establishing safety, hope, trust, collaboration, and healing (SAMHSA, 2014). Collaboration and mutuality begin with asking about priorities, values, and goals of care. *What would you like to discuss during this visit? What are your health goals? Which one is your priority? Who or what can support you to achieve and maintain that goal? Let's discuss the best ways that I can assist you.* The organization and staff practice a strengths-based resilience approach to empower and elevate the individual's voice and choices to engage in healing. The organization and clinician acknowledge their biases and actively work to move past their cultural, historical, and gendered assumptions to provide cultural and gender-affirming services that recognize and address historical trauma.

6 guiding principles to a trauma-informed approach

The CDC's Center for Preparedness and Response (CPR), in collaboration with SAMHSA's National Center for Trauma-Informed Care (NCTIC), developed and led a new training for CPR employees about the role of trauma-informed care during public health emergencies. The training aimed to increase responder awareness of the impact that trauma can have in the communities where they work.

Participants learned SAMHSA'S six principles that guide a trauma-informed approach, including:

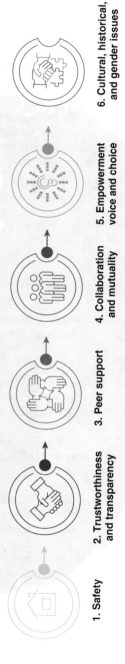

1. Safety

2. Trustworthiness and transparency

3. Peer support

4. Collaboration and mutuality

5. Empowerment voice and choice

6. Cultural, historical, and gender issues

Adopting a trauma-informed approach is not accomplished through any single particular technique or checklist. It requires constant attention, caring awareness, sensitivity, and possibly a cultural change at an organizational level. On-going internal organizational assessment and quality improvement, as well as engagement with community stakeholders, will help to imbed this approach which can be augmented with organizational development and practice improvement. The training provided by CPR and NCTIC was the first step for CDC to view emergency preparedness and response through a trauma-informed lens.

Figure 2-4 Six Guiding Principles to a Trauma-Informed Approach

Originally published in 2004, the Primary Care Post-Traumatic Stress Disorder (PC-PTSD) screen was developed and tested with 188 U.S. Veterans to detect PTSD in primary care clinics with limited time and resources (Prins et al., 2004). The screener includes four items with yes/no response options beginning with the following statement,

> In your life, have you ever had any experience that was so frightening, horrible, or upsetting that, in the past month, you:
>
> 1. Had nightmares about the event(s) or thought about the event(s) when you did not want to?
> 2. Tried hard not to think about the event(s) or went out of your way to avoid situations that reminded you of the event(s)?
> 3. Been constantly on guard, watchful, or easily startled?
> 4. Felt numb or detached from people, activities, or your surroundings?

(Prins et al., 2016) and colleagues updated the screener in 2016 to align with the DSM-5 (PC-PTSD-5). They added an introductory item,

> Sometimes things happen to people that are unusually or especially frightening, horrible, or traumatic. For example:
>
> - a serious accident or fire
> - a physical or sexual assault or abuse
> - an earthquake or flood
> - a war
> - seeing someone be killed or seriously injured
> - having a loved one die through homicide or suicide.
>
> Have you ever experienced this kind of event? YES / NO
> If no, screen total = 0. Please stop here.

If the respondent answers "Yes" they answer five items. Four of the items are consistent with the PC-PTSD, with the fifth item being,

> **In the past month, have you** . . . Felt guilty or unable to stop blaming yourself or others for the event(s) or any problems the event(s) may have caused?

If a respondent endorses a trauma exposure in the initial statement, they can score a 0–5 on the PC-PTSD-5, which is one point for each of the affirmative responses to the five subsequent items. Tested in a sample of approximately 400 primary care–seeking veterans, a cut-point of four balanced false negatives and false positives for the overall sample and for men (Bovin et al., 2021). However, for women, a cut-point of three resulted in a better fit. The researchers advised clinicians to adjust the cut-point depending on the sample characteristics and screening purposes (Bovin et al., 2021). For people who meet the cut-point, a referral to a mental health professional trained in trauma-informed care is warranted.

The PC-PTSD and PC-PTSD-5 have been tested in non-veteran populations. The PC-PTSD-5 maintained strong and similar diagnostic accuracy within a middle-aged (M=40.97 +/− 17.03 years) civilian primary care sample (Williamson et al., 2022).

However, the PC-PTSD had poor diagnostic accuracy among college-age students (Hawn et al., 2022). All people who have experiences trauma should be screened for suicidal ideation. Panagioti and colleagues (2009), in their narrative review explain the relationship between PTSD and suicidal thoughts and behaviors, cautioning clinicians to note that comorbid depression increases the effect of PTSD on ideation and behaviors.

The staff at the U.S. Department of Veteran's Affairs developed the tool, which is in the public domain and not copyrighted. You may access it and publications at the PTSD: National Center for PTSD (n.d.) website.

Implicit Bias as Related to Advanced Communication Skills and Person-Centered Engagement Materials

Implicit bias is a human condition where people unconsciously assign judgments to a person or group based on their overt or perceived characteristics and past experiences (Narayan, 2019). It occurs across professions, but when healthcare professionals hold negative implicit biases, they contribute to healthcare disparities (FitzGerald & Hurst, 2017). Care recipients also notice. Blair and colleagues (2013) evaluated providers' level of implicit ethnic/racial bias and patients' perceptions receiving person-centered care. Individuals who rated their provider lower on "person-centeredness" (e.g., interpersonal communication, trust, knowledge, and treatment) received care from providers who had more implicit bias. Bias may be experienced by members of the nondominant race, ethnic groups, or religious minorities (Narayan, 2019). Other populations may also experience discrimination based on sexual orientation, gender identification, (dis)ability, social class, level of education, or stigmatized diagnoses (e.g., obesity or mental illness) (Narayan, 2019). To fulfill the goal of providing person-centered care, nurses must be conscious of thoughts and actions that impart a negative evaluation of an individual who is connected to membership of a group or to a certain characteristic (FitzGerald & Hurst, 2017).

The first step is to recognize implicit bias and acknowledge the harms that arise when implicit bias occurs within the healthcare system. To recognize implicit bias, Project Implicit (n.d.) offers 15 Implicit Association Tests (IAT) that measure the strength of associations between concepts (e.g., dark skin, gender-career, young-old) and evaluations (e.g., good, bad, neutral) or stereotypes (e.g., athletic, smart, frail). The results may reveal unconscious biases that the participant holds. Once known, individuals can begin to resolve implicit biases by taking implicit bias training, mandated in some states for healthcare professionals (Cooper et al., 2022). There are many free implicit bias training opportunities for healthcare professionals. One example is the UnBIASED Project, which is funded by the National Library of Medicine (NLMR01LM013301) to help reduce health disparities by improving patient–clinician communication for low-income, racially diverse patients in primary care (Hartzler, 2019). The Think Cultural Health website from the National Institutes of Health provides a free 2-hour online training for healthcare providers and students to increase their skills and knowledge for cultural humility, person-centered care, and combating implicit bias across the care continuum of maternal health (Maternal Health Care, n.d.). The Kirwan Institute has a free online five-module course that assists participants with understanding the origins of implicit associations (The Ohio

State University, n.d.). The University of California–Los Angeles has an implicit bias video series (University of California Los Angeles, n.d.) and Project READY: Reimagining Equity & Access for Diverse Youth hosts a series of free, online professional development modules for people interested in improving their knowledge about race and racism, racial equity, and culturally sustaining pedagogy (Project READY: Reimagining Equity & Access for Diverse Youth – A Free Online Professional Development Curriculum, n.d.). APNs/DNPs can also develop evidence-based materials with diverse groups to ensure the person-centered materials are culturally affirming.

Implicit Bias Activity

Directions: Read the following five clinical scenarios and answer the reflection questions.

Scenario 1. Anita is a 30-year-old working single mother of a 3-year-old son and is expecting a second child (36 weeks pregnant). She needs to be screened for group B streptococcus (GBS) during this prenatal visit. Anita discloses that she has not felt the baby move in the last 24 hours. Anita is worried that there is something wrong with the baby.

Scenario 2. Jan, a 22-year-old, married woman, is 24 weeks pregnant, and presenting to the clinic today for a routine prenatal visit. She is 5 feet, 2 inches tall, and weighs 260 pounds. Her BMI is 48. Upon review of her electronic health record, you note her blood pressure was 150/111 mm Hg (normal <130/80) at her last visit 4 weeks ago and is 163/105 mm Hg today. You are concerned about a new diagnosis of pre-eclampsia and/or the potential to develop HELLP. Jan has difficulty transitioning from the chair to the exam table due to joint pain and lower extremity edema.

Scenario 3. Hailey, who is 29 weeks pregnant, received blunt-force trauma to her abdomen during an argument with her boyfriend. She has no obvious injuries and denies pain and vaginal bleeding. Hailey has two other children present at the visit, ages 2 and 4 years. She is not currently working and receives food supplements from the Women, Infants, and Children (WIC) program.

Scenario 4. Shafaq Zahra, a 24-year-old woman, presents to a mobile clinic for a postpartum visit six weeks after the birth of her third child. Her children are 24 months, 12 months, and 6 weeks. She immigrated to the United States four years ago from Iran and identifies as a devout woman of the Shia tradition. She is wearing a hijab and requests only female clinicians and an interpreter.

Scenario 5. Jenny (she/her/hers), a 25-year-old male-to-female transgender person, wants to investigate the services that you provide. She has not legally changed her name, so her documents display her birth name, James. She is new in transition, dressed in t-shirts and jeans, and still produces facial hair (which is exposed). She appears to be shy, jittery, and very nervous, and does not look anyone in the eyes. Jenny had unprotected sex one week prior and is concerned about her HIV status.

Implicit Bias Self-Reflection Questions

- What are my mental models and assumptions that I employed when reading the scenarios?
- Where do I derive my assumptions (previous healthcare interactions, social/political influences, parental/familial norms, media portrayals)?
- How can I view an individual as a "whole person"?

Integrate Assessment Skills in Practice

Patient-Centered Assessment Method to Demonstrate That One's Practice Is Informed by a Method Appropriate to Function in Advanced Nursing Practice

The Patient-Centered Assessment Method (PCAM) identifies an individual's bio-psychosocial complexities to facilitate referral to the appropriate services (Pratt et al., 2015; Scored, n.d.; Yoshida et al., 2017). It includes four domains: health and well-being, social environment, health literacy and communication, and service coordination. PCAM has good reliability and validity, tested internationally (Yoshida et al., 2017) and in primary and acute care settings (Pratt et al., 2015; Yoshida et al., 2017). In a Japan-based study, higher levels of biopsychosocial complexity were positively correlated to longer hospital lengths of stay. The researchers advised that addressing the biopsychosocial concerns early in the acute care stay may assist in a timely discharge (Yoshida et al., 2017). In primary care–based studies in Scotland, the implementation of the PCAM correlated with decreases in medical referrals and increases in psychological, social, and lifestyle referrals (Pratt et al., 2015). However, the researchers noted that the referral increases did not overburden the system. Nurses involved in the study reported feeling supported by a network of health systems and community-based organizations. People were forthright and willing to discuss their challenges and accepted referrals to organizations that may assist with their needs (Pratt et al., 2015).

Clinical Scenario. Rolonda is a 22-year-old who identifies as a Black woman. She presents to the clinic six days after giving birth via cesarean section. She reports feeling tired and warm and has little to no appetite. She brings her 6-day-old son with her, whom she is breastfeeding. Rolonda is concerned that he is not latching well. The APN notes that his birth weight was 8 lbs., 0 oz, and today he weighs 7 lbs., 1 oz. Rolonda does not have any help at home and is feeling overwhelmed and exhausted.

Using the four domains of PCAM—health and well-being, social environment, health literacy and communication, and service coordination—how should the APN begin the visit? It is essential that the clinician create a caring environment that provides privacy and builds trust. The APN should sit down and actively listen while acknowledging and validating Rolonda's feelings and concerns. As part of the therapeutic discourse, the clinician can ask how they may assist Rolonda to alleviate some of her sufferings. The APN can further explore Rolonda's social environment using the principles of SAMSHA's Trauma-Informed Care (TIC) framework (SAMSHA, 2014). Using a validated instrument, the care team can assess service coordination needs and referral to resources. During the physical exam, the APN can exemplify actions in the Person-Centered Nursing Index (McCance et al., 2009) by listening to Rolonda's questions and requests, explaining assessment techniques, involving Rolonda in the assessment, and respecting Rolonda's agency if she declines care.

Diagnose Actual or Potential Health Problems and Needs

Clinical Reasoning as Context-Driven Diagnostic Integration of Advanced Scientific Knowledge

Clinical reasoning is a process of thinking through various aspects of a clinical encounter, (e.g., presentation, clinical data, and diagnostic test results) to arrive at a reasonable decision regarding the prevention, diagnosis, or care plan for a given patient (Hawkins et al., 2019; Reinoso et al., 2018). Hawkins et al. (2019) delineated an eight-step clinical reasoning process. The following questions guide the clinician through the process:

1. What is the purpose of the clinical reasoning?
2. What clinical problem are you trying to solve?
3. Are the assumptions that you are making justified?
4. What are the strengths and weaknesses of your point of view?
5. Is there enough relevant data to support a conclusion?
6. How are you applying concepts and theories correctly to guide your clinical reasoning?
7. What inferences are you and should you be considering?
8. What are the implications of your conclusions?

Clinical Scenario. Consider the following clinical scenario. Allie, a 15-year-old Latina, presents to the mobile clinic with concerns of persistent fatigue. Her history reveals a 24-hour diet recall of a granola bar, chips, a box of corn starch, ice chips from the gas station, and a 20 oz. cup of soda. She also disclosed compulsive consumption of ice. She denies gastrointestinal (GI) symptoms, epistaxis, menorrhagia, melena, hematuria, hematemesis, surgical history, and a family history of GI malignancy. Her physical examination reveals a well-developed, slightly undernourished, pale female. During the exam, Allie shared that she slept on a friend's couch because her home was unsafe. She does not know how long she will be able to stay there. Her laboratory test results reveal a low mean corpuscular volume, low ferritin, increased total iron binding capacity, low serum iron level, and low transferrin saturation.

Use the clinical reasoning process to arrive at a reasonable care plan for Allie.

1. Purpose: To address Allie's chief complaints of fatigue.
2. Clinical problem: What is the most effective way to address the likely diagnosis of iron deficiency anemia?
3. Assumptions: Lab tests indicate iron deficiency anemia. The most effective treatment will be iron replacement therapy. The underlying cause of the anemia is a lack of nutritional intake of iron.
4. Point-of-view: A conservative approach would be to initiate a trial of iron therapy and educate Allie on iron-rich foods.

5. Relevant data: Lab results, patient history, and physical exam.
6. Concepts: Iron deficiency anemia is the most common nutritional disorder worldwide, characterized by decreased red blood cell production due to low iron stores.
7. Inferences: The laboratory data indicate a positive diagnosis of iron deficiency anemia. Since Allie has clinical symptoms and laboratory data indicative of iron deficiency anemia, iron replacement therapy should be initiated.
8. Conclusions: Failure to treat iron deficiency anemia may result in fatigue, headaches, restless legs syndrome, heart problems, and pregnancy complications. (Short & Domagalski, 2013)

Clinical Decision Making as Context-Driven Integration of Advanced Scientific Knowledge to Guide Decision Making

Clinical decision making, as defined by Reinoso and colleagues (2018), has the elements of clinical reasoning PLUS the person's unique circumstances, including social support, cultural beliefs, financial support, health beliefs, and practices. Using the clinical decision-making definition, how would Allie's plan of care be adjusted?

Raising awareness of and avoiding potential errors of diagnostic reasoning will increase an APN student's competency in diagnosing actual or potential health problems and needs (LaManna et al., 2019). During the data gathering phase, engage in empathetic listening to understand the concern from the individual and/or family's perspective. Also, systematically collect and interpret data to gain situational awareness of the concern. Generate a succinct but comprehensive list of the obvious hypotheses, not to be missed hypotheses, and hypotheses not influenced by the age or gender of the individual. As the APN evaluates the list of hypotheses, continue to use a systematic approach to gather more data to rule out or confirm a hypothesis. Self-reflect, *what else could this be?* Throughout the process, communicate with the healthcare team, engaging in consultation and referring the individual to specialty clinicians as needed. Furthermore, engage with the individual and/or family about the process, goals, priorities, capacity, and resources. Finally, evaluate care from the individual's and/or family's perspective.

Develop a Plan of Care

Cumulative Complexity Model to Prioritize Risk Mitigation Strategies for Prevention or Reduction of Adverse Outcomes

In 2012, Shippee and colleagues presented the Cumulative Complexity Model that illustrated the complicating factors that individuals may face when managing multiple chronic conditions (MCC). The model purports that an *individual's workload of demands* (e.g., employment, caretaker responsibilities, self-care, and healthcare system navigation) and an *individual's capacity* (e.g., physical and mental wellness, social connectedness, financial resources, and health literacy) to meet those demands may directly or indirectly influence outcomes.

Burden of Treatment Theory to Lead and Collaborate With an Interprofessional Team Considering Risk Mitigation as Well as Evidence-Based Interventions to Improve Outcomes and Safety

Similar to the Cumulative Complexity Model is the Burden of Treatment Theory (May et al., 2014) developed for individuals who seek to manage health rather than cure a condition. The model recognizes that plans of care may demand complex self-management regimens that assume a high level of individual knowledge, motivation, resources, and behaviors. People may struggle to balance the treatment regimens with daily life, leading to structurally induced non-adherence and/or over- or under-utilization of healthcare services. As self-care complexity increases (i.e., burden of treatment), some individuals and families become overwhelmed, leading to poor health outcomes, caregiver strain, healthcare services over-utilization, and rising healthcare costs (Boehmer et al., 2016; May et al., 2014).

Clinicians can lessen the burden of treatment by recognizing the plan of care demands and asking about treatment burden to address or prevent workload–capacity imbalances (Shippee et al., 2012). APNs can lead and collaborate with interprofessional teams to review and develop a comprehensive plan of care that reduces the burden of treatment. Articles from several authors (i.e., May et al., 2014; Shippee et al., 2012; Tinetti et al., 2019) informed the following clinical example.

Vanessa, a 42-year-old, married, working mother of five, presents to the clinic with concerns about not having a period for the last three months. She usually menstruates every 28-days. Her past medical history reveals type 2 diabetes, hypertension, and obesity. She ate lunch 1 hour ago and her glucose at the clinic today was 211 mg/dL (normal <180 mg/dL), BP 150/99 (normal <130/80), Ht 5 ft, 11 in., 275 pounds, BMI 38. She states that she is very stressed by the recent loss of her job and insurance. She requests a pregnancy test and help with her medications and glucose testing strips that she cannot afford to pay for out of pocket.

The Cumulative Complexity Model informs us that Vanessa's recent job loss may have simultaneous direct and indirect influences on care and outcomes (e.g., inability to pay and chronic stress), reflecting the amplification of structural vulnerabilities (Bourgois et al., 2017; Shippee et al., 2012). Additionally, capacity-limiting circumstances (e.g., physical and mental functioning, symptoms, and social support) may sensitize her, leaving her especially susceptible to a complex plan of care (Shippee et al., 2012).

A strengths-based approach may guide a plan of care that lessens Vanessa's workload demands and builds her capacity. Completing a social health screening tool may assist with identifying additional areas of need and lead to connecting Vanessa to resources. The tool may also identify areas of strength that must continue to be supported. Redesigning her care plan may include identifying goals, prioritizing care demands, integrating healthcare and community resources to support capacity, and engaging social support to lessen burdens (Shippee et al., 2012). For example, engaging Vanessa's social support in her care may assist with negotiating and navigating the healthcare system (May et al., 2014). It is important to document Vanessa's goals, values, and preferences in the EHR for the healthcare team.

A nonrandomized clinical trial that compared patients who identified care priorities and those who did not indicated that care priority identification increased patients' perceptions of goal-directed and less burdensome care. Results also indicate that care priority identification yielded fewer medications, self-management tasks, and diagnostic tests ordered when compared to usual care (Tinetti et al., 2019). Individuals and clinicians found the intervention feasible and acceptable with minimal implementation time or impact on the workflow.

Innovation and Design Thinking for Incorporation When Evidence Is Not Available

Central to developing a plan of care is the recognition that some care systems need to be redesigned to prevent or reduce adverse outcomes. The nursing profession holds in high esteem evidence-based practice (EBP) and clinical guidelines (Melnyk & Fineout-Overholt, 2019), yet current technologies, supplies, and processes may not serve nurses' practice needs and thus lead to inefficient and at times unsafe care (Debono et al., 2013; M. E. S. Glasgow et al., 2018; Risling & Risling, 2020; Westphal et al., 2014). In practice, this translates to nurses needing to adapt, adopt, and modify their workflow to "workaround" poorly designed technologies, products, or processes (Debono et al., 2013; Risling & Risling, 2020). Instead of circumventing current protocols and creating makeshift solutions, nurses need the innovation and design thinking skills to develop solutions to challenges in their daily practice.

Design thinking is a methodology that focuses on creating empathy for stakeholders (e.g., patients, families, nurses), working in collaborative teams, and employing an action-oriented approach to prototype and test solutions (Altman et al., 2018; MacFadyen, 2014; Roberts et al., 2016; Rowe, 1991). It is an iterative process that uses analytical, creative, critical, divergent, and convergent thinking to find effective, acceptable, and sustainable solutions, that is, *an innovation* (Rahemi et al., 2018). The goal of the design-thinking process is to foster innovation. Unlike the traditional linear approach to health intervention design, which is often led by healthcare leadership (Lyon & Koerner, 2016; MacFadyen, 2014; Roberts et al., 2016), in the design-thinking process, stakeholders are the experts, and innovation emerges from several cycles of ideation, prototyping, and testing. Holt and colleagues (2022b) described a pilot study that showed the feasibility and acceptability of graduate nursing students' participation in a 150-minute innovation and design thinking workshop as part of their curriculum. Reflections from students provided preliminary evidence that creative self-efficacy, design-thinking traits, and psychological empowerment may increase after engaging in innovation and design thinking experiential learning. The National Academy of Medicine (NAM, 2021) affirms that I&DT are competencies needed in nursing education so nurses can lead the redesign of safe, effective, and efficient person-centered care systems.

Demonstrate Accountability for Care Delivery

Nurse-Managed Health Centers as a Model of Best Care Practice and to Promote Care Delivery at Full Scope of Education

Silver Spring Neighborhood Center is in one of Wisconsin's largest housing developments (Westlawn Gardens) and has been in operation since 1958. The Silver Spring Community Nursing Center (SS CNC), now the Silver Spring Health and Wellness center, was opened in 1986 by Sally Lundeen, PhD, RN, FAAN, who intentionally sought a community partner who valued whole-person health. In her

1993 publication, Dr. Lundeen (Lundeen, 1993) referred to the SS CNC within the neighborhood center as a one-stop shop for food, education, recreation, health, childcare, and more. The Capuchin Community Services-House of Peace is in and has served the poorest population in the City of Milwaukee since 1968. Sandra Underwood, PhD, RN, FAAN, and a House of Peace founder, Br. Booker Ashe, noticed the need for health education for community members. The House of Peace Community Nursing Center (HOP CNC), now the House of Peace Health and Wellness center, began in 1992, when undergraduate nursing students provided health education to community residents. In these centers, health professions students, baccalaureate prepared, and APNs deliver continuous, comprehensive, coordinated, collaborative, community-based, and culturally relevant health and wellness care to individuals, families, and communities (Lundeen, 1999). They deliver care at the full scope of their education, practice, and expertise. However, to demonstrate success of these innovative healthcare delivery models, a standardized, systematic, and comprehensive documentation method was needed.

Dr. Lundeen and colleagues found what they were looking for in the Omaha System (Martin, 2005). The Omaha System is a standardized nursing taxonomy encompassing diagnoses, interventions, and outcomes that can be analyzed to produce practice-based evidence (Martin, 2005). The practice-based evidence may improve communication, healthcare quality, safety and outcomes, and interoperability among healthcare systems (Fennelly et al., 2021).

Omaha System for Monitoring Aggregate Metrics for Accountability of Care Outcomes, Applying Current and Emerging Evidence in Development of Care Guidelines/Tools, and Ensuring Accountability Throughout Transitions of Care

The Omaha System (Martin, 2005) is a healthcare taxonomy developed by nurses to capture systematically and comprehensively all of health and health care. In 1992, the American Nurses'Association endorsed the Omaha System as a taxonomy to identify, support, and represent nursing practice across settings (Rutherford, 2008). The Omaha System is a comprehensive set of health concepts, interventions, and outcomes supporting person-centered care, critical thinking, best practices, and safe and effective health care (American Nurses Association, 2018). Please see **Figure 2-5**. Tested and revised from 1978 to 1993, nurses developed it to track care and outcomes in a methodical and complete manner.

The Omaha System consists of three interrelated elements: the Problem Classification Scheme, Intervention Scheme, and Problem Rating Scale for Outcomes (Martin, 2005).

The Omaha System is available in the public domain and used across healthcare professions (Jurkovich et al., 2014; Kang et al., 2022; Kates, 2020), settings (Hobensack et al., 2022; Martin et al., 2011), and internationally (Ardic & Turan, 2021; Monsen et al., 2011, 2019). Clinicians can aggregate Omaha System data to account for care quality and outcomes among adults receiving nurse-led healthcare services (Holt et al., 2014), evaluate the integration of behavioral health services into nurse-led primary health care (Holt et al., 2022a), and develop strengths-based population health metrics to inform person-centered care, risk and protective factors, and improve health outcomes and value (Gao et al., 2018).

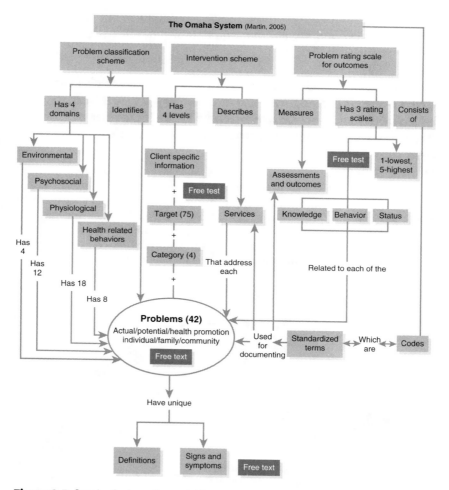

Figure 2-5 Omaha System Concept Map

Reproduced from Monsen, et al. (2011). Evidence-based Standardized Care Plans for Use Internationally to Improve Home Care Practice and Population Health. *Applied Clinical Informatics, 2*(3), 373–383. https://doi.org/10.4338/ACI-2011-03-RA-0023

The Omaha System has been used to assess changes in care delivery and scope of interventions of care. Recently, Kang et al. (2022) compared changes in interventions that RNs and Licensed interventions Nurses (LPNs)/Licensed Vocational Nurses (LVNs) employed from pre-pandemic to interventions used in response to COVID-19 (WHO, 2020). There was a 75% increase in the types of interventions used in response to the pandemic with a shift in intervention focus to infection precautions and sickness/illness care (Kang et al., 2022).

The Omaha System Guidelines website provides evidence-based practice guidelines and standardized care plans in coded, open access format, for clinicians and consumers. An international transdisciplinary group of scholars, clinical experts, and Omaha System experts have translated 31 evidence-based guidelines (e.g., sexual assault nurse examiner, transgender care management) to the Omaha

System, LOINC, and Sno-Med CT. The open access format allows for sharing and comparable data across settings and systems to improve the continuity of care (Omaha System Guidelines, n.d.).

Person-Centered Practice Framework to Model Best Care Practice, Promote Care Delivery at Full Scope of Education, and Contribute to Development of Transparency and Accountability in Policies and Practices

McCormack and McCance (2006) developed the Person-Centered Practice Framework (PCPF) to operationalize PCC in healthcare environments. Initially developed by nurses for nurses, the authors expanded the framework to encompass all healthcare workers (McCance et al., 2021). The PCPF embodies a systems-level approach to create an accountable person-centered healthcare system. Please see **Figure 2-6**. The PCPF figure depicts a flower surrounded by two concentric circles. At the center of the flower are person-centered outcomes, for example, satisfaction

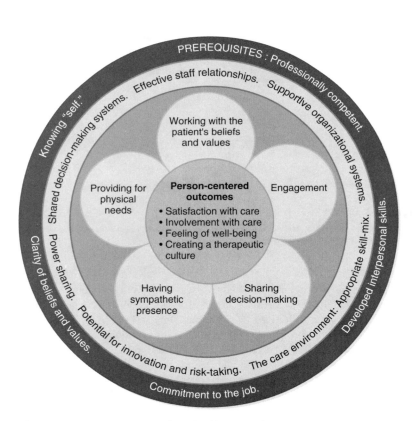

Figure 2-6 Person-Centered Practice Framework

Reproduced from McCormack, B., & McCance, T. V. (2006). Development of a framework for person-centred nursing. *Journal of Advanced Nursing, 56*(5), 472–479. https://doi.org/10.1111/j.1365-2648.2006.04042.x

and involvement with care, well-being, and therapeutic culture. The five petals depict the person-centered processes, various activities that actualize person-centered nursing engagement, shared decision-making, empathetic presence, providing for physical needs, and working with the patient's beliefs and values. The inner circle is the care environment, comprised of the appropriate skill mix, shared decision-making systems, effective staff relationships, supportive organizational systems, power sharing, and potential for innovation and risk-taking. The outer circle includes prerequisites of the healthcare worker: professional competence, interpersonal skills, job commitment, clarity of beliefs and values, and self-knowing (McCormack & McCance, 2006). APNs can use the PCPF to assess and model best practices and to deliver care using the full scope of their education and experience. The PCPF also supports the development of policies and processes that promote transparency and accountability of the person-centered healthcare system.

Evaluate Outcomes of Care
APN Quality of Care

Dr. Loretta Ford and Dr. Henry Silver developed the nurse practitioner role in 1965 to increase access to pediatric care (Ford, 2015). The role has expanded to four advanced practice registered nurse roles (Nurse Practitioner, Certified Nurse Midwife, Certified Nurse Anesthetists, and Clinical Nurse Specialist) and continues to address healthcare access limitations across the country (Brennan, 2020). As early as 1979, the U.S. Congress Congressional Budget Office recognized the value of APNs. Congress cited research demonstrating improved patient outcomes, appropriate diagnosis and management of medical conditions, patient satisfaction, and preliminary evidence of more cost-effective care comparable to physicians (U.S. Congressional Budget Office & Smith, 1979). Over the next four decades numerous original research studies (e.g., DesRoches et al., 2017; Kippenbrock et al., 2019), systematic reviews (e.g., Newhouse et al., 2011; Stanik-Hutt et al., 2013), meta-analyses (e.g., Brown & Grimes, 1995; Naylor & Kurtzman, 2010), and a Cochrane review (Laurant et al., 2005) came to the same conclusions. APNs provide care that is comparable or superior to physicians and physician assistants. A sentinel example is a randomized control trial conducted by Mundinger et al. (2000). The results indicated no statistically significant differences at 6 months in patient satisfaction, health status, physiological tests, and health service utilization of people who received primary care by nurse practitioners (NPs) or physicians after an emergency department or urgent care visit. Individuals randomly assigned to NPs had statistically significant lower diastolic blood pressure values at 6 months. Two years after the initial visit, study participants were contacted again. There continued to be no statistically significant differences found in patient satisfaction, self-reported health status, disease-specific physiologic measures, or use of specialist, emergency department, or acute care between NP or physician providers. However, individuals who received primary care from physicians had a higher primary care utilization when compared to individuals who received primary care from NPs (Lenz et al., 2004). The American Association of Nurse Practitioners (*Quality of Nurse Practitioner Practice*, n.d.) maintains a comprehensive list of quality nurse practitioner practice publications on their website.

Structure-Process-Outcome Model as Approach to Analyze Data for Identification of Gaps, Inequities, and Trends in Care and Monitoring Epidemiological and Systems-Level Aggregate Data for Outcomes and Trends and Synthesizing to Inform Evidence-Based Practice, Guidelines, and Policies

Santana and colleagues (2018) present practice guidance on how to implement PCC in healthcare settings using the Donabedian (1988) Structure, Process, and Outcomes model. At the healthcare system and organizational level, creating a PCC culture involves co-designing, implementing, and evaluating PCC education for clinicians, staff, and employees. Additionally, designing interoperable health information technology facilitates care across settings and organizations. Finally, create a feedback system for individuals and families to share their experiences in the system or organization. PCC processes occur at the individual and healthcare clinician level including creating culturally safe environments, providing compassionate care, empowering individuals to be active in achieving their health goals, and integrating care across the healthcare continuum. PCC outcomes are measured at the individual, clinician, and healthcare system/organization levels. Individuals provide outcome data through patient-reported outcome and patient experience measures. Systems can measure timely access to and cost-effective care and health outcomes at the population level (Santana et al., 2018).

Patient-Centered Outcomes Research Institute and Analysis of Data for Gaps and Inequities as Well as Monitoring Outcome Trends

The Patient-Centered Outcomes Research Institute (PCORI) began in 2011 as a governmentally supported, independent, nonprofit research institute. PCORI is dedicated to supporting comparative clinical effectiveness research (CER) to evaluate the outcomes of two or more treatments, interventions, or other therapeutic methods to improve health and health care and inform healthcare policy (Fischer & Asch, 2019; Patient-Centered Outcomes Research Institute, 2021). The U.S. Congress reauthorized the Institute in 2019 for another decade of funding. Published in June 2022, PCORI's strategic plan focuses on patient-centered CER; engagement with the community to ensure evidence is applicable, relevant, and trustworthy; disseminating results and implementation of proven treatments, interventions, or other therapeutic methods to improve health or health care; and developing and maintaining a CER research infrastructure (Greene et al., 2021). APNs/DNPs can use PCORI resources to measure outcomes in their setting.

Patient Experience as a Measure to Synthesize Outcome Data to Inform Evidence-Based Practice, Guidelines, and Policies

Another way to measure outcomes in care is from the care recipient. In a systematic review of the literature and concept analysis of patient experience, patient experience is "any process discernible by patients who receive healthcare, including subjective experiences, objective experiences, and observations of provider or staff behavior within the healthcare system" (Holt, 2018, p. 560). How the care recipient perceived the level of trust, communication, shared decision making, expectations, values, beliefs, knowledge, power, and acceptance mediated patient engagement (Holt, 2018). Therefore, this underlines the importance of critical tenets of person-centered care. Also noteworthy, patient experience is not the same as patient satisfaction, which only reflects if the healthcare exchange meets the patient's expectations (Cleary, 2016; Holt, 2018).

Patient engagement is "the desire and capability to actively choose to participate in care in a way uniquely appropriate to the individual" (Higgins, Larson, & Schnall, 2017, p. 33). Patient engagement includes the contextual, relational, organizational, and structural aspects that facilitate or hinder an individual's ability to drive health and interactions with healthcare systems (Barello et al., 2015). Engaged patients are more likely to collaborate with a healthcare provider or institution (Salgado et al., 2017), optimize outcomes (Sacks et al., 2017), and report improved care experiences (Higgins et al., 2017). Although researchers have proposed that increasing patient activation may be a critical link to lessening health disparities in populations who historically experience health disparities (Hibbard et al., 2008), there is a dearth of research to date testing interventions designed to improve patient engagement in these populations.

Reporting of Outcomes in Relationship to Analysis and Synthesis of Outcome Data

It is important to note how researchers, clinicians, and administrators report population-level outcomes. Researchers, clinicians, and administrators contribute to health disparities when they describe population-level outcomes that perpetuate biases or stereotypes. For example, *the majority of patients have uncontrolled hypertension because they are noncompliant with their medications, eat fried foods, and do not exercise*, instead of *the majority of patients have uncontrolled hypertension because the built environment lacks access to fruits and vegetables, safe places to exercise, and a pharmacy to pick up prescriptions*. One approach blames individuals, and the other acknowledges how social, economic, racialized, and political structures impact health (Bowen et al., 2022).

Promote Self-Care Management
Individual and Family Self-Management Theory as a Strategy to Promote Self-Care Management

Self-management is a multidimensional, complex phenomenon that includes condition-specific risk and protective factors, the built and social environment, and characteristics of individuals and family members (Ryan & Sawin, 2009). Self-management is influenced by knowledge, beliefs, priorities, goals, self-regulation skills and abilities, and social support (Ryan & Sawin, 2009). The degree to which individuals self-manage their health (i.e., chronic condition and health promotion activities) affects short- and long-term outcomes (Ryan & Sawin, 2009). Ryan and Sawin (2009) described how a nursing research team applied and modified (Schilling et al., 2002) a definition of self-management in a family-centered clinical example of juveniles with spina bifida. In their example, self-management is an active, daily process in which juveniles and their guardians share accountability and decision making for achieving optimal outcomes of their condition, health, and well-being using various knowledge, behaviors, and skills (Ryan & Sawin, 2009). Ryan and Sawin (2009) noted in their example that as the juveniles aged, they assumed more accountability and decision making regarding their daily health practices (Ryan & Sawin, 2009).

Shared Decision Making as a Strategy for Self-Care Management in Incorporating Current and Emerging Technologies, Counseling Techniques, Evaluation of Adequacy of Resources, and Fostering Community Partnerships

RJ, a 41-year-old man, presents to the clinic for help with his recently diagnosed type 2 diabetes (A1c 8.7%) when hospitalized for pneumonia. He is adamant that he does not want to take "shots" for his diabetes. An angiotensin-converting enzyme (ACE) inhibitor controls his blood pressure, and he is on statin therapy. He does not have renal insufficiency. He was treated with insulin while in the hospital and was discharged on monotherapy with metformin 1,000 mg twice daily. He was also given nutrition and exercise instructions and is trying to incorporate lifestyle modifications into his routine. He asks if you think the metformin will sufficiently treat his diabetes. You discuss with him that metformin would only be expected to reduce his A1c by 1% to 1.5%. Therefore, he wants to know what other treatment options can help him.

In this clinical scenario, RJ invites you to engage in a shared decision making (SDM) conversation. SDM is a collaborative way to make health decisions between a person and their health team, where pertinent and valid information is accessible to the individual, and the decision incorporates the person's circumstances, beliefs, and preferences (Elwyn et al., 2017).

There are over 40 SDM models comprising 53 elements (Bomhof-Roordink et al., 2019). Some SDM models can be applied across care settings (e.g., three-talk model [Elwyn et al., 2017]), while others were created for specific settings (e.g., primary care (Lenzen et al., 2018); emergency departments (Probst et al., 2017); and clinical situations, for example, lung cancer screening (Dobler et al., 2017). In a systematic review of SDM models, Bomhof-Roordink et al. (2019) found that most SDM models include decision making (75%), patient preferences (65%), individualized information (65%), deliberation (58%), overview of options (55%), and learning about the patient (53%). Interestingly, a third of SDMs did not identify the healthcare professional and patient as actors.

SDM models continue to evolve. As an exemplar, first published in 2012 (Elwyn et al., 2012), the three-talk model of shared decision making was critiqued for the omission of the coproduction of goals, patient preferences, and context (Elwyn et al., 2017). The revised model incorporates those concepts during the three phases: team talk, options talk, and decision talk (Elwyn et al., 2017). Team talk includes discussing choices and patient goals and offering support. Options talk focuses on weighing the potential benefits and drawbacks of the options. Decision talk moves the discussion to understand the person's values and priorities in the decision (Elwyn et al., 2017).

Motivational Interviewing as a Counseling Technique Strategy to Incorporate New and Emerging Technologies for Self-Care

Motivational interviewing is a collaborative, person-centered discourse method used in clinical practice to elicit and promote an individual's motivation for change (Miller & Rollnick, 2009). It honors autonomy and recognizes that only the individual has the agency to change. Clinicians can use motivational interviewing as part of a communication method that involves informing, asking, and reflective listening to guide the individual to resolve uncertainty about behavior change (Miller & Rollnick, 2009). Motivational interviewing can be delivered during traditional or telehealth clinical encounters and mHealth applications (Nurmi et al., 2020). It differs from the Transtheoretical Model (also known as the Stages of Change Model), a comprehensive conceptual model of how health behavior progresses through six stages of change (Prochaska & Velicer, 1997). In accordance with the Stages of Change Model, clinicians recognize which stage of change (i.e., precontemplation, contemplation, preparation, action, and maintenance) an individual is in and employ different intervention strategies to assist the person to the next stage (Prochaska et al., 1992; Prochaska & DiClemente, 1982, 1984).

The University of Connecticut's Rudd Center for Food Policy and Health's Toolkit for health professionals guided the following clinical exemplar to illustrate identifying a person's stage of change and tailoring discourse accordingly (University of Connecticut, 2020).

Clinical Scenario. Rosa, is a 34-year-old woman of Hispanic descent who comes to the clinic to discuss weight management. She is currently 62 inches, 265 lbs., with a BMI of 48.5. She says she always had a hard time managing her weight as a child, but she became very overweight during her college years. She has had two children in the past five years. She gained 50 lbs. with the first child and lost 30 lbs. With the second child, she gained 35 lbs. and lost 10 lbs. She has tried many diets where she initially loses weight but gains it back. She walks up to 30 minutes daily but is often limited by pain in her knees. She has thought about gastric bypass surgery but is fearful of undergoing a surgical procedure.

The APN can begin the weight management discourse with Rosa using the following questions: Would you like to talk about your weight or health today? Which words would you like me to use when talking about your weight? **Table 2-1** presents sample questions and clinician responses using intervention strategies from the Stages of Change Model (Prochaska et al., 1992; Prochaska & DiClemente, 1982, 1984).

5-A's Framework as an Evidence-Based Approach to Advance Wellness and Self-Care in Addition to Evaluating Adequacy of Resources

Another evidence-based behavior change model and person-centered way to develop a plan of care is the 5-A's Framework (i.e., Assess, Advise, Agree, Assist, Arrange) (R. E. Glasgow et al., 2006). It has been applied in various settings, behaviors, and health conditions (Friedman et al., 2017; Mateo et al., 2018; Pollak et al., 2016). First, the clinician *assesses* the individual's health behaviors, including individual-, environmental-, and structural-level risks and factors that may

Table 2-1 Stages of Change Model Applied to Weight Management

Stage of Behavior Change & Questions	Clinician Response
Precontemplation (Resistance, Reluctance, Overwhelmed, Resigned, Rationalizing)	
How ready do you feel to change your eating patterns and/or lifestyle behaviors?	I understand why you feel that way.
How does your weight affect you?	I believe that your lifestyle patterns are putting you at risk for conditions such as heart disease and type 2 diabetes. Making some lifestyle changes could help you improve your health substantially.
Are you considering/planning to make lifestyle changes soon?	It is your choice when you are ready to make lifestyle changes.
On a scale of 1–10, how ready are you to make lifestyle changes?	Everyone who's ever made lifestyle changes starts right where you are now. They start by seeing the reasons where they might want to make changes.
Contemplation (Ambivalent about change)	
For you, what is one benefit and one drawback to starting a lifestyle change?	I hear that you are thinking about making some lifestyle changes but are not ready right now.
Where are you on the scale of 1–10 as far as being ready for a change?	If "0" is not ready to make changes (in your eating habits/physical activity) and "10" is ready to make changes, what score would you give yourself? You gave yourself a score of X. Why do you think you are X, and not (a lower number)? OR You gave yourself a score of X. What would have to happen to move up to (higher #)?
How do you see me helping you in this process?	It is your decision if there are changes that you want to make now. I am here to help you and point you to other sources of support.
Arrange follow-up.	This is for you and I am here to help you. Can we talk about this at the next visit?
Preparation for and Making Changes	
Have you made some lifestyle changes?	It's great that you are taking important steps to improve your health. There are different ways that people successfully change their lifestyle behaviors. Can we spend a few moments discussing some strategies, and you can tell me what makes the most sense for you?

Stage of Behavior Change & Questions	Clinician Response
What is/are your lifestyle change priorities? What change would make the most impact on your health?	Help to set small lifestyle change goals based on priorities (e.g., nutrition, physical activity, and sleep).
Have you ever made lifestyle changes before? What makes you feel like you can continue to make progress if you decide to?	What was helpful? What kinds of problems would you expect in making those changes now? How do you think you could deal with them?
Are there people in your life who can support you in this change?	Identify support systems. How could they support you? Is there anything else I can do to help?
What do you feel about this change in lifestyle plan?	It's great that you feel good about your decision to make some lifestyle changes. It's common to feel scared/anxious/nervous about making changes.

Data from the University of Connecticut's Rudd Center for Food Policy and Health's *Toolkit for Health Providers*. Ha, E. (2020, April 20). Toolkit for Health Providers. University of Connecticut's Rudd Center for Food Policy and Health; UConn Rudd Center for Food Policy and Health. https://uconnruddcenter.org/research/weight-bias-stigma/healthcare-providers/

influence the behavior change goals and methods. Second, the clinician *advises* the individual on making a behavior change using clear, specific, and individualized information about health risks and benefits. Third, the clinician and individual *agree* on co-developed care goals and methods based on the individual's beliefs, values, resources, and motivation to change the behavior. Fourth, the clinician *assists* the individual in identifying barriers and facilitators of behavioral change. The clinician may assist the individual in acquiring new knowledge, skills, self-efficacy, and social, structural, and environmental supports for behavior change. Furthermore, the clinician may prescribe medications or refer the individual to medical treatments as appropriate. Finally, the clinician *arranges* follow-up in-person or telehealth visits to provide continued support, modify the care plan, or refer to specialty care (R. E. Glasgow et al., 2006).

Decision Aids as Technology to Support Self-Management

Decision aids are interventions designed to support individuals to make health decisions (Stacey et al., 2017). They provide information about choices and outcomes, and help to align decisions with personal values, goals, and health status (Munro et al., 2016). In a Cochrane review, the use of decision aids as part of the clinical exchange decreased decisional conflict related to feeling uninformed, reduced uncertainty about personal values, goals, and health status; increased active decision making; and positively affected patient–clinician communication when compared to usual care (Stacey et al., 2017). Moreover, people exposed to decision aids felt more informed, clearer about their goals, and equally or more satisfied with their decision compared to usual care. The use of a decision aid increased the clinical visit by a median of 2.6 minutes (Stacey et al., 2017). Research is needed to evaluate the effects of decision aids on the follow-through with the chosen option, cost-effectiveness, and use in populations with lower health literacy (Stacey et al., 2017). The Patient Decision Aids Research Group, part of the Ottawa Hospital Research Institute and affiliated with the University of Ottawa, maintains a comprehensive international list of decision aids by health condition and personal decision guide (*A to Z Inventory—Patient Decision Aids*, 2022). As APNs achieve competency in promoting self-care management, they may find decision aids a useful tool to attain goal-concordant care. Goal-concordant care has been associated with stronger medication self-management behaviors (Ellis et al., 2019).

Fostering Partnerships With Community Organizations Through Social Capital in Evaluation of Adequacy of Available Resources for Self-Care Management

Webel and colleagues (2013) researched the self-management behaviors of individuals who self-reported an HIV diagnosis, were ≥ 18 years, self-identified as female, and were fluent in English. They selected predictor variables of self-management behaviors of social roles, race, income, housing stability, education, individual-level social capital, and healthcare access. Webel and colleagues (2013) found that the strongest predictor of self-management behaviors was individual-level social capital measured as the level of local community participation, social agency, feelings of trust and safety, neighborhood relations, friends and family relationships, tolerance of diversity, and value of life, measured using the Social Capital Scale (Onyx & Bullen, 2000). The research reported social capital significantly predicated daily health practices ($F = 5.40$, adjusted R2 = 0.27, $p<0.01$), HIV social support ($F = 4.50$, adjusted R2 = 0.22, $p<0.01$), and accepting the chronicity of HIV ($F = 5.57$, adjusted R2 = 0.27, $p<0.01$). Strikingly, a one-point increase in total social capital score yielded a 13% increase in the self-management score. The authors concluded that the predictor models indicate that supporting or increasing a person with HIV's social capital may be among the most effective interventions to enhance HIV self-management (Webel et al., 2013).

Reflect on how you may assess and foster a person's level of local community participation, social agency, feelings of trust and safety, neighborhood relations, friends and family relationships, tolerance of diversity, and value of life.

Provide Care Coordination

Nurse Care Coordinators for Evaluation of Communication Pathways, Development of Strategies to Optimize Care (as Well as Transitions of Care), and Guidance of Coordination Across Health Systems as Well as Analysis of Systems-Level and Public Policy Influence on Care Coordination

The U.S. healthcare system is fragmented and difficult to navigate (NAM, 2021). The complex system often leaves consumers confused regarding how to access the right level of care for prevention, treatment, and urgent health needs. However, well-designed and targeted care coordination by a knowledgeable healthcare professional can assist the individual and family to effectively use the resources of complex health systems and multiple providers in harmony with their needs and preferences (American Nurses Association, 2021). APN and RN care coordinators may provide general care management to all individuals but often with a special focus on medium- and high-risk or high-complexity populations. Actions of APN care coordinators may include creating a care plan that lessens treatment burden; revising treatment plans in response to changes in health status; supporting self-management goals; referral to specialty providers and community resources; and working to realign resources to restore or improve individual, family, and population needs (Campagna et al., 2022). Effective care coordination is sensitive to the strengths, challenges, and needs of individuals, families, and populations. The nature of the interventions must be tailored to match the schedules, language, health literacy level, safety issues, and limited resources of these individuals and families (Anderson & Hewner, 2021).

The APN care coordinator can mobilize the appropriate interdisciplinary care team members based on individual and caregiver input and the identified social and medical needs. Nurses can coordinate interdisciplinary care and make referrals to internal or external community resources. The individual's plan of care is updated regularly to assure it addresses continuing healthcare and social needs. Follow-up care and outcomes are tracked using an electronic registry with touchpoints to affirm and revise self-management strategies (Manalili et al., 2022). Care coordination may be less burdensome to the care recipient when delivered using telehealth services, which facilitates continuity of care, eliminates the burdens of travel and transportation, and lowers the risk of disease transmission (Dhaliwal et al., 2021).

A person-centered nurse-led coordination model is a response to the call to action outlined in 2021, the NAM report titled, *The Future of Nursing 2020-2030: Charting a Path to Achieve Health Equity.* The report cites compelling evidence supporting the role nurses can and should play in addressing the inequities in health care resulting from uneven access to conditions needed for good health. The report's authors recognized that professional nurses have seen firsthand the inequitable impact that COVID-19 has had on those they have served and the profession itself. The report articulates a vision to leverage nurses' capacity and unique expertise across the United States to contribute more comprehensively to creating equitable health care designed to work for everyone. Innovative models fully leveraging nursing roles targeted to support health equity will be one way to realize that vision (NAM, 2021).

Participation in Person-Centered Care Coordination at Systems Level to Improve Care Coordination Across Settings

A person-centered care coordination model utilizes the unique skills of nurses to connect and coordinate a population of individuals served by a healthcare system and strategically positions nurses at different points of care. The model is person-centric and engages the individual and their identified caregivers as the center of the care team (Manalili et al., 2022). The care recipient chooses the care team members, identifies their health goals, and works with the nurse to derive strategies to accomplish those goals. The assembled team will surround the individual to educate, support, and guide them in reaching their health goals in a culturally safe manner. This coordinated, team-based approach to care is a departure from the traditional disease-oriented approach (Farre & Rapley, 2017) where a physician provider dictated the care plan. Patient engagement is essential to success as individuals activated in the self-management process are more likely to follow their care plan and participate in evidence-based preventative services (Alvarez et al., 2016).

The impact of care coordination can be evaluated using process and outcome measures. The person-centric, individualized approach is anticipated to result in improvements in these measures for all patients, but most notably for those with the greatest number of social needs and most negatively impacted by structural racism and structural and social determinants of health (e.g., people of color, LGBTQ+ community, people with disabilities, those with low income, and those living in rural areas) (Yearby et al., 2022). The overall effect will reduce health disparities for the population served. Outcomes to be measured will include but not be limited to the following:

- Increased number of new and recurring primary care visits across services because of improved access to care.
- Increased percentage of individuals who complete annual medical and dental preventative care visits.
- Increased percentage of individuals who receive recommended screenings for cancer (oral, breast, colon, cervical, prostate, etc.) and other health conditions.
- Improved self-management with recommended chronic care testing and treatments for hypertension, diabetes, heart failure, and others.
- Increased satisfaction in communication between the care team and the care recipient.
- Decreased emergency department visits and hospital readmission rates.

Summary

To achieve the domain of PCC, a nurse must co-develop person-centered interventions and evaluate those interventions at the personal level. The personal level includes the context of an individual's life including strengths, challenges, needs, and resources. The person must determine the success of the care. This may conflict with the nurse's or healthcare system's view of improving health outcomes. Slater (2006) supports this ideal, saying that "pathways of healing are designed for the individual, saluting the individual's right to not only receive care but to have choices in how it is perceived and provided" (p. 42). As nurses gain competency in PCC, the health care system needs to reconcile evaluating and valuing PCC from the perspective of the recipient, not the provider of PCC. When we recognize, value, and prioritize an individual as a holistic being, competence in PCC will be actualized (Zhao et al., 2016).

References

Abulebda, K., Auerbach, M., & Limaiem, F. (2022). Debriefing techniques utilized in medical simulation. In *StatPearls*. StatPearls Publishing. https://www.ncbi.nlm.nih.gov/pubmed/31536266

Agency for Healthcare Research and Quality. (2013, March). 3. What is the Clinical-Community Relationships Measurement Framework? Socioecological Model. https://www.ahrq.gov/prevention/resources/chronic-care/clinical-community-relationships-measures-atlas/ccrm-atlas3.html

Altman, M., Huang, T. T. K., & Breland, J. Y. (2018). Design thinking in health care. *Preventing Chronic Disease*, *15*, E117. https://doi.org/10.5888/pcd15.180128

Alvarez, C., Greene, J., Hibbard, J., & Overton, V. (2016). The role of primary care providers in patient activation and engagement in self-management: A cross-sectional analysis. *BMC Health Services Research*, *16*, 85. https://doi.org/10.1186/s12913-016-1328-3

American Association of Colleges of Nursing. (2021). *AACN Essentials*. https://www.aacnnursing.org/AACN-Essentials

American Nurses Association. (2021). *Care coordination and registered nurses' essential role*. Position Statement. https://www.nursingworld.org/practice-policy/nursing-excellence/official-position-statements/id/care-coordination-and-registered-nurses-essential-role/

American Nurses Association. (2018). *Inclusion of Recognized Terminologies Supporting Nursing Practice within Electronic Health Records and Other Health Information Technology Solutions*. ANA Position Statement. https://www.nursingworld.org/practice-policy/nursing-excellence/official-position-statements/id/Inclusion-of-Recognized-Terminologies-Supporting-Nursing-Practice-within-Electronic-Health-Records/

Anderson, A., & Hewner, S. (2021). Care coordination: A concept analysis. *The American Journal of Nursing*, *121*(12), 30–38. https://doi.org/10.1097/01.NAJ.0000803188.10432.e1

Anderson, A., Mills, C. W., Willits, J., Lisk, C., Maksut, J. L., Khau, M. T., & Scholle, S. H. (2022). Follow-up post-discharge and readmission disparities among medicare fee-for-service beneficiaries, 2018. *Journal of General Internal Medicine*, *37*(12), 3020–3028. https://doi.org/10.1007/s11606-022-07488-3

Ardic, A., & Turan, E. (2021). Nursing care management based on the Omaha system for inpatients diagnosed with COVID-19: An electronic health record study. *Journal of Advanced Nursing*, *77*(6), 2709–2717. https://doi.org/10.1111/jan.14793

A to Z Inventory—Patient Decision Aids. (2022). Ottawa Hospital Research Institute. https://decisionaid.ohri.ca/azlist.html

Austin, R. R., Martin, C. L., Jones, C. R., Lu, S.-C., Jantraporn, R., Nestrasil, I., Martin, K. S., & Monsen, K. A. (2022). Translation and validation of the Omaha System into English language simplified Omaha System terms. *Kontakt*, *24*(1), 48–54. https://doi.org/10.32725/kont.2022.007

Austin, R. R., Mathiason, M. A., Lindquist, R. A., McMahon, S. K., Pieczkiewicz, D. S., & Monsen, K. A. (2021). Understanding women's cardiovascular health using mystrengths+myhealth: a patient-generated data visualization study of strengths, challenges, and needs differences. *Journal of Nursing Scholarship: An Official Publication of Sigma Theta Tau International Honor Society of Nursing / Sigma Theta Tau*, *53*(5), 634–642. https://doi.org/10.1111/jnu.12674

Bailey, Z. D., Krieger, N., Agénor, M., Graves, J., Linos, N., & Bassett, M. T. (2017). Structural racism and health inequities in the USA: Evidence and interventions. *The Lancet*, *389*(10077), 1453–1463. https://doi.org/10.1016/S0140-6736(17)30569-X

Barello, S., Graffigna, G., Vegni, E., Savarese, M., Lombardi, F., and Bosio, A. C. (2015). "Engage me in taking care of my heart": a grounded theory study on patient-cardiologist relationship in the hospital management of heart failure. *BMJ Open* 5:e005582 https://doi.org/10.1136/bmjopen-2014-005582

Baur, C., & Prue, C. (2014). The CDC Clear Communication Index is a new evidence-based tool to prepare and review health information. *Health Promotion Practice*, *15*(5), 629–637. https://doi.org/10.1177/1524839914538969

Blair, I. V., Steiner, J. F., Fairclough, D. L., Hanratty, R., Price, D. W., Hirsh, H. K., Wright, L. A., Bronsert, M., Karimkhani, E., Magid, D. J., & Havranek, E. P. (2013). Clinicians' implicit ethnic/racial bias and perceptions of care among Black and Latino patients. *Annals of Family Medicine*, *11*(1), 43–52. https://doi.org/10.1370/afm.1442

Boehmer, K. R., Gionfriddo, M. R., Rodriguez-Gutierrez, R., Dabrh, A. M. A., Leppin, A. L., Hargraves, I., May, C. R., Shippee, N. D., Castaneda-Guarderas, A., Palacios, C. Z., Bora, P., Erwin, P., & Montori, V. M. (2016). Patient capacity and constraints in the experience of chronic disease: A qualitative systematic review and thematic synthesis. *BMC Family Practice*, *17*, 127. https://doi.org/10.1186/s12875-016-0525-9

Bolster, D., & Manias, E. (2010). Person-centred interactions between nurses and patients during medication activities in an acute hospital setting: Qualitative observation and interview study. *International Journal of Nursing Studies*, *47*(2), 154–165. https://doi.org/10.1016/j.ijnurstu.2009.05.021

Bomhof-Roordink, H., Gärtner, F. R., Stiggelbout, A. M., & Pieterse, A. H. (2019). Key components of shared decision making models: A systematic review. *BMJ Open*, *9*(12), e031763. https://doi.org/10.1136/bmjopen-2019-031763

Bourgois, P., Holmes, S. M., Sue, K., & Quesada, J. (2017). Structural vulnerability: Operationalizing the concept to address health disparities in clinical care. *Academic Medicine: Journal of the Association of American Medical Colleges*, *92*(3), 299–307. https://doi.org/10.1097/ACM.0000000000001294

Bovin, M. J., Kimerling, R., Weathers, F. W., Prins, A., Marx, B. P., Post, E. P., & Schnurr, P. P. (2021). Diagnostic accuracy and acceptability of the primary care posttraumatic stress disorder screen for the *Diagnostic and Statistical Manual of Mental Disorders* (Fifth Edition) among US veterans. *JAMA Network Open*, *4*(2), e2036733. https://doi.org/10.1001/jamanetworkopen.2020.36733

Bowen, F. R., Epps, F., Lowe, J., & Guilamo-Ramos, V. (2022). Restoring trust in research among historically underrepresented communities: A call to action for antiracism research in nursing. *Nursing Outlook*. https://doi.org/10.1016/j.outlook.2022.06.006

Braveman, P. A., Arkin, E., Proctor, D., Kauh, T., & Holm, N. (2022). Systemic and structural racism: Definitions, examples, health damages, and approaches to dismantling. *Health Affairs*, *41*(2), 171–178. https://doi.org/10.1377/hlthaff.2021.01394

Brennan, C. (2020). Tracing the history of the nurse practitioner profession in 2020, the Year of the Nurse. *Journal of Pediatric Health Care: Official Publication of National Association of Pediatric Nurse Associates & Practitioners*, *34*(2), 83–84. https://doi.org/10.1016/j.pedhc.2019.12.005

Bronfenbrenner, U. (1977). Toward an experimental ecology of human development. *The American Psychologist*, *32*(7), 513–531. https://doi.org/10.1037/0003-066X.32.7.513

Brown, S. A., & Grimes, D. E. (1995). A meta-analysis of nurse practitioners and nurse midwives in primary care. *Nursing Research*, *44*(6), 332–339. https://www.ncbi.nlm.nih.gov/pubmed/7501486

Campagna, V., Mitchell, E., & Krsnak, J. (2022). Addressing social determinants of health: A care coordination approach for professional case managers. *Professional Case Management*, *27*(6), 263–270. https://doi.org/10.1097/NCM.0000000000000590

Capp, A. I. (2022). "They make you feel less of a human being": Understanding and responding to Milwaukee's racial disparity in infant mortality. *Maternal and Child Health Journal*, *26*(4), 736–746. https://doi.org/10.1007/s10995-021-03281-6

Chae, D. H., Snipes, S. A., Chung, K. W., Martz, C. D., & LaVeist, T. A. (2021). Vulnerability and resilience: Use and misuse of these terms in the public health discourse. *American Journal of Public Health*, *111*(10), 1736–1740. https://doi.org/10.2105/AJPH.2021.306413

Chagin, K., Choate, F., Cook, K., Fuehrer, S., Misak, J. E., & Sehgal, A. R. (2021). A framework for evaluating social determinants of health screening and referrals for assistance. *Journal of Primary Care & Community Health*, *12*, 21501327211052204. https://doi.org/10.1177/21501327211052204

Chinn, P. L. (2018). Critical theory and emancipatory knowing. In J. B. Butts & K. L. Rich (Eds.), *Philosophies and theories for advanced nursing practice* (3rd ed., pp. 143–162). Jones & Bartlett Learning.

Chinn, P. L., & Kramer, M. K. (2014). *Knowledge development in nursing* (9th ed.). Mosby.

Christianson-Silva, P., Russell-Kibble, A., & Shaver, J. (2021). A nurse practitioner-led care bundle approach for primary care of patients with complex health needs. *Journal of the American Association of Nurse Practitioners*. https://doi.org/10.1097/JXX.0000000000000628

Cleary, P. D. (2016). Evolving concepts of patient-centered care and the assessment of patient care experiences: Optimism and opposition. *Journal of Health Politics, Policy and Law*, *41*(4), 675–696. https://doi.org/10.1215/03616878-3620881

Cooper, L. A., Saha, S., & van Ryn, M. (2022). Mandated implicit bias training for health professionals—A step toward equity in health care. *JAMA Health Forum*, *3*(8), e223250. https://doi.org/10.1001/jamahealthforum.2022.3250

Dagher, R. K., & Linares, D. E. (2022). A critical review on the complex interplay between social determinants of health and maternal and infant mortality. *Children*, *9*(3). https://doi.org/10.3390/children9030394

Dawkins, D. J., & Daum, D. N. (2022). Person-first language in healthcare: The missing link in healthcare simulation training. *Clinical Simulation In Nursing, 71*, 135–140. https://doi .org/10.1016/j.ecns.2022.03.002

Debono, D. S., Greenfield, D., Travaglia, J. F., Long, J. C., Black, D., Johnson, J., & Braithwaite, J. (2013). Nurses' workarounds in acute healthcare settings: A scoping review. *BMC Health Services Research, 13*, 175. https://doi.org/10.1186/1472-6963-13-175

DesRoches, C. M., Clarke, S., Perloff, J., O'Reilly-Jacob, M., & Buerhaus, P. (2017). The quality of primary care provided by nurse practitioners to vulnerable Medicare beneficiaries. *Nursing Outlook, 65*(6), 679–688. https://doi.org/10.1016/j.outlook.2017.06.007

Devine, P. G., Forscher, P. S., Austin, A. J., & Cox, W. T. L. (2012). Long-term reduction in implicit race bias: A prejudice habit-breaking intervention. *Journal of Experimental Social Psychology, 48*(6), 1267–1278. https://doi.org/10.1016/j.jesp.2012.06.003

Dhaliwal, J. K., Hall, T. D., LaRue, J. L., Maynard, S. E., Pierre, P. E., & Bransby, K. A. (2021). Expansion of telehealth in primary care during the COVID-19 pandemic: Benefits and barriers. *Journal of the American Association of Nurse Practitioners, 34*(2), 224–229. https://doi .org/10.1097/JXX.0000000000000626

Dobler, C. C., Midthun, D. E., & Montori, V. M. (2017). Quality of shared decision making in lung cancer screening: The right process, with the right partners, at the right time and place. *Mayo Clinic Proceedings. Mayo Clinic, 92*(11), 1612–1616. https://doi.org/10.1016/j .mayocp.2017.08.010

Donabedian, A. (1988). The quality of care. *JAMA: The Journal of the American Medical Association, 260*(12), 1743. https://doi.org/10.1001/jama.1988.03410120089033

Dzau, V. J., McClellan, M. B., McGinnis, J. M., Marx, J. C., Sullenger, R. D., & ElLaissi, W. (2021). Vital directions for health and health care: Priorities for 2021. *Health Affairs*, 101377hlthaff202002204. https://doi.org/10.1377/hlthaff.2020.02204

Ellenbecker, C. H., Fawcett, J., Jones, E. J., Mahoney, D., Rowlands, B., & Waddell, A. (2017). A staged approach to educating nurses in health policy. *Policy, Politics & Nursing Practice, 18*(1), 44–56. https://doi.org/10.1177/1527154417709254

Ellis, J. L., Kovach, C. R., Fendrich, M., Olukotun, O., Baldwin, V. K., Ke, W., & Nichols, B. (2019). Factors related to medication self-management in African American older women. *Research in Gerontological Nursing, 12*(2), 71–79. https://doi.org/10.3928/19404921-20190206-01

Elwyn, G., Durand, M. A., Song, J., Aarts, J., Barr, P. J., Berger, Z., Cochran, N., Frosch, D., Galasiński, D., Gulbrandsen, P., Han, P. K. J., Härter, M., Kinnersley, P., Lloyd, A., Mishra, M., Perestelo-Perez, L., Scholl, I., Tomori, K., Trevena, L., …& Van der Weijden, T. (2017). A three-talk model for shared decision making: Multistage consultation process. *BMJ, 359*, j4891. https://doi.org/10.1136/bmj.j4891

Elwyn, G., Frosch, D., Thomson, R., Joseph-Williams, N., Lloyd, A., Kinnersley, P., Cording, E., Tomson, D., Dodd, C., Rollnick, S., Edwards, A., & Barry, M. (2012). Shared decision making: A model for clinical practice. *Journal of General Internal Medicine, 27*(10), 1361–1367. https:// doi.org/10.1007/s11606-012-2077-6

Engel, G. L. (1977). The need for a new medical model: a challenge for biomedicine. *Science, 196*(4286), 129–136. https://www.ncbi.nlm.nih.gov/pubmed/847460

Everson, N., Levett-Jones, T., Lapkin, S., Pitt, V., van der Riet, P., Rossiter, R., Jones, D., Gilligan, C., & Courtney-Pratt, H. (2015). Measuring the impact of a 3D simulation experience on nursing students' cultural empathy using a modified version of the Kiersma-Chen Empathy Scale. *Journal of Clinical Nursing, 24*(19–20), 2849–2858. https://doi.org/10.1111/jocn.12893

Farre, A., & Rapley, T. (2017). The new old (and old new) medical model: Four decades navigating the biomedical and psychosocial understandings of health and illness. *Healthcare (Basel, Switzerland), 5*(4). https://doi.org/10.3390/healthcare5040088

Felitti, V. J., Anda, R. F., Nordenberg, D., Williamson, D. F., Spitz, A. M., Edwards, V., Koss, M. P., & Marks, J. S. (1998). Relationship of childhood abuse and household dysfunction to many of the leading causes of death in adults: The Adverse Childhood Experiences (ACE) study. *American Journal of Preventive Medicine, 14*(4), 245–258. https://doi.org/10.1016/s0749-3797(98)00017-8

Fennelly, O., Grogan, L., Reed, A., & Hardiker, N. R. (2021). Use of standardized terminologies in clinical practice: A scoping review. *International Journal of Medical Informatics, 149*, 104431. https://doi.org/10.1016/j.ijmedinf.2021.104431

Fischer, M. A., & Asch, S. M. (2019). The future of the patient-centered outcomes research institute (PCORI). *Journal of General Internal Medicine, 34*(11), 2291–2292. https://doi.org/10.1007/s11606-019-05324-9

FitzGerald, C., & Hurst, S. (2017). Implicit bias in healthcare professionals: A systematic review. *BMC Medical Ethics, 18*(1), 19. https://doi.org/10.1186/s12910-017-0179-8

Ford, L. C. (2015). Reflections on 50 years of change. *Journal of the American Association of Nurse Practitioners, 27*(6), 294–295. https://doi.org/10.1002/2327-6924.12271

Fredrickson, B. L., Cohn, M. A., Coffey, K. A., Pek, J., & Finkel, S. M. (2008). Open hearts build lives: Positive emotions, induced through loving-kindness meditation, build consequential personal resources. *Journal of Personality and Social Psychology, 95*(5), 1045–1062. https://doi.org/10.1037/a0013262

Freij, M., Dullabh, P., Lewis, S., Smith, S. R., Hovey, L., & Dhopeshwarkar, R. (2019). Incorporating social determinants of health in electronic health records: Qualitative study of current practices among top vendors. *JMIR Medical Informatics, 7*(2), e13849. https://doi.org/10.2196/13849

Friedman, J. L., Lyna, P., Sendak, M. D., Viera, A. J., Silberberg, M., & Pollak, K. I. (2017). Use of the 5 As for teen alcohol use. *Clinical Pediatrics, 56*(5), 419–426. https://doi.org/10.1177/0009922816655884

Gao, G., Kerr, M. J., Lindquist, R. A., Chi, C.-L., Mathiason, M. A., Austin, R. R., & Monsen, K. A. (2018). A strengths-based data capture model: Mining data-driven and person-centered health assets. *JAMIA Open, 1*(1), 11–14. https://doi.org/10.1093/jamiaopen/ooy015

Gee, G. C., & Ford, C. L. (2011). Structural racism and health inequities: Old Issues, New Directions. *Du Bois Review: Social Science Research on Race, 8*(1), 115–132. https://doi.org/10.1017/S1742058X11000130

Giordano, G. N., Björk, J., & Lindström, M. (2012). Social capital and self-rated health—a study of temporal (causal) relationships. *Social Science & Medicine, 75*(2), 340–348. https://doi.org/10.1016/j.socscimed.2012.03.011

Glasgow, M. E. S., Colbert, A., Viator, J., & Cavanagh, S. (2018). The nurse-engineer: A new role to improve nurse technology interface and patient care device innovations. *Journal of Nursing Scholarship: An Official Publication of Sigma Theta Tau International Honor Society of Nursing / Sigma Theta Tau, 50*(6), 601–611. https://doi.org/10.1111/jnu.12431

Glasgow, R. E., Emont, S., & Miller, D. C. (2006). Assessing delivery of the five "As" for patient-centered counseling. *Health Promotion International, 21*(3), 245–255. https://doi.org/10.1093/heapro/dal017

Gottlieb, L., Fichtenberg, C., & Adler, N. (2017). *Introducing the social interventions research and evaluation network*. San Francisco, CA: SIREN. https://sirenetwork.ucsf.edu/sites/default/files/SIREN_Issue_Brief_Updt.pdf

Gottlieb, L. N. (2014). Strengths-based nursing. *The American Journal of Nursing, 114*(8), 24–32; quiz 33, 46. https://doi.org/10.1097/01.NAJ.0000453039.70629.e2

Gottlieb, L. N., & Gottlieb, B. (2017). Strengths-based nursing: A process for implementing a philosophy into practice. *Journal of Family Nursing, 23*(3), 319–340. https://doi.org/10.1177/1074840717717731

Greene, S. M., P. Embi, M. Gaines, B. Johnson, N. Powe, J. Schiff, B. Siegel, E. Stewart, C. Wilkins (Eds.). (2021). *Priorities on the health horizon: Informing PCORI's strategic plan*. National Academy of Medicine. https://nam.edu/wp-content/uploads/2021/11/Priorities-on-the-Health-Horizon_final_prepub.pdf

Hardeman, R. R., Karbeah, J. 'mag, & Kozhimannil, K. B. (2020). Applying a critical race lens to relationship-centered care in pregnancy and childbirth: An antidote to structural racism. *Birth, 47*(1), 3–7. https://doi.org/10.1111/birt.12462

Hartzler, A. L. (2019). *UnBIASED*: A Study by University of Washington and University of California San Diego. https://www.unbiased.health/home

Hawkins, D., Elder, L., & Paul, R. (2019). *The thinker's guide to clinical reasoning: Based on critical thinking concepts and tools*. Rowman & Littlefield. https://play.google.com/store/books/details?id=GDWbDwAAQBAJ

Hawn, S. E., Cusack, S. E., George, B., Sheerin, C. M., Spit for Science Working Group, Dick, D., & Amstadter, A. B. (2022). Diagnostic validity of the PC-PTSD screen in college students. *Journal of American College Health: J of ACH, 70*(6), 1909–1919. https://doi.org/10.1080/07448481 .2020.1841768

Healthy People 2030. (2020). *Social determinants of health.* U.S. Department of Health and Human Services, Office of Disease Prevention and Health Promotion. https://health.gov/healthypeople /priority-areas/social-determinants-health

Hibbard, J. H., Greene, J., Becker, E. R., Roblin, D., Painter, M. W., Perez, D. J., Burbank-Schmitt, E., & Tusler, M. (2008). Racial/ethnic disparities and consumer activation in health. *Health Affairs, 27*(5), 1442–1453. https://doi.org/10.1377/hlthaff.27.5.1442

Higgins, T., Larson, E., & Schnall, R. (2017). Unraveling the meaning of patient engagement: A concept analysis. *Patient Education and Counseling, 100*(1), 30–36. https://doi.org/10.1016/j .pec.2016.09.002

Hobbs, L. J. (2009). A dimensional analysis of patient-centered care. *Nursing Research, 58*(1), 52–62. doi:10.1097/NNR.0b013e31818c3e79

Hobensack, M., Ojo, M., Barrón, Y., Bowles, K. H., Cato, K., Chae, S., Kennedy, E., McDonald, M. V., Rossetti, S. C., Song, J., Sridharan, S., & Topaz, M. (2022). Documentation of hospitalization risk factors in electronic health records (EHRs): A qualitative study with home healthcare clinicians. *Journal of the American Medical Informatics Association: JAMIA, 29*(5), 805–812. https://doi.org/10.1093/jamia/ocac023

Holt, J., Zabler, B., & Baisch, M. J. (2014). Evidence-based characteristics of nurse-managed health centers for quality and outcomes. *Nursing Outlook, 62*(6), 428–439. https://doi.org/10.1016/j .outlook.2014.06.005

Holt, J. M. (2018). An evolutionary view of patient experience in primary care: A concept analysis. *Nursing Forum, 53*(4), 555–566. https://doi.org/10.1111/nuf.12286

Holt, J. M., Cusatis, R., Winn, A., Asan, O., Spanbauer, C., Williams, J. S., Flynn, K. E., Somai, M., Laud, P., & Crotty, B. H. (2020). The impact of previsit contextual data collection on patient-provider communication and patient activation: Study protocol for a randomized controlled trial. *JMIR Research Protocols, 9*(9), e20309. https://doi.org/10.2196/20309

Holt, J. M., Kibicho, J., & Bell-Calvin, J. (2022a). Factors that sustained the integration of behavioral health into nurse-led primary care. *Community Mental Health Journal.* https://doi.org /10.1007/s10597-022-00976-0

Holt, J. M., Talsma, A., Woehrle, L. M., Klingbeil, C., & Avdeev, I. (November/December, 2022b). Fostering innovation and design thinking in graduate programs. *Nurse Educator, 47*(6), 356–357. https://doi.org/10.1097/NNE.0000000000001206

Imran, A., Rawal, M. D., Botre, N., & Patil, A. (2022). Improving and promoting social determinants of health at a system level. *Joint Commission Journal on Quality and Patient Safety / Joint Commission Resources, 48*(8), 376–384. https://doi.org/10.1016/j.jcjq.2022.06.004

Institute of Medicine. (2001). *Crossing the quality chasm: A new health system for the 21st century.* The National Academies Press. https://www.nap.edu/catalog/10027/crossing-the-quality-chasm -a-new-health-system-for-the

Johnson, C. B., Luther, B., Wallace, A. S., & Kulesa, M. G. (2022). Social determinants of health: What are they and how do we screen? *Orthopaedic Nursing / National Association of Orthopaedic Nurses, 41*(2), 88–100. https://doi.org/10.1097/NOR.0000000000000829

Jurkovich, M. W., Ophaug, M., Salberg, S., & Monsen, K. (2014). Investigation of the Omaha System for dentistry. *Applied Clinical Informatics, 5*(2), 491–502. https://doi.org/10.4338/ACI -2014-01-RA-0001

Kang, Y. J., Monsen, K., Jeppesen, B., Hanson, C., Nichols, K., O'Neill, K., & Lundblad, J. (2022). Interprofessional roles and collaborations to address COVID-19 pandemic challenges in nursing homes. *Interdisciplinary Journal of Partnership Studies, 9*(1), 7–7. https://doi.org/10.24926 /ijps.v9i1.4644

Kates, B. J. (2020). Ten years after: How the Omaha System helped save Colorado Springs community centers from closure. *Computers, Informatics, Nursing: CIN, 38*(4), 174–175. https://doi .org/10.1097/CIN.0000000000000633

Kippenbrock, T., Emory, J., Lee, P., Odell, E., Buron, B., & Morrison, B. (2019). A national survey of nurse practitioners' patient satisfaction outcomes. *Nursing Outlook, 67*(6), 707–712. https:// doi.org/10.1016/j.outlook.2019.04.010

Kitson, A., Marshall, A., Bassett, K., & Zeitz, K. (2013). What are the core elements of patient-centered care? A narrative review and synthesis of the literature from health policy, medicine and nursing. *Journal of Advanced Nursing, 69*(1), 4–15. https://doi.org/10.1111/j.1365-2648.2012.06064.x

LaManna, J. B., Guido-Sanz, F., Anderson, M., Chase, S. K., Weiss, J. A., & Blackwell, C. W. (2019). Teaching diagnostic reasoning to advanced practice nurses: Positives and negatives. *Clinical Simulation In Nursing, 26*, 24–31. https://doi.org/10.1016/j.ecns.2018.10.006

Landis, P. (2021). Think health literacy to improve the patient experience. *Holistic Nursing Practice, 35*(2), 57–59. https://doi.org/10.1097/HNP.0000000000000409

Laurant, M., Reeves, D., Hermens, R., Braspenning, J., Grol, R., & Sibbald, B. (2005). Substitution of doctors by nurses in primary care. *Cochrane Database of Systematic Reviews, 2*, CD001271. https://doi.org/10.1002/14651858.CD001271.pub2

Lauver, D. R., Ward, S. E., Heidrich, S. M., Keller, M. L., Bowers, B. J., Brennan, P. F., Kirchhoff, K. T., & Wells, T. J. (2002). Patient-centered interventions. *Research in Nursing & Health, 25*(4), 246–255. https://doi.org/10.1002/nur.10044

Lenzen, S. A., Daniëls, R., van Bokhoven, M. A., van der Weijden, T., & Beurskens, A. (2018). Development of a conversation approach for practice nurses aimed at making shared decisions on goals and action plans with primary care patients. *BMC Health Services Research, 18*(1), 891. https://doi.org/10.1186/s12913-018-3734-1

Lenz, E. R., Mundinger, M. O., Kane, R. L., Hopkins, S. C., & Lin, S. X. (2004). Primary care outcomes in patients treated by nurse practitioners or physicians: Two-year follow-up. *Medical Care Research and Review: MCRR, 61*(3), 332–351. https://doi.org/10.1177/1077558704266821

Levett-Jones, T., & Cant, R. (2020). The empathy continuum: An evidenced-based teaching model derived from an integrative review of contemporary nursing literature. *Journal of Clinical Nursing, 29*(7–8), 1026–1040. https://doi.org/10.1111/jocn.15137

Levinson, W., Lesser, C., & Epstein, R. (2010). Developing physician communication skills for patient-centered care. *Health Affairs, 29*(7), 1310–1318. doi:10.1377/hlthaff.2009.0450

Lundeen, S. P. (1993). Comprehensive, collaborative, coordinated, community-based care: A community nursing center model. *Family & Community Health, 16*(2), 57. https://journals.lww.com/familyandcommunityhealth/Citation/1993/07000/Comprehensive,_collaborative,_coordinated,.10.aspx

Lundeen, S. P. (1999). An alternative paradigm for promoting health in communities: The Lundeen Community Nursing Center model. *Family & Community Health, 21*(4), 15. https://journals.lww.com/familyandcommunityhealth/abstract/1999/01000/an_alternative_paradigm_for_promoting_health_in.4.aspx

Lyon, A. R., & Koerner, K. (2016). User-centered design for psychosocial intervention development and implementation. *Clinical Psychology: A Publication of the Division of Clinical Psychology of the American Psychological Association, 23*(2), 180–200. https://doi.org/10.1111/cpsp.12154

MacFadyen, J. S. (2014). Design thinking. *Holistic Nursing Practice, 28*(1), 3–5. https://doi.org/10.1097/HNP.0000000000000008

Makoul, G., Krupat, E., & Chang, C.-H. (2007). Measuring patient views of physician communication skills: Development and testing of the Communication Assessment Tool. *Patient Education and Counseling, 67*(3), 333–342. https://doi.org/10.1016/j.pec.2007.05.005

Manalili, K., Lorenzetti, D. L., Egunsola, O., O'Beirne, M., Hemmelgarn, B., Scott, C. M., & Santana, M. J. (2022). The effectiveness of person-centred quality improvement strategies on the management and control of hypertension in primary care: A systematic review and meta-analysis. *Journal of Evaluation in Clinical Practice, 28*(2), 260–277. https://doi.org/10.1111/jep.13618

Martínez, N., Connelly, C. D., Pérez, A., & Calero, P. (2021). Self-care: A concept analysis. *International Journal of Nursing Sciences, 8*(4), 418–425. https://doi.org/10.1016/j.ijnss.2021.08.007

Martin, K. S. (2005). *The Omaha System: A key to practice, documentation, and information management* (Reprinted 2nd ed.). Health Connections Press.

Martin, K. S., Monsen, K. A., & Bowles, K. H. (2011). The Omaha system and meaningful use: Applications for practice, education, and research. *Computers, Informatics, Nursing: CIN, 29*(1), 52–58. https://doi.org/10.1097/NCN.0b013e3181f9ddc6

Mateo, K. F., Berner, N. B., Ricci, N. L., Seekaew, P., Sikerwar, S., Tenner, C., Dognin, J., Sherman, S. E., Kalet, A., & Jay, M. (2018). Development of a 5As-based technology-assisted weight management intervention for veterans in primary care. *BMC Health Services Research*, 18(1), 47. https://doi.org/10.1186/s12913-018-2834-2

Maternal Health Care. (n.d.). Think Cultural Health. Retrieved December 30, 2022, from https://thinkculturalhealth.hhs.gov/education/maternal-health-care

Maternal Mortality Rates in the United States, 2020. (2022, November 7). https://www.cdc.gov/nchs/data/hestat/maternal-mortality/2020/maternal-mortality-rates-2020.htm

May, C. R., Eton, D. T., Boehmer, K., Gallacher, K., Hunt, K., MacDonald, S., Mair, F. S., May, C. M., Montori, V. M., Richardson, A., Rogers, A. E., & Shippee, N. (2014). Rethinking the patient: Using Burden of Treatment Theory to understand the changing dynamics of illness. *BMC Health Services Research*, 14, 281. https://doi.org/10.1186/1472-6963-14-281

McCance, T., McCormack, B., Slater, P., & McConnell, D. (2021). Examining the theoretical relationship between constructs in the person-centred practice framework: A structural equation model. *International Journal of Environmental Research and Public Health*, 18(24). https://doi.org/10.3390/ijerph182413138

McCance, T., Slater, P., & McCormack, B. (2009). Using the caring dimensions inventory as an indicator of person-centred nursing. *Journal of Clinical Nursing*, 18(3), 409–417. https://doi.org/10.1111/j.1365-2702.2008.02466.x

McCormack, B., McCance, T., & Brown, D. (2020). The future of person-centred practice—a call to action! *Of Person-Centred ....* https://books.google.ca/books?hl=en&lr=&id=uOQSEAAAQBAJ&oi=fnd&pg=PT362&ots=7CJzZdbAJ2&sig=g-zNjvjbF6DxyboDg2bv25_rgdU

McCormack, B., McCance, T., Bulley, C., & Brown, D. (2021). *Fundamentals of person-centred healthcare practice*. https://books.google.ca/books?hl=en&lr=&id=KnYOEAAAQBAJ&oi=fnd&pg=PA17&ots=3rsIfzNkmN&sig=-xS6MGrq9TLYn8r1T90R2emsyhU

McCormack, B., & McCance, T. V. (2006). Development of a framework for person-centred nursing. *Journal of Advanced Nursing*, 56(5), 472–479. https://doi.org/10.1111/j.1365-2648.2006.04042.x

McCormack, B. (2003a). A conceptual framework for person-centered practice with older people. *International Journal of Nursing Practice*, 9(3), 202–209. doi:10.1046/j.1440-172X.2003.00423.x

McCormack, B. (2003b). Researching nursing practice: does person-centredness matter? *Nursing Philosophy*, 4(3), 179–188. doi:10.1046/j.1466-769X.2003.00142.x

McCormack, L., Thomas, V., Lewis, M. A., & Rudd, R. (2017). Improving low health literacy and patient engagement: A social ecological approach. *Patient Education and Counseling*, 100(1), 8–13. https://doi.org/10.1016/j.pec.2016.07.007

McFarlane, J., Soroya, Occa, A., Peng, W., Awonuga, O., & Morgan, S. E. (2022). Community-Based Participatory Research (CBPR) to enhance participation of racial/ethnic minorities in clinical trials: A 10-year systematic review. *Health Communication*, 37(9), 1075–1092. https://doi.org/10.1080/10410236.2021.1943978

Medicaid Coverage of Pregnancy-Related Services: Findings From a 2021 State Survey - Report. (2022, May 19). KFF. https://www.kff.org/report-section/medicaid-coverage-of-pregnancy-related-services-findings-from-a-2021-state-survey-report/

Medicaid Postpartum Coverage Extension Tracker. (2022, October 27). KFF. https://www.kff.org/medicaid/issue-brief/medicaid-postpartum-coverage-extension-tracker/

Mead, N., & Bower, P. (2002). Patient-centred consultations and outcomes in primary care: A review of the literature. *Patient Education and Counseling*, 48(1), 51–61. doi:10.1016/S0738-3991(02)00099-X

Melnyk, B. M., & Fineout-Overholt, E. (2019). *Evidence-based practice in nursing & healthcare: A guide to best practice* (4th ed.). Wolters Kluwer.

Miller, W. R., & Rollnick, S. (2009). Ten things that motivational interviewing is not. *Behavioural and Cognitive Psychotherapy*, 37(2), 129–140. https://doi.org/10.1017/S1352465809005128

Monsen, K. A., Chatterjee, S. B., Timm, J. E., Poulsen, J. K., & McNaughton, D. B. (2015). Factors explaining variability in health literacy outcomes of public health nursing clients [Review of *Factors explaining variability in health literacy outcomes of public health nursing clients*]. *Public Health Nursing*, 32(2), 94–100. https://doi.org/10.1111/phn.12138

Monsen, K. A., Foster, D. L., Gomez, T., Poulsen, J. K., Mast, J., Westra, B. L., & Fishman, E. (2011). Evidence-based standardized care plans for use internationally to improve home care practice and population health. *Applied Clinical Informatics*, 2(3), 373–383. https://doi.org/10.4338/ACI-2011-03-RA-0023

Monsen, K. A., Rudenick, J. M., Kapinos, N., Warmbold, K., McMahon, S. K., & Schorr, E. N. (2019). Documentation of social determinants in electronic health records with and without standardized terminologies: A comparative study. *Proceedings of Singapore Healthcare*, *28*(1), 39–47. https://doi.org/10.1177/2010105818785641

Morgan, S., & Yoder, L. H. (2012). A concept analysis of person-centered care. *Journal of Holistic Nursing*, *30*(1), 6–15. doi:10.1177/0898010111412189

Morris, J. H., Irvine, L. A., Dombrowski, S. U., & McCormack, B. (2022). We Walk: A person-centred, dyadic behaviour change intervention to promote physical activity through outdoor walking after stroke—an intervention. *BMJ Open*. https://bmjopen.bmj.com/content/12/6/e058563.abstract

Mukerjee, R., Wesp, L., & Singer, R. (2021). *Clinician's guide to LGBTQIA+ care: Cultural safety and social justice in primary, sexual, and reproductive healthcare* (D. Menkin (Ed.)). Springer Publishing Company. https://play.google.com/store/books/details?id=JxL5DwAAQBAJ

Mundinger, M. O., Kane, R. L., Lenz, E. R., Totten, A. M., Tsai, W. Y., Cleary, P. D., Friedewald, W. T., Siu, A. L., & Shelanski, M. L. (2000). Primary care outcomes in patients treated by nurse practitioners or physicians: A randomized trial. *JAMA: The Journal of the American Medical Association*, *283*(1), 59–68. https://doi.org/10.1001/jama.283.1.59

Munro, S., Stacey, D., Lewis, K. B., & Bansback, N. (2016). Choosing treatment and screening options congruent with values: Do decision aids help? Sub-analysis of a systematic review. *Patient Education and Counseling*, *99*(4), 491–500. https://doi.org/10.1016/j.pec.2015.10.026

Narayan, M. C. (2019). CE: Addressing implicit bias in nursing: A review. *The American Journal of Nursing*, *119*(7), 36–43. https://doi.org/10.1097/01.NAJ.0000569340.27659.5a

National Academies of Sciences, Engineering, and Medicine. (NAM) (2021). *The future of nursing 2020–2030: Charting a path to achieve health equity*. The National Academies Press. https://doi.org/10.17226/25982

National Academies of Sciences, Engineering, and Medicine, Health and Medicine Division, Board on Health Care Services, & Committee on Integrating Social Needs Care into the Delivery of Health Care to Improve the Nation's Health. (NAM) (2020). *Integrating social care into the delivery of health care: Moving upstream to improve the nation's health*. National Academies Press. https://doi.org/10.17226/25467

National Institutes of Health. (2015, May 8). *Clear & simple*. Clear Communication. https://www.nih.gov/institutes-nih/nih-office-director/office-communications-public-liaison/clear-communication/clear-simple

Naylor, M. D., & Kurtzman, E. T. (2010). The role of nurse practitioners in reinventing primary care. *Health Affairs* , *29*(5), 893–899. https://doi.org/10.1377/hlthaff.2010.0440

Nethers, S. B., & Milstead, J. A. (2022). Future perspectives on nursing policy, technology, education, and practice. *The Nursing Clinics of North America*, *57*(4), 627–638. https://doi.org/10.1016/j.cnur.2022.06.010

Newhouse, R. P., Stanik-Hutt, J., White, K. M., Johantgen, M., Bass, E. B., Zangaro, G., Wilson, R. F., Fountain, L., Steinwachs, D. M., Heindel, L., & Weiner, J. P. (2011). Advanced practice nurse outcomes 1990-2008: A systematic review. *Nursing Economics*, *29*(5), 230–250; quiz 251. https://www.ncbi.nlm.nih.gov/pubmed/22372080

Nickitas, D. M., Emmons, K. R., & Ackerman-Barger, K. (2022). A policy pathway: Nursing's role in advancing diversity and health equity. *Nursing Outlook*, *70*(6S1), S38–S47. https://doi.org/10.1016/j.outlook.2022.03.013

Nightingale, Florence. *Notes on Nursing: What It Is, and What It Is Not*. Appleton-Century, 1873.

Nurmi, J., Knittle, K., Ginchev, T., Khattak, F., Helf, C., Zwickl, P., Castellano-Tejedor, C., Lusilla-Palacios, P., Costa-Requena, J., Ravaja, N., & Haukkala, A. (2020). Engaging users in the behavior change process with digitalized motivational interviewing and gamification: Development and feasibility testing of the precious app. *JMIR mHealth and uHealth*, *8*(1), e12884. https://doi.org/10.2196/12884

Omaha System Guidelines. (n.d.). *Welcome to Omaha System Guidelines*. Omaha System Guidelines, from https://sites.google.com/view/omahasystemguidelines

Onyx, J., & Bullen, P. (2000). Measuring social capital in five communities. *The Journal of Applied Behavioral Science*, *36*(1), 23–42. https://doi.org/10.1177/0021886300361002

Osakwe, Z. T., Barrón, Y., McDonald, M. V., & Feldman, P. H. (2021). Effect of nurse practitioner interventions on hospitalizations in the community transitions intervention trial. *Nursing Research*, *70*(4), 266–272. https://doi.org/10.1097/NNR.0000000000000508

Panagioti, M., Gooding, P., & Tarrier, N. (2009). Post-traumatic stress disorder and suicidal behavior: A narrative review. *Clinical Psychology Review, 29*(6), 471–482. https://doi.org/10.1016/j.cpr.2009.05.001

Papps, E., & Ramsden, I. (1996). Cultural safety in nursing: the New Zealand experience. *International Journal for Quality in Health Care: Journal of the International Society for Quality in Health Care / ISQua, 8*(5), 491–497. https://doi.org/10.1093/intqhc/8.5.491

Parker, M., Wallerstein, N., Duran, B., Magarati, M., Burgess, E., Sanchez-Youngman, S., Boursaw, B., Heffernan, A., Garoutte, J., & Koegel, P. (2020). Engage for equity: Development of community-based participatory research tools. *Health Education & Behavior: The Official Publication of the Society for Public Health Education, 47*(3), 359–371. https://doi.org/10.1177/1090198120921188

Patient-Centered Outcomes Research Institute. (2021, October 28). *About PCORI.* About PCORI. https://www.pcori.org/about/about-pcori

Peplau, H. E. (1997). Peplau's theory of interpersonal relations. *Nursing Science Quarterly, 10*(4), 162. doi:10.1177/089431849701000407

Peters, E. (2018). Compassion fatigue in nursing: A concept analysis. *Nursing Forum, 53*(4), 466–480. https://doi.org/10.1111/nuf.12274

Pollak, K. I., Tulsky, J. A., Bravender, T., Østbye, T., Lyna, P., Dolor, R. J., Coffman, C. J., Bilheimer, A., Lin, P.-H., Farrell, D., Bodner, M. E., & Alexander, S. C. (2016). Teaching primary care physicians the 5 A's for discussing weight with overweight and obese adolescents. *Patient Education and Counseling, 99*(10), 1620–1625. https://doi.org/10.1016/j.pec.2016.05.007

Prather, C., Fuller, T. R., Marshall, K. J., & Jeffries, W. L., 4th. (2016). The impact of racism on the sexual and reproductive health of African American women. *Journal of Women's Health, 25*(7), 664–671. https://doi.org/10.1089/jwh.2015.5637

Pratt, R., Hibberd, C., Cameron, I. M., & Maxwell, M. (2015). The Patient-Centered Assessment Method (PCAM): Integrating the social dimensions of health into primary care. *Journal of Comorbidity, 5*(1), 110–119. https://doi.org/10.15256/joc.2015.5.35

Premier, Inc. (2019, February 7). *Premier Inc. Identifies $8.3B Savings Opportunity in the ED with More Preventative and Coordinated Ambulatory Care.* Premier, Inc. https://www.premierinc.com/newsroom/press-releases/premier-inc-identifies-8-3b-savings-opportunity-in-the-ed-with-more-preventative-and-coordinated-ambulatory-care

Prins, A., Bovin, M. J., Smolenski, D. J., Marx, B. P., Kimerling, R., Jenkins-Guarnieri, M. A., Kaloupek, D. G., Schnurr, P. P., Kaiser, A. P., Leyva, Y. E., & Tiet, Q. Q. (2016). The Primary Care PTSD Screen for DSM-5 (PC-PTSD-5): Development and evaluation within a veteran primary care sample. *Journal of General Internal Medicine, 31*(10), 1206–1211. https://doi.org/10.1007/s11606-016-3703-5

Prins, A., Ouimette, P., Kimerling, R., Camerond, R. P., Hugelshofer, D. S., Shaw-Hegwer, J., Thrailkill, A., Gusman, F. D., & Sheikh, J. I. (2004). The primary care PTSD screen (PC–PTSD): development and operating characteristics. *Primary Care Psychiatry, 9*(1), 9–14. https://doi.org/10.1185/135525703125002360

Probst, M. A., Kanzaria, H. K., Schoenfeld, E. M., Menchine, M. D., Breslin, M., Walsh, C., Melnick, E. R., & Hess, E. P. (2017). Shared decision making in the Emergency Department: A guiding framework for clinicians. *Annals of Emergency Medicine, 70*(5), 688–695. https://doi.org/10.1016/j.annemergmed.2017.03.063

Prochaska, J. O., & DiClemente, C. C. (1982). Transtheoretical therapy: Toward a more integrative model of change. *Group Dynamics: Theory, Research, and Practice: The Official Journal of Division 49, Group Psychology and Group Psychotherapy of the American Psychological Association, 19*(3), 276–288. https://doi.org/10.1037/h0088437

Prochaska, J. O., & DiClemente, C. C. (1984). Self change processes, self efficacy and decisional balance across five stages of smoking cessation. *Progress in Clinical and Biological Research, 156*, 131–140. https://www.ncbi.nlm.nih.gov/pubmed/6473420

Prochaska, J. O., DiClemente, C. C., & Norcross, J. C. (1992). In search of how people change: Applications to addictive behaviors. *The American Psychologist, 47*(9), 1102–1114. https://doi.org/10.1037//0003-066x.47.9.1102

Prochaska, J. O., & Velicer, W. F. (1997). The transtheoretical model of health behavior change. *American Journal of Health Promotion: AJHP, 12*(1), 38–48. https://doi.org/10.4278/0890-1171-12.1.38

Project Implicit. (n.d.). Retrieved December 30, 2022, from https://www.projectimplicit.net/

Project READY: Reimagining Equity & Access for Diverse Youth – A free online professional development curriculum. (n.d.). Retrieved January 14, 2023, from https://ready.web.unc.edu/

PTSD: National Center for PTSD. (n.d.). Retrieved December 22, 2022, from https://www.ptsd.va.gov/professional/assessment/screens/pc-ptsd.asp

Quality of Nurse Practitioner Practice. (n.d.). American Association of Nurse Practitioners. Retrieved October 26, 2022, from https://www.aanp.org/advocacy/advocacy-resource/position-statements/quality-of-nurse-practitioner-practice

Rahemi, Z., D'Avolio, D., Dunphy, L. M., & Rivera, A. (2018). Shifting management in healthcare: An integrative review of design thinking. *Nursing Management, 49*(12), 30–37. https://doi.org/10.1097/01.NUMA.0000547834.95083.e9

Ramsden, I. M. (n.d.). *Cultural Safety and Nursing Education in Aotearoa and Te Waipounamu.* Retrieved December 11, 2022, from https://www.croakey.org/wp-content/uploads/2017/08/RAMSDEN-I-Cultural-Safety_Full.pdf

Rasanathan, K. (2018). 10 years after the Commission on Social Determinants of Health: Social injustice is still killing on a grand scale. *The Lancet, 392*(10154), 1176–1177. https://doi.org/10.1016/S0140-6736(18)32069-5

Rashid, T., Anjum, A., Chu, R., Stevanovski, S., Zanjani, A., & Lennox, C. (2014). Strength based resilience: Integrating risk and resources towards holistic well-being. In G. A. Fava & C. Ruini (Eds.), *Increasing psychological well-being in clinical and educational settings: Interventions and cultural contexts* (pp. 153–176). Springer Netherlands. https://doi.org/10.1007/978-94-017-8669-0_10

Ravi, A., & Little, V. (2017). Providing trauma-informed care. *American Family Physician, 95*(10), 655–657. https://www.ncbi.nlm.nih.gov/pubmed/28671409

Reinoso, H., Bartlett, J. L., & Bennett, S. L. (2018). Teaching differential diagnosis to nurse practitioner students. *The Journal for Nurse Practitioners: JNP, 14*(10), e207–e212. https://doi.org/10.1016/j.nurpra.2018.08.028

Risling, T. L., & Risling, D. E. (2020). Advancing nursing participation in user-centred design. *Journal of Research in Nursing: JRN, 25*(3), 226–238. https://doi.org/10.1177/1744987120913590

Roberts, J. P., Fisher, T. R., Trowbridge, M. J., & Bent, C. (2016). A design thinking framework for healthcare management and innovation. *Healthcare (Amsterdam, Netherlands), 4*(1), 11–14. https://doi.org/10.1016/j.hjdsi.2015.12.002

Robinson, J. H., Callister, L. C., Berry, J. A., & Dearing, K. A. (2008). Patient-centered care and adherence: Definitions and applications to improve outcomes. *Journal of the American Association of Nurse Practitioners, 20*(12), 600–607. https://doi.org/10.1111/j.1745-7599.2008.00360.x

Roe, L., & Galvin, M. (2021). Providing inclusive, person-centred care for LGBT+ older adults: A discussion on health and social care design and delivery. *Journal of Nursing Management, 29*(1), 104–108. https://doi.org/10.1111/jonm.13178

Rooney, M. K., Santiago, G., Perni, S., Horowitz, D. P., McCall, A. R., Einstein, A. J., Jagsi, R., & Golden, D. W. (2021). Readability of patient education materials from high-impact medical journals: A 20-year analysis. *Journal of Patient Experience, 8*, 2374373521998847. https://doi.org/10.1177/2374373521998847

Rowe, P. G. (1991). *Design thinking.* MIT Press. https://play.google.com/store/books/details?id=ZjZ3mflzJtUC

Rush, K. L., Seaton, C., Li, E., Oelke, N. D., & Pesut, B. (2021). Rural use of health service and telemedicine during COVID-19: The role of access and eHealth literacy. *Health Informatics Journal, 27*(2), 14604582211020064. https://doi.org/10.1177/14604582211020064

Rutherford, M. A. (2008). Standardized nursing language: What does it mean for nursing practice? *OJIN: The Online Journal of Issues in Nursing, 13*(1). https://doi.org/10.3912/OJIN.Vol13No01PPT05

Ryan, P., & Sawin, K. J. (2009). The individual and family self-management theory: Background and perspectives on context, process, and outcomes. *Nursing Outlook, 57*(4), 217–225.e6. https://doi.org/10.1016/j.outlook.2008.10.004

Sacks, R. M., Greene, J., Hibbard, J., Overton, V., & Parrotta, C. D. (2017). Does patient activation predict the course of type 2 diabetes? A longitudinal study. *Patient Education and Counseling, 100*(7), 1268–1275. https://doi.org/10.1016/j.pec.2017.01.014

Salgado, T. M., Mackler, E., Severson, J. A., Lindsay, J., Batra, P., Petersen, L., & Farris, K. B. (2017). The relationship between patient activation, confidence to self-manage side effects, and adherence to oral oncolytics: a pilot study with Michigan oncology practices. *Supportive Care in Cancer, 25*, 1797–1807.

Salmond, E., Salmond, S., Ames, M., Kamienski, M., & Holly, C. (2019). Experiences of compassion fatigue in direct care nurses: A qualitative systematic review. *JBI Evidence Synthesis, 17*(5), 682. https://doi.org/10.11124/JBISRIR-2017-003818

Santana, M. J., Manalili, K., Jolley, R. J., Zelinsky, S., Quan, H., & Lu, M. (2018). How to practice person-centred care: A conceptual framework. *Health Expectations: An International Journal of Public Participation in Health Care and Health Policy, 21*(2), 429–440. https://doi.org/10.1111/hex.12640

Saulnier, D. D., Dixit, A. M., Nunes, A. R., & Murray, V. (n.d.). *3.2 Disaster risk factors— hazards, exposure and vulnerability.* https://extranet.who.int/kobe_centre/sites/default/files/pdf/WHO%20Guidance_Research%20Methods_Health-EDRM_3.2.pdf

Schilling, L. S., Grey, M., & Knafl, K. A. (2002). The concept of self-management of type 1 diabetes in children and adolescents: An evolutionary concept analysis. *Journal of Advanced Nursing, 37*(1), 87–99. https://doi.org/10.1046/j.1365-2648.2002.02061.x

Schimmels, J., & Cunningham, L. (2021). How do we move forward with trauma-informed care? *The Journal for Nurse Practitioners: JNP, 17*(4), 405–411. https://doi.org/10.1016/j.nurpra.2020.12.005

Scored, P. (n.d.). *Patient-Centered Assessment Method (PCAM) Sample Training Cases.* https://med.umn.edu/sites/med.umn.edu/files/scored_sample_training_cases.pdf

Sharp, S., McAllister, M., & Broadbent, M. (2016). The vital blend of clinical competence and compassion: How patients experience person-centred care. *Contemporary Nurse, 52*(2–3), 300–312. https://doi.org/10.1080/10376178.2015.1020981

Shippee, N. D., Shah, N. D., May, C. R., Mair, F. S., & Montori, V. M. (2012). Cumulative complexity: A functional, patient-centered model of patient complexity can improve research and practice. *Journal of Clinical Epidemiology, 65*(10), 1041–1051. https://doi.org/10.1016/j.jclinepi.2012.05.005

Short, M. W., & Domagalski, J. E. (2013). Iron deficiency anemia: Evaluation and management. *American Family Physician, 87*(2), 98–104. https://www.ncbi.nlm.nih.gov/pubmed/23317073

Sinclair, S., Beamer, K., Hack, T. F., McClement, S., Raffin Bouchal, S., Chochinov, H. M., & Hagen, N. A. (2017). Sympathy, empathy, and compassion: A grounded theory study of palliative care patients' understandings, experiences, and preferences. *Palliative Medicine, 31*(5), 437–447. https://doi.org/10.1177/0269216316663499

Singer, T., & Klimecki, O. M. (2014). Empathy and compassion. *Current Biology: CB, 24*(18), R875–R878. https://doi.org/10.1016/j.cub.2014.06.054

Singh Ospina, N., Phillips, K. A., Rodriguez-Gutierrez, R., Castaneda-Guarderas, A., Gionfriddo, M. R., Branda, M. E., & Montori, V. M. (2019). Eliciting the patient's agenda—secondary analysis of recorded clinical encounters. *Journal of General Internal Medicine, 34*(1), 36–40. https://doi.org/10.1007/s11606-018-4540-5

Slater, L. (2006). Person-centredness: A concept analysis. *Contemporary Nurse, 23*(1), 135–144. https://doi.org/10.5172/conu.2006.23.1.135

Stacey, D., Légaré, F., Lewis, K., Barry, M. J., Bennett, C. L., Eden, K. B., Holmes-Rovner, M., Llewellyn-Thomas, H., Lyddiatt, A., Thomson, R., & Trevena, L. (2017). Decision aids for people facing health treatment or screening decisions. *Cochrane Database of Systematic Reviews, 4*(4), CD001431. https://doi.org/10.1002/14651858.CD001431.pub5

Stanik-Hutt, J., Newhouse, R. P., White, K. M., Johantgen, M., Bass, E. B., Zangaro, G., Wilson, R., Fountain, L., Steinwachs, D. M., Heindel, L., & Weiner, J. P. (2013). The quality and effectiveness of care provided by nurse practitioners. *The Journal for Nurse Practitioners: JNP, 9*(8), 492–500.e13. https://doi.org/10.1016/j.nurpra.2013.07.004

Steeves-Reece, A. L., Totten, A. M., Broadwell, K. D., Richardson, D. M., Nicolaidis, C., & Davis, M. M. (2022). Social needs resource connections: A systematic review of barriers, facilitators, and evaluation. *American Journal of Preventive Medicine, 62*(5), e303–e315. https://doi.org/10.1016/j.amepre.2021.12.002

Stewart, M. A. (1995). Effective physician-patient communication and health outcomes: A review. *CMAJ: Canadian Medical Association Journal = Journal de l'Association Medicale Canadienne*, 152(9), 1423–1433. https://www.ncbi.nlm.nih.gov/pubmed/7728691

Stewart, M., Brown, J. B., Donner, A., McWhinney, I. R., Oates, J., Weston, W. W., & Jordan, J. (2000). The impact of patient-centered care on outcomes. *Journal of Family Practice*, 49(9), 796.

Street, R. L., Jr., Makoul, G., Arora, N. K., & Epstein, R. M. (2009). How does communication heal? Pathways linking clinician-patient communication to health outcomes. *Patient Education and Counseling*, 74(3), 295–301. https://doi.org/10.1016/j.pec.2008.11.015

Substance Abuse and Mental Health Services Administration. (2014). *SAMHSA's Concept of Trauma and Guidance for a Trauma-Informed Approach* (HHS Publication No. (SMA) 14-4884). SAMHSA. https://store.samhsa.gov/sites/default/files/d7/priv/sma14-4884.pdf

The Fenway Institute. (2015, January 20). *Education & Training—Fenway Health: Health Care Is a Right, Not a Privilege*. Fenway Health: Health Care Is a Right, Not a Privilege. https://fenwayhealth.org/the-fenway-institute/education/

The Ohio State University. (n.d.). *Implicit bias module series*. Kirwan Institute for the Study of Race and Ethnicity. https://kirwaninstitute.osu.edu/implicit-bias-training

Tinetti, M. E., Naik, A. D., Dindo, L., Costello, D. M., Esterson, J., Geda, M., Rosen, J., Hernandez-Bigos, K., Smith, C. D., Ouellet, G. M., Kang, G., Lee, Y., & Blaum, C. (2019). Association of patient priorities-aligned decision-making with patient outcomes and ambulatory health care burden among older adults with multiple chronic conditions: A nonrandomized clinical trial. *JAMA Internal Medicine*, 179(12), 1688–1697. https://doi.org/10.1001/jamainternmed.2019.4235

Trost, S., Beauregard, J., Chandra, G., Njie, F., Berry, J., Harvey, A., & Goodman, D. A. (2022). *Pregnancy-related deaths: Data from maternal mortality review committees in 36 US states, 2017–2019*. Centers for Disease Control and Prevention. https://www.cdc.gov/reproductivehealth/maternal-mortality/docs/pdf/Pregnancy-Related-Deaths-Data-MMRCs-2017-2019-H.pdf

United States Congressional Budget Office, & Smith, C. L. (1979). *Physician extenders: Their current and future role in medical care delivery*. Congress of the United States, Congressional Budget Office. https://play.google.com/store/books/details?id=W0XjdRUoMOMC

University of California Berkeley. (2022). *Loving-kindness meditation*. The Greater Good Science Center. https://ggia.berkeley.edu/practice/loving_kindness_meditation

University of California Los Angeles. (n.d.). *Implicit bias*. UCLA Equity, Diversity & Inclusion. https://equity.ucla.edu/know/implicit-bias/

University of Connecticut. (2020, April 20). *Research—weight bias & stigma: Healthcare providers*. Rudd Center for Food Policy and Health; UConn Rudd Center for Food Policy and Health. https://uconnruddcenter.org/research/weight-bias-stigma/healthcare-providers/

Webel, A. R., Cuca, Y., Okonsky, J. G., Asher, A. K., Kaihura, A., & Salata, R. A. (2013). The impact of social context on self-management in women living with HIV. *Social Science & Medicine*, 87, 147–154. https://doi.org/10.1016/j.socscimed.2013.03.037

Westphal, J., Lancaster, R., & Park, D. (2014). Work-arounds observed by fourth-year nursing students. *Western Journal of Nursing Research*, 36(8), 1002–1018. https://doi.org/10.1177/0193945913511707

Williams, D. R., & Collins, C. (2001). Racial residential segregation: A fundamental cause of racial disparities in health. *Public Health Reports*, 116(5), 404–416. https://doi.org/10.1093/phr/116.5.404

Williams, D. R., Lawrence, J. A., & Davis, B. A. (2019). Racism and health: Evidence and needed research. *Annual Review of Public Health*, 40, 105–125. https://doi.org/10.1146/annurev-publhealth-040218-043750

Williams, D. R., & Mohammed, S. A. (2013). Racism and health I: Pathways and scientific evidence. *The American Behavioral Scientist*, 57(8), 1152–1173. https://doi.org/10.1177/0002764213487340

Williamson, M. L. C., Stickley, M. M., Armstrong, T. W., Jackson, K., & Console, K. (2022). Diagnostic accuracy of the Primary Care PTSD Screen for DSM-5 (PC-PTSD-5) within a civilian primary care sample. *Journal of Clinical Psychology*, 78(11), 2299–2308. https://doi.org/10.1002/jclp.23405

Wisconsin Department of Health Services. (2019). *Annual Wisconsin Birth and Infant Death Report*. https://www.dhs.wisconsin.gov/stats/births/index.htm

Wong, Y. J., Owen, J., Gabana, N. T., Brown, J. W., McInnis, S., Toth, P., & Gilman, L. (2018). Does gratitude writing improve the mental health of psychotherapy clients? Evidence from a randomized controlled trial. *Psychotherapy Research: Journal of the Society for Psychotherapy Research, 28*(2), 192–202. https://doi.org/10.1080/10503307.2016.1169332

World Health Organization. (2007). People-centered health care: A policy framework. Retrieved from http://www.wpro.who.int/health_services/people_at_the_centre_of_care/documents/ENG-PCIPolicyFramework.pdf

World Health Organization. (2020). *Coronavirus disease (COVID-19) pandemic.* Emergencies. https://www.who.int/europe/emergencies/situations/covid-19

World Health Organization. (2021). Strategic toolkit for assessing risks: A comprehensive toolkit for all-hazards health emergency risk assessment. https://www.who.int/publications/i/item/9789240036086

World Health Organization: Europe. (2003). *Social Determinants of Health: The solid facts* (R. Wilkinson & M. Marmot (Eds.), 2nd ed. http://www.euro.who.int/__data/assets/pdf_file/0005/98438/e81384.pdf

Wright, N., Wilson, L., Smith, M., Duncan, B., & McHugh, P. (2017). The BROAD study: A randomised controlled trial using a whole food plant-based diet in the community for obesity, ischaemic heart disease or diabetes. *Nutrition & Diabetes, 7*(3), e256. https://doi.org/10.1038/nutd.2017.3

Yearby, R., Clark, B., & Figueroa, J. F. (2022). Structural racism in historical and modern US health care policy. *Health Affairs, 41*(2), 187–194. https://doi.org/10.1377/hlthaff.2021.01466

Yoshida, S., Matsushima, M., Wakabayashi, H., Mutai, R., Murayama, S., Hayashi, T., Ichikawa, H., Nakano, Y., Watanabe, T., & Fujinuma, Y. (2017). Validity and reliability of the Patient Centred Assessment Method for patient complexity and relationship with hospital length of stay: A prospective cohort study. *BMJ Open, 7*(5), e016175. https://doi.org/10.1136/bmjopen-2017-016175

Zhao, J., Gao, S., Wang, J., Liu, X., & Hao, Y. (2016). Differentiation between two healthcare concepts: Person-centered and patient-centered care. *International Journal of Nursing Sciences, 3*(4), 398–402. https://doi.org/10.1016/j.ijnss.2016.08.009

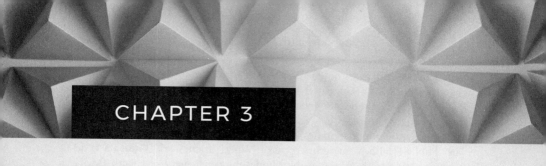

CHAPTER 3

Population Health

Carol Flaten, DNP, RN, PHN, Clinical Associate Professor
Stephanie Gingerich, DNP, RN, CPN, Clinical Assistant Professor

Grounded in social justice, equipped in the art and science of nursing, DNP prepared nurses impact health and well being of populations locally and globally.

—Carol Flaten

Introduction

The *American Association of Colleges of Nursing (AACN) Essentials* (2021, p. 33) describe population health as

> Population health spans the healthcare delivery continuum from public health prevention to disease management of populations and describes collaborative activities with both traditional and non-traditional partnerships from affected communities, public health, industry, academia, health care, local government entities, and others for the improvement of equitable population health outcomes. (Kindig & Stoddart, 2003; Kindig, 2007; Swartout & Bishop, 2017; CDC, 2020)

This definition is expansive in that it approaches health from multiple perspectives and moves beyond an individual approach to improving health through actions that impact vast numbers of people, environmental issues that affect health, and the health of the planet. Alongside this description of population health, the American Public Health Association (APHA, 2013) defines public health nursing as "the practice of promoting and protecting the health of populations using knowledge from nursing, social, and public health sciences" (p. 2). Roux (2016) states the following:

> Improving and protecting the health of the population is a key social goal that requires a broad interdisciplinary science and many different kinds of actions. The more synonyms we have to refer to approaches that will allow us to do this, and the more disciplines and sectors that identify with this approach, the better. (p. 619)

Expert nurse leaders at the doctoral level are in a prime position to lead and participate in this work. Population health work involves complex systems with multiple perspectives and traditions represented. This chapter will put forward approaches that align with the *AACN Essentials* (2021) for Level II competencies, acknowledging that the foundation lies in Level I competencies.

The "Public Health Nursing Intervention Wheel" framework (**Figure 3-1**) developed by public health nurses at the Minnesota Department of Health (MDH, 2019) is used nationally and globally to describe the complex work of individual/family, community, and systems level interventions. Although the framework was designed to delineate what public health nurses as a specialty do, the interventions are not exclusive to public health nurses. As described in the definitions above, addressing the assets and gaps in population-based needs at local, state, tribal, national, and global levels requires an interdisciplinary approach and team members. This framework is well suited to this work.

The National Academies of Science, Engineering and Medicine, Consensus Report, *The Future of Nursing 2020–2030, Charting a Path to Achieve Health Equity* (2021), emphasizes the goal of health equity and healthcare equity in diverse populations and settings through structural changes in payment systems,

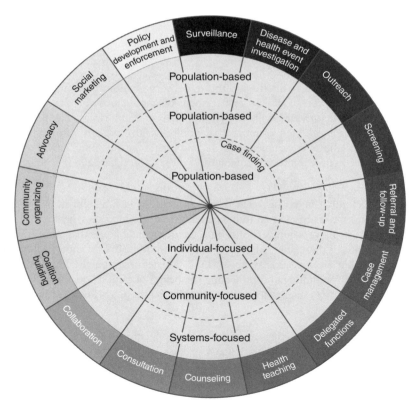

Figure 3-1 Public Health Nursing Intervention Wheel

Minnesota Department of Health. (2019). *Public health interventions: Applications for public health nursing practice* (2nd ed.) p. 11

laws, policies, and regulation. These are all population/system-level changes that nurses are well positioned to influence from a population health perspective. The *AACN Essentials* (2021) description of population health, the APHA definition of the public health nurse and the *Future of Nursing 2020–2030* (National Academies of Sciences, Engineering, and Medicine, 2021) report provide synergy for the DNP-prepared nurse in advanced practice or leadership roles to develop sustainable interventions to impact the health of populations that are based in equity and social justice.

Selected Concepts for Nursing Practice Represented in the Domain

The *AACN Essentials* (2021) concepts of communication, diversity, equity and inclusion, ethics, health policy, and social determinant of health are woven throughout this chapter. Other *AACN Essentials* concepts, of course, may also apply but the concepts identified seem to be most pertinent to the competencies and subcompetencies for this domain. In addition, the authors of this chapter have included an additional concept, planetary health, which affects the health of all. DNP-prepared nurses are in a key position to impact population interventions and outcomes. Nurses have a unique understanding of the individual experience of wellness and illness and the devastating consequences of poor health conditions. Advanced-level education allows the nurse to conceptualize and act to assess and manage population interventions that produce health outcomes at the individual level and at the systems level. At the systems level, opportunity exists to change structures that address diversity, equity and inclusion; affect health policy; and create a voice for marginalized populations, while practicing from a social justice perspective guided by ethics of the nursing profession. Communication, including listening, is embedded in the competencies. All DNP-prepared nurses need to know the population they serve, recognize the social determinants of health that impact that population and make strides through collaboration to improve health outcomes. Listening to individuals and communities, assessing needs, and working through collaboration and partnerships to achieve mutual and measurable goals is the work of all DNP-prepared nurses at the local, state, national, and global levels.

An additional factor in advocating for the health of populations is to recognize the health of the planet and the reciprocal nature of human health and the health of the planet. Planetary health is an emerging field that aims to understand how changes happening to the planet threaten our health and how to protect people and the earth (Meyers & Frumpkin, 2020). An example of a planetary health issue is to think of drinking water and groundwater contamination. Groundwater can be contaminated in a variety of ways due to human impacts on the environment such as chemical spills from train derailments, agricultural runoff, or improper hazardous waste disposal. If contaminants enter the community drinking water supply and remain undetected, the health of the community may be put in jeopardy. Li et al. (2021), describe the presence of contaminants in groundwater that impact human health when ingested and land/soil quality leading to a poor environment for vegetation growth. Such contaminants affect the nutrient value of crops that adversely impacts nutrient sources for human health.

Level II Competencies

Manage Population Health

In order to achieve Level II subcompetencies it is expected that the nurse has the Level I subcompetencies met. These Level I subcompetencies include defining a target population, assessing population health data, accessing community priorities (if they exist), and having the ability to compare and contrast benchmarks to identify health patterns (*AACN Essentials*, 2021) and are all part of the nursing process at the community/population level. Managing population health has been a focus of public health nursing practice and is now emphasized further in the recent *Future of Nursing 2020–2030* (National Academies of Sciences, Engineering, and Medicine, 2021, p. 27).

Assess the Efficacy of a System's Capability to Serve a Target Subpopulation's Healthcare Needs

Initial questions that are crucial to consider related to the efficacy of a system are:

What are the system's assets?

Are there personnel who can fill the roles needed for the program or the work?

Is there financial capacity for supplies, personal, messaging, and so on?

Is there the desire by the system to meet this need?

Will additional training be required for personnel?

Is there the political will to move forward?

These questions and others are important to begin to understand what the system can contribute to meeting the need and whether there is there a need for additional partners. Are there potential partners? Determining answers to these questions is a phase of exploration at the systems level to understand how a system can support, be involved in, and ultimately sustain the intervention for the population's healthcare needs.

Analyze Primary and Secondary Population Health Data for Multiple Populations Against Relevant Benchmarks

Population health data supports an informed process of decision making related to the current status of an issue, what resources are available, and where gaps and opportunities to improve outcomes may lie. Knowledge of basic statistical values and necessary analysis of the data, that is "making sense" of that data within the context of the population to be served as well as the broader community or environment of interest, is core to this work.

An understanding of biostatistical and epidemiological methods qualifies the DNP-prepared nurse to analyze health statistics and environmental and other scientific data. The ability to analyze census data, morbidity and mortality reports, data from the National Center for Health Statistics, and other sources of public health data in relation to population health is part of the work of the DNP-prepared nurse. Knowledge of how to perform rate adjustments, to determine the number needed to treat (NNT), and to interpret confidence intervals as well as knowledge of epidemiological principles of risk are also vital when considering prevention activities. An understanding of the difference between relative risk and attributable risk is necessary when working on the population health level to develop appropriate interventions and decrease any potential for causing harm by inappropriate prevention activities (Gévas, Starfield, & Heath, 2008). The DNP graduate is well prepared to do this.

Data regarding the negative impact of environmental changes and toxins on health are becoming more prevalent, and analysis of these data may provide the basis for prevention interventions developed for use by the DNP in program project planning (Ashton & Green, 2008; Barrett, 2015; Liu & Lewis, 2014; Stanhope & Lancaster, 2016; Trasande, 2014). The DNP's ability to perform analysis of data is further enhanced by developing proficiency in the practice of evidence-based nursing. DiCenso, Guyatt, and Ciliska (2005) have provided a framework for utilization of evidence-based nursing in a text on implementation of evidence-based nursing in clinical practice. The development of any nursing intervention always begins with assessment. To practice evidence-based nursing, however, it is also necessary to develop a properly formulated question about the patient population, the intervention, a comparison, and outcome (PICO) to facilitate gathering the available evidence. Adding the element of time (PICOT) to the question formulation, if indicated by the condition or population of interest, has been suggested by others (Fineout-Overholt & Johnston, 2005; Flemming, 2008). Next, the evidence gathered in answer to these questions needs to be analyzed to determine whether it is appropriate to use for the particular individual or population of interest. This is where additional background from coursework in statistics and epidemiology is so vital for the DNP graduate. By developing skill in these areas, all DNP graduates will be prepared to analyze data at individual, aggregate, and population health levels in order to use such data appropriately when developing interventions.

The United Nations Sustainable Development Goals (United Nations, n.d.a.) provide a set of goals from a very broad perspective. In the United States one may also look to the *Healthy People 2030* goals (Office of Disease Prevention and Health Promotion, n.d.) that set 10-year goals for the nation. In addition, state, regional, and tribal goals are also crucial to understand. A collaborative approach in this process is required.

Use Established or Evolving Methods to Determine Population-Focused Priorities for Care, Develop a Collaborative Approach With Relevant Stakeholders to Address Population Healthcare Needs, Including Evaluation Methods, and Collaborate With Appropriate Stakeholders to Implement a Sociocultural and Linguistically Responsive Intervention Plan

These three subcompetencies connect to create a holistic approach for determining priorities and implementing a plan. Engaging in effective partnerships will be discussed in depth below. Diving deep into the community or population of interest is at the heart of this process. As discussed previously, collecting the data is important; analyzing and evaluating the data is a beginning. However, then progressing on to listening to the community needs and desires, learning about their priorities, identifying stakeholders, determining needs, considering evaluation plans, and including the communication needs, language, and cultural framework of the community bring together the many components that will be part of the work.

Attending community events and meetings is a beginning. Meet with stakeholders such as the mayor, elders, school leaders, faith leaders, workers on their breaks, and so on. Look for the gathering places in the community, learn from what your senses (eyes, ears, nose, touch, taste) might indicate, and learn where you could find the voices of those that may not be easily heard. Always strive for inclusion.

Engage in Effective Partnerships

Riane Eisler, a systems scientist, attorney, and theorist, developed the study of relational dynamics which focuses on societies throughout history, researching the relationships and unique characteristics within them. Her research yielded the understanding that cultures and societies fall on a continuum identified as a *partnership/domination continuum* (Eisler, 1987; Eisler & Potter, 2014). This research concluded that how far a society's families, education, religion, politics, economics and other institutions orient to either end of the continuum can have a profound impact on life, including health care (Eisler & Potter, 2014). The partnership versus domination characteristics permeate all aspects of the society and should be considered as DNP students and educators engage in direct patient care, nursing leadership, systems change, and educator roles.

While Eisler developed a list of unique characteristics that comprise a partnership model versus a domination model, she argues that societies fall within a continuum where they may exhibit varying degrees of the partnership or domination characteristics (Eisler & Potter, 2014). Within societies based in more of a domination model, characteristics such as rigid hierarchies, subordination of females to males, culturally accepted abuse and violence, and beliefs that justify domination and violence exist. Within societies based in a partnership model, these characteristics are challenged and instead include a culture with flattened hierarchies, equal valuing of males and females, mutual respect and trust, and values promoting empathy and caring relations (Eisler & Potter, 2014). See **Figure 3-2**.

As a DNP student, you must understand the benefits of engaging and promoting partnership-based models and relationships. Consider in a domination system the voices and ideas that are not valued and thus missed due to the rigid hierarchies and emphasis placed on gender or role domination. In these systems, it is also likely that minority cultures, races, and opinions will continue to be devalued. Rather, in a partnership system, the beliefs and stories of empathy and caring perpetuate a culture of care and safety for others to speak up. In such a partnership system, voices who are not represented may have a higher likelihood of speaking up and also being heard. This presents more opportunity to hear new ideas, perspectives, proposals, and change for improving health around the world.

Educators can assist DNP students to identify partnership versus domination models as well as engage in and participate in promoting partnership-based systems. DNP leaders can work to ensure that organizational culture is based on partnership

The partnership system

Democratic and
economically
equitable structure

Mutual respect and
trust with low degree
of violence

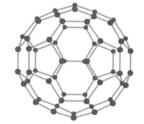

Equal valuing of males
and females and high
regard for stereotypical
feminine values

Beliefs and stories
that give high value
to empathic and
caring relations

The domination system

Authoritarian and
inequitable social
and economic
structure

High degree of abuse
and violence

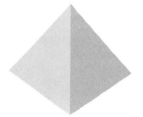

Subordination of women
and "femininity" to men
and "masculinity"

Beliefs and stories that
justify and idealize
domination and violence

Figure 3-2 The Partnership and Domination Systems

Reproduced from Eisler, R. (2007) The real wealth of nations: Creating a caring economy. Berrett-Koehler.

models. Leaders should identify the current status of their organizational culture and how the organization falls within the partnership/domination continuum. That information can then support leaders to promote appropriate action to encourage and model partnership systems, hold people accountable when engaging in abusive or domination behaviors that detract from the culture, and provide resources and tools for people to successfully maintain a partnership culture within teams and across the organization.

Ascertain Collaborative Opportunities for Individuals and Organizations to Improve Population Health

The DNP-prepared nurse should consider opportunities for partnership that may benefit individuals and work across systems for population health. Given a culture of partnership as described above, the DNP-prepared nurse can create a culture where key partners from various backgrounds, disciplines, experiences, and knowledge can collaborate to create solutions for population health.

In New Mexico, a partnership was developed to offer medical screening for miners in an effort to address high rates of hypertension and diabetes among the miners. The New Mexico Mobile Screening Program for Miners offers screenings for respiratory conditions, hearing loss, musculoskeletal, and respiratory conditions in addition to assessing risk factors for cancer, cardiovascular disease, diabetes, and hypertension, among others (Rural Health Information Hub, 2022). The mobile clinic is equipped to perform x-rays and examinations, assess current conditions and risk factors for health concerns, and complete follow-up calls following the miner's visit (Rural Health Information Hub, 2022). In addition to services offered within the mobile clinic, specialty services are offered via telemedicine scheduled for the same day as needed. As a result, "In a convenience-sample survey, all miners reported their care as good (8%) or very good (92%), and 100% would recommend the mobile screening clinic to others" (Rural Health Information Hub, 2022, para. 8). The program has expanded to Montana, Utah, and Wyoming.

The DNP-prepared nurse can consider partnerships such as the New Mexico Mobile Screening Program for miners which included an innovative approach to bringing interdisciplinary team members together to address health within the miners' environment. Working in collaboration within a partnership culture, DNP graduate nurses can impact health for the individual and across systems by bringing together key partners to address health in new and unique ways.

Challenge Biases and Barriers That Impact Population Health Outcomes

In order to challenge biases and stereotypes that exist within systems, one must first acknowledge the internal biases and stereotypes that exist within oneself. As such, it is valuable to become familiar with the terminology and concepts that permeate systems and perpetuate inequities within health care. Review the terminology of biases in **Table 3-1**.

Table 3-1 Terminology of Biases

Term	Definition
Cultural Racism	"Cultural systems that visibly and invisibly ground assumptions of white superiority and power across institutional, cultural, and social environments" (Cogburn, 2019, p. 741).
Discrimination	Discrimination is "the result of either implicit or explicit biases and is the inequitable treatment and/or impact of general policies, practices, and norms on individuals and communities based on social group membership" (Matteo & Williams, 2020, p. S5).
Ethnicity	Ethnicity is "a social system defining a group that shares a common ancestry, history or culture with some combination of shared geographic origins, family patterns, language, or cultural norms, religious traditions, or other cultural and social characteristics" (Williams, 1997, p. 325).
Explicit bias	Explicit forms of bias include "preferences, beliefs, and attitudes of which people are generally consciously aware, endorsed, and can be identified and communicated" (Daumeyer et al., 2019, p. 1).
Hidden curriculum	Lessons taught through socialization of learners especially as it pertains to professionalism, humanism, and accountability, as opposed to explicitly taught in the classroom or bedside (Rajput et al., 2017).

Term	Definition
Implicit bias	Implicit biases are "unconscious mental processes that lead to associations and reactions that are automatic and without intention and actors have no awareness of the associations with a stimulus. Implicit bias goes beyond stereotyping to include favorable or unfavorable evaluations toward groups of people." While we are not aware these implicit biases exist, they have a significant impact on decision making (Staats et al., 2015, p. 14).
Institutional racism	Institutional racism (structural) "... laws (local, state and federal), policies, and practices of society ... that provide advantages to racial groups deemed superior while ... oppressing, disadvantaging or otherwise neglecting racial groups viewed as inferior." (Williams et al., 2019, p. 107).
Race	Race is "... a social category, based on nationality, ethnicity, phenotypic or other markers ... It ... socializes people to accept as true the inferiority of nondominant racial groups leading to negative normative beliefs (stereotypes) and attitudes (prejudice)." (Williams et al., 2019, p. 106).
Racism	Racism is "... an organized social system in which the dominant racial group, ... categorizes and ranks people into social groups ... 'races' and uses its power to devalue, disempower, and differentially allocate ... resources and opportunities to groups defined as inferior ..." (Williams et al., 2019, p. 106).
Role modeling	Role modeling is a mechanism for teaching behavior through learning by observation (Jochemsen-van der Leeuw et al., 2013, p. 26).
Stereotype	When a set of beliefs lead an individual to make judgment about another related to or in association with a group whether that assumption is true or not (Puddifoot, 2019).
Stereotype threat	Stereotype threat "occurs when cues in the environment make negative stereotypes associated with an individual's group status salient, triggering physiological and psychological processes that have detrimental consequences for behavior" and performance of the individual who identifies as a member of the stereotyped group (Burgess et al., 2010, p. S169).

Data from Cogburn, C. (2019). Culture, race, and health: Implications for racial inequities and population health. *The Milbank Quarterly, 97*(3); 736–761. https://doi.org/10.1111/1468-0009.12411; Puddifoot, K. (2019). Stereotyping patients. *Journal of Social Philosophy, 50*(1); 1–126. https://doi.org/10.1111/josp.12269; Vela, M.B. et al., (2022). Eliminating explicit and implicit biases in health care: Evidence and research needs. *Annual Review of Public Health, 43*; 477–501. doi: 10.1146/annurev-publhealth-052620-103528

The DNP graduate must consider their unique biases and stereotypes in order to challenge them and begin to address the inequities that exist within health care. Consider the ways in which you have witnessed, been a recipient of, or perpetuated discrimination, stereotypes, and bias. How have those examples impacted the way in which people were served in the community or within healthcare settings? By removing the biases and stereotypes, how could the care provided be rewritten to better serve the individual for improved health outcomes or health experiences?

As a DNP educator, using examples in which DNP students can challenge their biases and stereotypes in the classroom and practicum settings will support them to continue to challenge systems throughout their career. These examples and experiences can vary from the individual care level through the systemic and global levels.

Evaluate the Effectiveness of Partnerships for Achieving Health Equity

To address ways in which to achieve health equity, one must first understand the concepts of equality versus equity and how they impact people. Equality, as noted in **Figure 3-3**, is when everyone receives the same treatment, care, or product regardless of whether it is the most appropriate for that individual (Robert Wood Johnson Foundation, 2022). Equity, on the other hand, is when people and systems understand the barriers, issues, and unique situations to address disparities and ensure that everyone is able to receive care based on their unique needs (Campaign for Action, n.d.; Robert Wood Johnson Foundation, 2022). "For the purposes of measurement, health equity means reducing and ultimately eliminating disparities in health and its determinants that adversely affect excluded or marginalized groups" (Braveman et al., 2017, p. 2). If healthcare systems focus on equality rather than equity, valuable resources may be wasted as they will be used unnecessarily without advancing the health of those whom they may be attempting to serve. Focusing

EQUALITY:
Everyone gets the same regardless if it's needed or right for them.

EQUITY:
Everyone gets what they need — understanding the barriers, circumstances, and conditions.

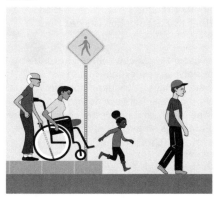
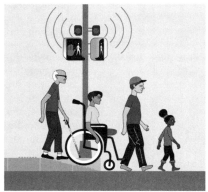

Figure 3-3 Equality Versus Equity

on health equity means would be an intentional focus on eliminating disparities to address the needs at hand and thus not wasting resources in solving issues that are not of concern.

With health equity in mind, DNP-prepared practitioners, leaders, and educators can be forward thinking by including the necessary steps for program evaluation from the onset of the project or intervention. Evaluation of any program requires clear and thoughtful communication from the onset of the program. From the beginning, the key partners should identify what will be evaluated, what criteria will be used to determine effectiveness, what standards of performance must be met to be deemed successful, what evidence will be measured, and what conclusions can be made based on the evidence and measurements obtained (Community Tool Box, n.d.).

The Future of Nursing: Campaign for Action toolkit was developed specifically to address health equity using the nursing process: assessment, diagnosis, planning, implementation, and evaluation (Ackerman-Barger et al., 2022). This toolkit guides individuals through actionable strategies and steps to address health disparities and inequities in practice. In addition, it offers methods to evaluate the work completed through a series of questions including:

- What has changed in the issues of the community you hoped to address?
- What policy suggestions could you make as a result of your effort?
- What health outcome/s or health behaviors have changed as a result of your work?
- Could your strategy be replicated by another community? If so, how? (Ackerman-Barger et al., 2022)

In addition, the DNP-prepared nurse can follow the six steps noted within the Framework for Program Evaluation (see **Figure 3-4**). This framework contains steps in evaluation practice as well as standards for "good" evaluation, guiding the individual to work through the steps while allowing for flexibility as needed within any project or program (Community Tool Box, n.d.). The six steps include: "engage stakeholders, describe the program, focus the evaluation design, gather credible evidence, justify conclusions, and ensure use and share lessons learned" (Community Tool Box, n.d., para. 18).

Lead Partnerships to Improve Population Health Outcomes

The nursing scope and standards of practice identifies *Collaboration* as standard #11 and *Leadership* as standard #12 (ANA, 2021). Competencies within both of these standards address the role of the nurse as partnering with the consumer and key stakeholders as well as leading initiatives within nursing and across practice (ANA, 2021). According to the National Academies of Sciences, Engineering, and Medicine (2021), nurses are

> well positioned to bring [their] expertise to working in partnership with other disciplines and sectors to leverage contemporary opportunities and address deep-seated health and social challenges . . . all nurses, at all levels, and no matter the setting in which they work, have a duty and responsibility to work with other health professionals and sectors to address SDOH and help achieve health equity. (p. xvii)

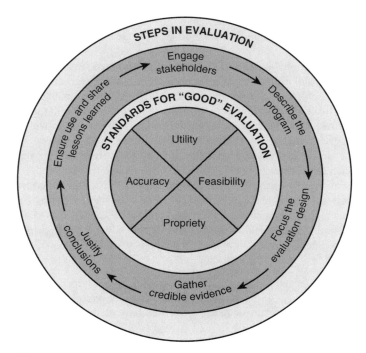

Figure 3-4 Framework for Program Evaluation

Reproduced from Recommended Framework for Program Evaluation in Public Health Practice, by Bobby Milstein, Scott Wetterhall, and the CDC Evaluation Working Group.

DNP students should not only be prepared to voice opinions and expertise in order to improve health outcomes, but should also be ready to lead this work. Nurses carry the unique stories of patients and communities throughout healthcare settings and can bring this knowledge along with evidence from research and practice to lead partnerships for health improvement. While nurses should partner with interdisciplinary colleagues, it is vital to also incorporate the voice of the community being served, whether at the individual level such as a patient or at a systems level such as a specific population or geographic area. As such, DNP educators should incorporate these opportunities for DNP leaders to navigate leading interdisciplinary work as well as ensuring that all key partners are included at the table.

Co-Design, Co-Production, and Co-Creation Methodologies. Traditionally, quality improvement work has focused with independent systems in place: the user encountering a process or environment, the individual observing the process or environment for potential changes, and the designer who develops a new process or environment as a result of the observations made (Sanders & Stappers, 2008). This method of change limits innovation as the input of the user is often reduced to simply demonstrating how they encounter the space or process. By functioning in a more partnership-based model, the co-design method to change would incorporate the voices and perspectives of the user, observer, and designer to facilitate change (Sanders & Stappers, 2008). Co-design methodology promotes partnership approaches where the user, observer, and designer work cohesively to co-design a new solution by strategizing together rather than working in silos. This partnership can yield a new, often innovative approach.

While co-design is the intentional focus of working in collaboration with all parties involved, such as key partners (Sanchez, et al, 2017; Sanders & Stappers, 2008), co-production is characterized as implementing the agreed-upon solution developed in the co-design process (Ansell & Torfing, 2021; Etgar, 2008; Sanchez, et al., 2017; Vargas et al., 2022). The co-creation concept was developed by incorporating these two methodologies into a streamlined process for implementing change designed with users rather than for users (de Koning et al., 2016; Vargas et al., 2022). See **Figure 3-5**.

The DNP-prepared nurse should consider the qualities unique to a partnership-based system as discussed previously (flattened hierarchies, equal valuing of males and females, mutual respect and trust, and values promoting empathy and caring relations) (Eisler & Potter, 2014). These qualities align with those identified in order to support a co-creation model. Within co-design principles, equal partnership, openness, respect, and empathy are identified as necessary for this process to be effective (NSW Government Agency for Clinical Innovation, 2019). Co-production principles include the sharing of power, inclusion of perspectives, respect, and building relationships (Hickey et al., 2018). The overarching principles of co-creation (including both processes and principles of co-design and co-production) include inclusion of all stakeholders and creation of space where stakeholders can continue the creative and collaborative process (Ramaswamy &

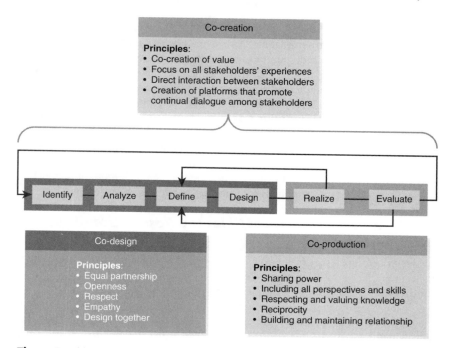

Figure 3-5 Model for Co-Creation of Public Health Initiatives

Ozcan, 2014). In essence, a partnership-based approach for the culture of the team should be present in order for the co-design and co-production processes to be effective within the co-creation model.

The DNP student should be prepared to promote a partnership-based approach in leading change. In doing so, the DNP student can effectively partner with key stakeholders to facilitate change through models such as co-design, co-production, and co-creation to ensure an inclusive method for change identification, implementation, and measurement.

Assess Preparation and Readiness of Partners to Organize During Natural and Manmade Disasters

Ideally, partnerships will be formed and preparedness plans will be widely disseminated to key stakeholders prior to an actual event. However, based on unique factors such as available supplies, change in availability of workers, and so on, the foundation of the partnerships in place "in the moment," during the disaster need to be reassessed quickly. These factors should already have been set in motion and based on an established trustworthy working relationship. DNP-prepared nurses should be equipped to be creative problem solvers in the context of known risks and decisions based on evidence and best practices as they seek consultation with others on the team. Collaboration, teamwork, and communication are vital to this process. See "Advance Preparedness to Protect Population Health During Disasters and Public Health Emergencies."

Consider the Socioeconomic Impact of the Delivery of Health Care

The United States currently ranks last overall when compared to 10 other high-income industrialized countries around the world in their delivery of health care (Schneider et al., 2021). Schneider et al. compared 11 countries across 5 domains in health care, including access to care, care process, administrative efficiency, equity, and healthcare outcomes. Within this report, the United States not only ranked last overall (see **Figure 3-6**), but also ranked last in all domains except for care process, for which it ranked as #2 overall.

In addition, the United States spends significantly more on health care despite poorer outcomes (Schneider et al., 2021). As the DNP-prepared nurse identifies ways to address health for individuals and populations, it is important to consider the successes noted internationally for learnings to address issues locally.

Analyze Cost–Benefits of Selected Population-Based Interventions

A cost–benefit analysis can be done to determine whether the benefit outweighs the cost or vice versa. With a cost–benefit analysis, one subtracts the total costs of the decision or project from the projected benefits (Stobierski, 2019). Benefits for a cost–benefit analysis in health care can include "medical costs averted, productivity gains, and monetized value of health improvements" (CDC, 2021). While cost alone should not guide interventions, it should be a consideration to ensure proper allocation of resources.

While in some cases, the immediate costs of an intervention may outweigh the initial benefits, the DNP-prepared nurse should consider the future implication

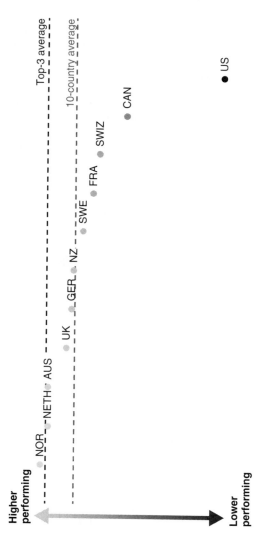

Higher performing

Lower performing

Note: To normalize performance scores across countries, each score is the calculated standard deviation from a 10-country average that excludes the US.

Figure 3-6 Comparative Healthcare System Performance Scores

or potential benefits that may result from the intervention. DNP educators can enhance the curriculum to challenge DNP students to consider financial responsibility from an ethical and logistical standpoint.

Collaborate With Partners to Secure and Leverage Resources Necessary for Effective, Sustainable Interventions

Collaboration refers to the process of working alongside individuals to achieve a common goal while partnership furthers that mission by developing a relationship with key stakeholders and colleagues to achieve a common goal with the potential of creating something new that otherwise may not have been achieved individually (World Health Organization, 2010). This distinction is necessary as the process and the relationships are key to ensuring that a common goal may be achieved. Working within a partnership culture, as discussed previously, allows for creativity and ideas to emerge given that individuals and perspectives are valued and respected and allows for the collaboration process and partnership relationships to exist.

Once the culture of partnership, collaboration process, and partner relationships have been established, the DNP graduate should consider the resources (necessary and available) needed for initiatives, interventions, programs, and so on to be successful in practice. Whether it be at the individual care level as a DNP-prepared practitioner or at the systems level as a DNP-prepared nurse leader, resources should be identified early in any process.

The DNP nurse graduate should be prepared to partner and collaborate with individuals across nursing and other disciplines, locally and around the world, to best address the needs of the population they are serving. Key partners to consider may include, but are not limited to community members and leaders, subject matter experts, those impacted by the issue at hand or the proposed change, those with financial and resource support, and strategy and thought leaders. One individual alone will not have all the tools and resources needed to make an impact across a population, but rather, working in collaboration and in partnership with others with a common goal and strategy in mind, the DNP nurse graduate may begin to identify and pull together resources to address the inequities that exist in health care.

Advocate for Interventions That Maximize Cost-Effective, Accessible, and Equitable Resources for Populations

With any change, one must consider the resources available for sustainment. If necessary resources are not considered, there is a risk that the project may extend beyond the initial budget or that the project will not be sustained if the resources are not accessible. As such, DNP graduates should be prepared to complete a needs assessment for a specific community or population, identify the gap in practice, review the literature for available knowledge regarding recommended interventions, survey available resources, identify key partners, identify the intervention for change, design the implementation and change process, measure the impact of change, and finally, disseminate knowledge learned. Throughout this process, it is also key to continually assess the impact of change and to make the necessary incremental changes for success.

With keen eyes, observations, and an openness to learning the successes and weaknesses of any system, the DNP graduate may be able to identify the positive deviants, or those who achieve positive results in a system when others are struggling and achieving negative results with the same resources (Positive Deviance Collaborative, n.d.). DNP graduates may use intentional observation and curiosity during the needs assessment to identify those who are able to use local and accessible resources to achieve better results than their colleagues. In doing so, they can combine this knowledge with the knowledge obtained from research and available literature to support an intervention that would be most appropriate and best suited for the community for success and sustainment.

Incorporate Ethical Principles in Resource Allocation in Achieving Equitable Health

Obligations are often specified in terms of principles such as beneficence or doing good; nonmaleficence or doing no harm; justice or treating people fairly; reparations, or making amends for harm; fidelity, and respect for persons. Nurses in all roles, must create a culture of excellence and maintain practice environments that support nurses and others in the fulfillment of their ethical obligations.

— **ANA**, 2021, pp. 23–24

As nurses, we have an ethical commitment to do good and perform no harm. As part of this ethical commitment, we need to consider the individual we are caring for as well as the systems we engage in and create. In achieving equitable health, we must consider not only the end goal, but the process in which we engage to achieve the goal. Simply achieving good results or improving health is not enough, but rather, nurses must consider how to ethically engage with the individual and systems to ensure that no harm is done along the way.

In 2015, 17 Sustainable Development Goals were created to guide initiatives to drive "peace and prosperity for people and the planet, now and into the future" (United Nations, n.d.a, para. 1). These goals include focus on ending poverty and hunger, improving health and well-being for all, and creating sustainable cities and communities. Mindful and ethical initiatives should be made to address each of the 17 goals. An unethical or unstructured approach to resource allocation in any one of the goals may lead to less resources to address another area.

Some considerations that should be made when determining resources for allocation to achieve equitable health include:

- Assess and address individual and systemic biases and stereotypes
- Incorporate co-design, co-production, and co-creation to develop, implement, and sustain meaningful interventions (Vargas et al., 2022)
- Identify the positive deviants within the environment (Positive Deviance Collaborative, n.d.)
- Involve key stakeholders in partnership to address equitable health
- Cost-effectiveness: Ensure that the intervention does not spend more than the available resources (Munthe et al., 2021; Norheim, 2016)
- Consider positive versus negative dynamics of resource allocation
  - Positive dynamics of resource allocation: "more resources per health need become available for future allocations" (Munthe et al., 2021, p. 92)
  - Negative dynamics of resource allocation: "a justified resource allocation has the effect that less value can be generated through a future justified resource allocation" (Munthe et al., 2021, p. 92)

Nurses have the ethical responsibility and commitment to address health concerns for the individual, community, and broader. To do so, they must identify the biases and stereotypes which may impact their ability to address health needs and also pursue and lead interventions in an ethical and mindful manner.

Advance Equitable Population Health Policy

History provides a wealth of information that can support the work of DNP leaders to move forward in advocating and advancing health policy. When changes and advances in health policy are implemented, immense change in health outcomes can be achieved. Historically, the passing of seat belt laws in the 1980s decreased the number of fatalities in motor vehicle crashes (CDC, n.d.). In 2019, half of fatalities in motor vehicle crashes occurred when occupants were not wearing a seat belt. More recently, the Affordable Care Act (ACA) of 2010, required expansions in health care coverage. Buchmuller and Levy (2020) found that healthcare coverage in Black and Hispanic populations did increase following the ACA passing into law in 2010. Soni et al. (2020) report improved early-stage cancer diagnosis, improved cardiovascular health, and reduced mortality for certain groups of nonelderly adults related to increased access and healthcare coverage. Developing and advocating for policies that affect health outcomes serves large sections of the population that then impact overall health and well-being of communities and the individual. Some examples of nurses impacting health policy are included in the following three paragraphs.

Lillian Wald (1867–1940), who coined the term "Public Health Nurse," was a nurse and pioneer in serving refugees and immigrants in New York City. *The Henry Settlement* in NYC, which continues to exist today, was established by Wald to provide health and social services to support those in need. Wald also created space within the Henry Street Settlement for the National Negro Conference to meet and worked to secure the right of women to vote. Wald also supported Margaret Sanger in her work to give women the right to birth control. Wald fought for peace, leading several marches in protest of World War I. During the influenza epidemic of 1918, Wald worked with the American Red Cross and represented the United States at International Red Cross meetings. In addition, Wald also took on major industries, lobbying for health inspections of the workplace in order to protect workers. Wald was highly respected. In 1922, the *New York Times* named Wald one of the 12 greatest living American women (Rotheberg, n.d.). Wald exemplifies the knowledge and power that nurses are able to put forward to create change.

At the national level, Mary Wakefield, PhD, RN, FAAN, has been a practicing nurse, educator, and an advocate and leader in health policy. Her focus has been on increased health equity and improved well-being for vulnerable populations. Dr. Wakefield served as the Acting Deputy Secretary of the U.S. Department of Health and Human Services (HHS) under President Barack Obama, from March 2015 through January 2017, and as Administrator of the Health Resources and Services Administration (HRSA) from March 2009 through April 2015 (NDNA, n.d.). Dr. Wakefield is also one of the contributors to National Academies of Sciences, Engineering, and Medicine, *The Future of Nursing 2020–2030: Charting a Path to Achieve Health Equity* (2021). She has also served as a member of the Medicare Payment Advisory Commission, chaired the Institute of Medicine (IOM) Committee on Health Care Quality for Rural America and the Catholic Health Initiatives Board of Trustees, served on the editorial board for the *Journal of Rural Health*, and was a subcommittee chair for President Clinton's Advisory Commission on Consumer Protection and Quality in the Health Care Industry.

In Minnesota, Erin Murphy, RN, has served in state government as representative and currently is a state senator. Ms. Murphy has supported a bill requiring medical assistance coverage for gender-affirming care and authored a bill to support environmental state purchasing that would require specific standards for construction materials based on evolving impacts due to global warming. This impacts building materials for structures and road construction materials.

Identify Opportunities to Influence the Policy Process

Collaborating with organizations supporting nursing initiatives and raising a collective voice provides a platform to influence policy. Locally and nationally, organizations such as the Minnesota Organization of Leaders in Nursing (MOLN) or nationally, American Organization for Nursing Leadership (AONL), provide opportunities for nurses to organize and intentionally support policy initiatives. The AONL is putting forward the Home Health Care Planning Act (AONL, 2023). This Act would allow advanced practice registered nurses (APRN) to be recognized as Medicare providers. With this recognition, APRNs would be able to certify patient eligibility for nursing home care without having a physician also certify eligibility. The result of needing this additional layer of physician certification leads to extended hospital stays and nursing home admissions, resulting in the inability to return or remain home without home care services. This is an unnecessary barrier in the healthcare system (AOLN, 2023).

Design Comprehensive Advocacy Strategies to Support the Policy Process

The following strategies are from the Community Tool Box, Workgroup for Community Health and Development (http://communityhealth.ku.edu, n.d.). This tool box provides guidance for nursing and other collaborators in serving and advocating for populations.

Step 1: Gather Your Allies
- *There is strength in numbers.*

Step 2: Create a Coordinated Structure
- *Consider forming a coalition or defined group.*

Step 3: Do Your Pre-Work
- *Know your issue inside and out.*
- *Know the other side.*

Step 4: Define Your Message
- *Be specific and clear.*

Step 5: Create a Communication Network That Works
- *An individual or small group responsible for coordinating communication.*
- *A fast and reliable way of getting information out.*
- *A feedback loop. Messages to the whole group originate at the central point, so there will be no doubt about their content or accuracy.*
- *Links not only to the advocacy group or coalition.*
- *Regular updates.*
- *A crisis management plan.*

Step 6: Cultivate the Media
- *Maintain relationships both with newspapers and radio and TV stations and with individual editors, columnists, reporters, producers, and broadcasters, so that you can get your message out quickly and at the right time.*

Step 7: Take the Long View
- *This will take time.*

Engage in Strategies to Influence Policy Change

In practice and leadership roles, DNP-prepared nurses have the unique education and experience to influence policy. Below are key points from the University of North Carolina, Wilmington (2021), that support shaping health policy (https://onlinedegree.uncw.edu/articles/nursing/how-nurses-shape-health-policy.aspx).

1. Learn how policy is made.
2. Know who makes policy at your workplace and in your community.
3. Explore which health policies matter most to you.
4. Investigate which legislators support policies of interest to you.
5. Write to your legislator about issues impacting patient care.
6. Inform colleagues about opportunities to influence policy change.
7. Join organizations that lobby on behalf of patients or nurses.

Nurses are essential advocates for health policy. As frontline team members trying to meet multiple patients' unique needs, nurses are key to relating personal experiences of how health policy impacts patient care. Nurse leaders can use their sphere of influence to shape policy within their organization and encourage nursing staff's health policy involvement.

Contribute to Policy Development at the System, Local, Regional, or National Levels

Nursing is grounded in social justice (ANA, 2021). Please see **Figure 3-7**. This statement is further elaborated on in the *Code of Ethics for Nurses with Interpretive Statements*, American Nurses Association (2015). A grounding in social justice demands that DNP-prepared nurses use their knowledge, leadership skills, and influence to participate in policy development. **Table 3-2** provides examples of how nurses create, partner with others, or advocate for policy development that will impact populations.

Assess the Impact of Policy Changes and Evaluate the Ability of Policy to Address Disparities and Inequities Within Segments of the Population

Disparities in health and health care occur across a broad range of dimensions (Ndugga & Artiga, 2021). These dimensions include but are not limited to, socioeconomic status, age, gender, sexual identity, language, disability status, and more. Please see **Figure 3-8**.

Ndugga and Artiga (2021, para. 6) report that prior to the COVID-19 pandemic, people of color "fared worse compared to their White counterparts across a range of health measures, including infant mortality, pregnancy-related deaths, prevalence of chronic conditions, and overall physical and mental health status." The impact of the COVID-19 pandemic highlighted these disparities. Ndugga and

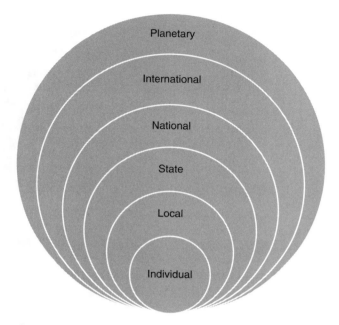

Figure 3-7 Spheres of Policy Development Guided by Nursing Practice: Grounded in Social Justice

Carol Flaten & Stephanie Gingerich

Table 3-2 Nursing Policy Development Aligned With Levels or Impact

Individual	Vote: In all parts of the political process. From local to national levels. Write letters: Credentials and stories matter.
Local	Attend or run for a seat on a city council. What impacts the community? Sidewalk ordinances, play structure safety requirements, drinking water regulations, etc.
State or Tribal	Work with state and tribal leaders to educate leaders and write policies to impact state areas of need.
National	Advocate, work with congressional representatives, write policy briefs, etc.
International	Work across boundaries to learn from other systems of health care.
Planetary	Advocate, educate, and develop partnerships worldwide that focus on the connectedness of planetary and human health.

Carol Flaten & Stephanie Gingerich

Artiga (2021) move on to describe the disparities in COVID vaccination rates among Black and Hispanic people compared to their White counterparts. Consistently Blacks and Hispanics have received fewer vaccinations compared to their shares of cases and COVID deaths in the population. These disparities continue to reinforce

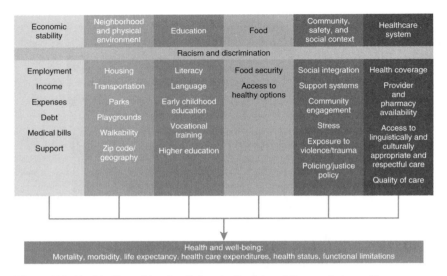

Figure 3-8 Health Disparities Are Driven by Social and Economic Inequities

Reproduced from Ngudda, N. Artiga, S. (2021). Disparities in health and health care: 5 questions and answers. Kaiser Family Foundation. https://www.kff.org/racial-equity-and-health-policy/issue-brief/disparities-in-health-and-health-care-5-key-question-and-answers/

long-standing inequities in health care. From a cost perspective, this results in excess Medicare costs, lost productivity, and economic losses due to premature deaths.

In 2010, the Affordable Care Act (ACA) was enacted, reducing the number of uninsured Americans by more than 20 million, extending critical consumer protections to more than 100 million people, and strengthening and improving the nation's healthcare system (the White House, 2021). In January 2021, the Biden administration noted that millions of people eligible for health coverage under the ACA were not receiving benefits. That data prompted the Biden administration to strengthen Medicaid and the ACA to improve access and affordability to high-quality health care. This example demonstrates that policies do impact health outcomes.

Seat belt laws in cars is a classic example of public health policy impacting health. The laws were enacted in the mid-1980s. In 2011, the Centers for Disease Control and Prevention (CDC, para. 4) reported, "People not wearing a seat belt are 30 times more likely to be ejected from a vehicle during a crash. More than 3 out of 4 people who are ejected during a fatal crash die from their injuries."

Evaluate the Risks to Population Health Associated With Globalization

The United Nations Sustainable Development Goals (UNSDGs) (2015) and The Rockefeller Foundation–Lancet Commission on Planetary Health (Whitmee et al., 2015) identify numerous factors that are affecting the health of populations worldwide. A global economy, global travel, and weather events that cross geographic and human-designed boundaries lead to impacts on human health locally and globally, including planetary health.

DNP-prepared nurses must be knowledgeable about the 17 UNSDGs (see **Figure 3-9**) and the Lancet Commission to fully use their voices to advocate for the needs of those they serve. All populations are affected by global events. The

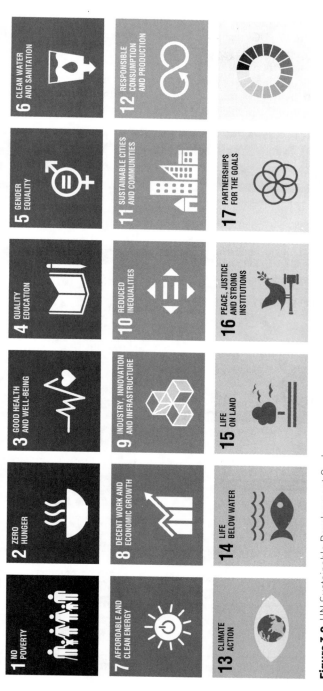

Figure 3-9 UN Sustainable Development Goals

UNSDGs goals identified for 2030 grew out of the June 1992 Earth Summit in Rio de Janeiro, Brazil. Through the past decades this initiative has grown within the United Nations as the Division for Sustainable Development Goals (DSDGs). Currently there are 17 SDGs that provide structure to move toward peace and prosperity for both people and the planet. These goals are meant to be an urgent call to action with global partnerships and take a holistic approach to understanding the factors that impact ending poverty and supporting our natural resources.

Figure 3-10 shows goal #2: No Hunger. This infographic provides an overview of the impact of the problem and some of the root causes. The next step for

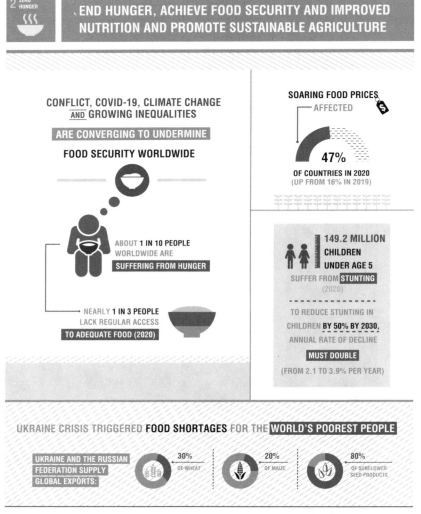

Figure 3-10 UN Sustainable Development Goal #2: End Hunger

practitioners and leaders who are DNP prepared is to delve deeply into the community and populations that they serve to learn the specific details of the needs. In a broadcast, *The Hidden Faces of Hunger in America* (National Public Radio, 2022), the challenges of two college-educated parents trying to supply food for their children and themselves on a limited budget were described. They discussed the need to ration food, learn to live without other supplies, and the detrimental effects on their physical and mental health. This same report states that in the Washington, DC, area, the Children's National Hospital and the Capital Area Food Bank have set up a food pharmacy so that doctors can prescribe healthy food to complement medical and clinical care.

Additional examples of globalization and impacts on health include infectious diseases (ebola, COVID), climate change (melting glaciers, flooding, fires), and food access (distribution, change in soil and weather patterns), as well as demographic changes (migration, urbanization, aging, etc.) and economic factors (labor conditions, wealth distribution, etc.).

Demonstrate Advocacy Strategies

People need to be convinced in order to make a change or transformation; without being convinced to change, they will maintain a status quo. As such, it is important that messaging is intentional to include the varying methods and strategies which will capture the listener's attention so they can hear the message in the unique way they listen.

One such strategy is to incorporate the message in a framework of "Head, Heart, Wallet" (Theprimes.com, n.d., para. 4). This framework incorporates "three basic ways that people listen: analytical people listen with their *Heads*, emotional people listen with their *Hearts*, financially motivated people listen with their *Wallets*" (Theprimes.com, n.d., para. 4). In addressing individuals in professional settings, the DNP graduate will want to incorporate these various aspects into their case for change: the *Head, Heart,* and *Wallet.* In doing so, the DNP graduate can capture the audience's attention and have a better chance of influencing the group for the call to action.

Appraise Advocacy Priorities for a Population and Strategize With an Interdisciplinary Group and Others to Develop Effective Advocacy Approaches

The DNP graduate can promote the voices of a population to identify unique needs by supporting a culture of partnership where hierarchy is flattened and voices are all heard equally (Eisler & Potter, 2014). In addition, the DNP graduate can use the co-design approach to actively engage the users, researchers, and designer to be part of the solution-building process (Sanders & Stappers, 2008). When voices are heard from within the community and those within the community are encouraged to be part of the solution, advocacy priorities will be identified and developed. DNP graduates can work alongside these populations to address the unique needs of the community through advocacy.

Engage in Relationship-Building Activities With Stakeholders at Any Level of Influence, Including System, Local, State, National, and/or Global

Engaging in the different circles in Figure 3-11 is crucial and expected of the DNP-prepared nurse. At the foundation of this figure is the premise that nurses are listening to and learning from their communities. What the nurse learns in one area of this figure may lead to impacting advocacy in another area. Examples of how nurses can engage in advocacy at various levels of impact are listed in **Table 3-3**.

The following points are a combination of strategies from experts in the field of advocacy (Pickover et al., 2020; American Library Association [ALA], n.d.):

- Do your homework. What issues are important?
- Attend regular events to show so that they can put a face with a name on all your communications with them.
- Make it easy for the leader or stakeholder to get to know you.
- What other committees or organizations do the leaders serve on?
- Sign up to receive regular email updates from your legislators and organizations to stay current on their messaging and activities.
- Prepare materials prior to a meeting that show your area of interest.

Demonstrate Leadership Skills to Promote Advocacy Efforts That Include Principles of Social Justice, Diversity, Equity, and Inclusion

The American Nurses Association (ANA) *Nursing Scope and Standards of Practice* (2021) describes the social contract that nursing enters into with society. This contract includes the need to address the Social Determinants of Health (SDOH). This work intersects with efforts to address social justice, diversity, equity, and inclusion. DNP-prepared nurses need to learn the history, understand how structures have supported inequity, and then move to use their knowledge and voice to impact change at the systems level.

Table 3-3 Nurses' Engagement in Advocacy

Local	Establish relationships with individuals/families and communities. Participate in "grass roots" organizations and local meetings.
State or Tribal	Meet with representatives and elders.
National	Join and participate in national nursing organizations.
International	Join and participate in international nursing organizations (i.e., International Council of Nurses).
Planetary	Join organizations that focus on the connectedness of planetary and human health.

Carol Flaten & Stephanie Gingerich

The ANA Nursing Scope and Standards of Practice state:

Social justice is a critical component related to respect, equity, and inclusion. Social justice is a form of justice that engages social criticism and social change. Its focus is on the analysis, critique, and change of social structures, policies, laws, customs, power, and privilege that disadvantage or harm vulnerable social groups through marginalization, exclusion, exploitation, and voicelessness. (ANA, *Nursing Scope and Standards of Practice*, 2021, p. 25)

Standard #12 of the ANA *Nursing Scope and Standards of Practice* (ANA, 2021, p. 98), *Leadership*, specifically calls on the DNP-prepared nurse in practice and leadership roles to

- Engage in decision-making bodies implementing an effective interprofessional environment that improves health care, consumer outcomes, and satisfaction.
- Interpret advanced practice nursing roles of policymakers and healthcare consumers.
- Model expert nursing practices to interprofessional team members and consumers.
- Mentor colleagues in professional growth and participation in succession planning.

These calls to action are the foundation for nurses to carry out their professional roles and obligations.

Advance Preparedness to Protect Population Health During Disasters and Public Health Emergencies

A disaster as defined by the United Nations International Strategy for Disaster Reduction is "a serious disruption of the functioning of a community or a society at any scale due to hazardous events interacting with conditions of exposure, vulnerability and capacity, leading to one or more of the following: human, material, economic and environmental losses and impacts" (UNISDR, 2017, para 1). *The Future of Nursing 2020–2030* brief document states, "nurses are bridge builders and collaborators who engage and connect with people, communities, and organizations to ensure people from all backgrounds have what they need to be healthy and well" (National Academies of Sciences, Engineering, & Medicine, 2021). This definition of "disaster" and the knowledge nurses bring to the work of advancing preparedness is clear and crucial to support positive outcomes.

DNP-prepared nurses with their expertise across many sectors of the healthcare system must be ready to take on the challenges of protecting the health of the public in times of disaster, natural or human created, and public health emergencies. This is a daunting component of the expectations of the DNP-prepared nurse. However, this work is not done in isolation. The work of *preparedness* is about teamwork and collaboration with multiple stakeholders in local communities, and at the national, international, and global level to protect the public and the health of the planet.

The National Response Framework (NRF), from the Office of Homeland Security, Federal Emergency Management (2019), provides the foundation for preparedness and response in the United States. The NRF provides structures and procedures to respond to incidents appropriate for the scale and type of disaster. In each of the subcompetencies below, components of the NRF will be discussed as they apply to the subcompetencies. However, wherever the DNP-prepared nurse is situated in practice or leadership, the detail and nuance of that unique setting will need to be understood and the specific role of the nurse will need to be identified. As advanced practice nurses and leaders participate in the work of advanced preparedness, they will require additional training. Such training is available on government websites through the Federal Emergency Management Agency (2018) at https://training.fema.gov/nims/ and https://training.fema.gov/nrfres.aspx. Training is designed to pertain to specific roles and the collaborative, interdisciplinary teamwork approach required in the emergency preparedness cycle.

Collaboratively Initiate Rapid Response Activities to Protect Population Health

An understanding of the National Incident Command System (NICS) is crucial for DNP-prepared nurses to be aware of and understand the scope of NICS. DNP-prepared nurses must be able to apply the principles of NICS to a variety of events that require multiple sectors to work together in interdisciplinary teams. These principles are used in times of disasters and emergencies, but can also be used in events to support prevention and wellness initiatives. The DNP-prepared nurse has in-depth knowledge in a specialty area of practice and has knowledge of the community in which they serve. This knowledge includes resources, accessibility of resources, economic needs, educational levels, transportation and housing status, informal and formal structures in the community, language, unique needs of specific groups, and so on. These are valuable insights of the community that the DNP nurse brings to the interdisciplinary team in times of urgent need.

Participate in Ethical Decision Making That Includes Diversity, Equity, and Inclusion in Advanced Preparedness to Protect Populations

Through partnerships developed earlier in the process of assessing the community, the DNP-prepared nurse will have knowledge of community factors that embed inclusion in preparedness plans. Ethical decision making in disasters is complex and likely involves unpredictable circumstances. Aung et al. (2017) suggest the importance of understanding ethical concepts such as, utility, justice, and fairness. However, healthcare providers will also need to go beyond standard bioethical principles and consider codes of ethics that guide ethical conduct in decision making at patient, provider, and societal levels (Aung et al., 2017). Attention to detail in the planning phases of preparedness that include ethical dilemmas that could develop, and training of healthcare workers regarding ethical principles that are supported by guidelines and protocols are all components of advanced preparedness that the DNP-prepared nurses are ready to inform at local, state, tribal, and national levels.

Collaborate With Interdisciplinary Teams to Lead Preparedness and Mitigation Efforts to Protect Population Health With Attention to the Most Vulnerable Populations

Collaboration in relation to preparedness and mitigation are met through knowledge of the community and engaging in partnerships with a wide range of stakeholders. Interdisciplinary teams may include fire chiefs, police officers, librarians, local leaders of nonprofit organizations, school officials, city managers, business owners, and so on. Each of these community members has a unique vantage point to know the community and contribute to a well-developed plan for preparedness and mitigation.

Coordinate the Implementation of Evidence-Based Infection Control Measures and Proper Use of Personal Protective Equipment

Nursing knowledge of infection prevention control practices and the use of personal protective equipment situates the DNP-prepared nurse in a crucial role to identify the need for equipment or measures to support infection prevention. Such measures include who needs to receive the equipment and/or who will be trained and how training will be implemented. Nurses have point-of-care knowledge and knowledge of the systems within which implementation of evidence-based practices are applied and therefore can lead coordination of such implementation.

Contribute to Systems-Level Planning, Decision Making, and Evaluation for Disasters and Public Health Emergencies

Through each of the five stages of preparedness planning, the DNP-prepared nurse is expected to contribute to the system-level planning that will support the needs of the population served. A DNP-prepared nurse with advanced knowledge of systems and population health needs grounded in a holistic and inclusive assessment of the population is required for systems-level planning that will support the complexities of preparedness planning and also dismantle structures of inequity.

Summary

Population health work and approaches are complex, interdisciplinary, strive for inclusion, and have the potential to impact thousands. The DNP-prepared nurse is well suited for this work with advanced practice knowledge and/or advanced leadership skills. Grounded in the nursing process and in a discipline that is grounded in social justice, nurses prepared with a DNP degree are able to advance health and wellness for populations and recognize the intersectionality of social determinants of health, planetary health, complex physical and mental health needs of communities; small or global.

References

Ackerman-Barger, K., Cooper, J., Eddie, R., Gualtieri, C., Martin, L., Nichols, B., & Perez, G. A. (2022). *Building coalitions to promote health equity: A toolkit for action*. https://campaignforaction.org /wp-content/uploads/2022/05/Building-Coalitions-To-Promote-Health-Equity-Toolkit-12-16 -22.pdf

American Association of Colleges of Nursing (AACN). (2021). *The essentials: Core competencies for professional nursing education*. Author.

American Library Association (ALA). (n.d.). *Issues and advocacy: Build relationships*. https://www.ala .org/advocacy/build-relationships

American Nurses Association. (2015). *Code of ethics for nurses with interpretive statements*. ANA.

American Nurses Association. (2021). *Nursing: Scope and standards of practice* (4th ed.). ANA.

American Public Health Association, Public Health Nursing Section. (2013). *The definition and practice of public health nursing: A statement of the public health nursing section*. Washington, DC: Author.

American Organization for Nursing Leadership (AONL). (2023). *Home health care planning act*. https://www.aonl.org/advocacy/key-issues/home-health-care-planning

Ansell, C., & Torfing, J. (2021). *Public governance as co-creation: A strategy for revitalizing the public sector and rejuvenating democracy*. Cambridge University Press.

Ashton, K., & Green, E. S. (2008). *The toxic consumer: Living healthy in a hazardous world*. Sterling.

Aung, K., Inayatibt, N, Rahman, A., Nurumal, M. S., & Ahayalimudin, N. A. (2017). Ethical disaster or natural disaster? Importance of ethical issue in disaster management. *IOSR Journal of Nursing and Health Science, 6*(2), 90–93.

Barrett, J. R. (2015). Seeds of toxicity? *Environmental Health Perspectives, 123*(3), A42.

Braveman, P., Arkin, E., Orleans, T., Proctor, D., & Plough, A. (2017, May 1). *What is health equity?* Robert Wood Johnson Foundation. https://www.rwjf.org/en/insights/our-research/2017/05 /what-is-health-equity-.html#:~:text=In%20a%20report%20designed%20to,be%20as%20 healthy%20as%20possible

Buckmueller, T. C., & Levy, H. G. (2020). The ACA's impact on racial and ethnic disparities in health insurance coverage and access to care. *Health Affairs, 39*(3). https://doi.org/10.1377 /hlthaff.2019.01394

Burgess, D. J., Warren, J., Phelan, S., Dovidio, J., & van Ryn, M. (2010). Stereotype threat and health disparities: What medical educators and future physicians need to know. *Journal of General Internal Medicine, 25*(Suppl. 2), 169–177. doi: 10.1007/s11606-009-1221-4

Campaign for Action. (n.d.). *Improving health equity*. https://campaignforaction.org/issue/improving -health-equity/

Campaign for Action. (2023, January 25). *A trauma-informed approach provides framework for achieving health equity*. https://campaignforaction.org/trauma-informed-approach-provides-framework/

Centers for Disease Control and Prevention. (2011). *Policy impact: Seat belts*. https://www.cdc.gov /transportationsafety/seatbeltbrief/index.html#:~:text=People%20not%20wearing%20a%20 seat,crash%20die%20from%20their%20injuri

Centers for Disease Control and Prevention. (2021). *Cost-benefit analysis*. https://www.cdc.gov /policy/polaris/economics/cost-benefit/index.html

Centers for Disease Control and Prevention. (n.d.). *Primary enforcement of seat belt laws*. https:// www.cdc.gov/transportationsafety/calculator/factsheet/seatbelt.html

Cogburn, C. (2019). Culture, race, and health: Implications for racial inequities and population health. *The Milbank Quarterly, 97*(3), 736–761. https://doi.org/10.1111/1468-0009.12411

Community Tool Box. (n.d.). *A framework for program evaluation: A gateway to tools*. https://ctb .ku.edu/en/table-of-contents/evaluate/evaluation/framework-for-evaluation/main

Daumeyer, N., Onyeador, I., Brown, X., & Richeson, J. (2019). Consequences of attributing discrimination to implicit versus explicit bias. *Journal of Experimental Social Psychology, 84*, 103812. https://doi.org/10.1016/j.jesp.2019.04.010

DiCenso, A., Guyatt, G., & Ciliska, D. (2005). *Evidenced-based nursing: A guide to clinical practice*. Elsevier Mosby.

De Koning, J. I., Crul, M. R., & Wever, R. (2016). Models of co-creation. In Service Design Geographies (Ed.). Proceedings of the Service Design Conference: Linköping University Electronic Press. pp. 266–278. www.researchgate.net/publication/303541138_ Models_of_Co-creation

Executive Order on Strengthening Medicaid and the Affordable Care Act. (2011). The White House. https://www.whitehouse.gov/briefing-room/presidential-actions/2021/01/28/executive-order-on-strengthening-medicaid-and-the-affordable-care-act/

Eisler, R. (1987). *The chalice and the blade: Our history, our future.* HarperCollins.

Eisler, R. (2007). *The real wealth of nations: Creating a caring economy.* Berrett-Koehler.

Eisler, R., & Potter, T. (2014). *Transforming interprofessional partnerships: A new framework for nursing and partnership-based health care.* Sigma Theta Tau International.

Etgar, M. (2008). A descriptive model of the consumer co-production process. *Journal of the Academy of Marketing Science, 36*(1), 97–108. https://doi.org/10.1007/s11747-007-0061-1

Federal Emergency Management Agency. (2018). Emergency Management Institute—National Incident Management System (NIMS). https://training.fema.gov/nims/

Federal Emergency Management Agency. (2018). National Response Framework Resource. (NRF). https://training.fema.gov/nrfres.aspx

Fineout-Overholt, E., & Johnston, L. (2005). Teaching EBP: Asking searchable, answerable clinical questions. *Worldviews on Evidence Based Nursing, 2,* 157–160.

Flemming, K. (2008). Asking answerable questions. In N. Cullum, D. Ciliska, R. B. Haynes, & S. Marks (Eds.), *Evidence-based nursing: An introduction* (pp. 18–23). Blackwell.

Freire, Paulo, et al. *Pedagogy of the Oppressed.* Bloomsbury Academic, 2020.

Gervais J., Starfield, B., & Health, I. (2008). Is clinical prevention better than cure? *Lancet, 372,* 1997–1999.

Hickey, G., Brearley, S., Coldham, T., Denegri, S., Green, G., Staniszewska, S., Tembo, D., Torok, K., and Turner, K. (2018). Guidance on co-producing a research project. Southampton: INVOLVE. www.invo.org.uk/wp-content/uploads/2019/04/Copro_Guidance_Feb19.pdf

Hinton, P. R. (1993). *The perception of people.* Psychology Press.

Jochemsen-van der Leeuw, H. G., van Dijk, N., van Etten-Jamaludin, F. S., & Wieringa-de Waard, M. (2013). The attributes of the clinical trainer as a role model: A systematic review. *Academic Medicine, 88*(1), 26–34. doi: 10.1097/ACM.0b013e318276d070

Kaiser Family Foundation. (n.d.). *Health disparities are driven by social and economic inequities.* https://www.kff.org/racial-equity-and-health-policy/issue-brief/disparities-in-health-and-health-care-5-key-question-and-answers/

LeClair, J., & Potter, T. (2022). Planetary health nursing. *American Journal of Nursing, 122*(4), 47–52. doi: 10.1097/01.NAJ.0000827336.29891.9b

Li, P., Karunanidhi, D., Subramani, T., & Srinivasamoorthy, K. (2021). Sources and consequences of groundwater contamination. *Archives of Environmental Contamination and Toxicology, 80*(1), 1–10. doi: 10.1007/s00244-020-00805-z

Liu, J., & Lewis, G. (2014). Environmental toxicity and poor cognitive outcomes in children and adults. *Journal of Environmental Health, 76*(6), 130–138.

Mateo, C. M., & Williams, D. R. (2020). Addressing bias and reducing discrimination: The professional responsibility of health care providers. *Academic Medicine, 95,* S5–S10. doi: 10.1097/ACM.0000000000003683

McMicheal, A. J. (2013). Globalization, climate change, and human health. *New England Journal of Medicine, 368,* 1335–1343. doi: 10.1056/NEJMra1109341

Meyers, S., & Frumpkin, H. (2020). *Planetary health: Protecting nature to protect ourselves.* Island Press.

Minnesota Department of Health. (2019). *Public health interventions: Applications for public health nursing practice* (2nd ed.).

Munthe, C., Fumagalli, D., & Malmqvist, E. (2021). Sustainability principle for the ethics of healthcare resource allocation. *Journal of Medical Ethics, 47*(2), 90–97. doi: 10.1136/medethics-2020-106644

National Academies of Sciences, Engineering, and Medicine. (2021). *The future of nursing 2020–2030: Charting a path to achieve health equity.* The National Academies Press. https://doi.org/10.17226/25982

National Public Radio. (2022). *The hidden faces of hunger in America.* https://www.npr.org/2022/10/02/1125571699/hunger-poverty-us-dc-food-pantry

Ndugga, N., & Artiga, S. (2021, May 11). *Disparities in health and health care: 5 key questions and answers.* https://www.kff.org/racial-equity-and-health-policy/issue-brief/disparities-in-health-and-health-care-5-key-question-and-answers/

Norheim, O. F. (2016). Ethical priority setting for universal health coverage: Challenges in deciding upon fair distribution of health services. *BMC Medicine, 14*(75). doi: 10.1186/s12916-016
-0624-4

North Dakota Nurses Association. (n.d.). *NURSING INSPIRATION ALERT for ALL—Especially
Students and Rural Nurses! NDNA Member Dr. Mary Wakefield Named Living Legend by the
American Academy of Nursing.* https://ndna.nursingnetwork.com/nursing-news/176677-nursing
-inspiration-alert-for-all-especially-students-and-rural-nurses-ndna-member-dr-mary-wakefield
-named-living-legend-by-the-american-academy-of-nursing

NSW Government Agency for Clinical Innovation. (2019). Patient experience and consumer engagement: A guide to build co-design. https://aci.health.nsw.gov.au/__data/assets/pdf_file/0013
/502240/Guide-Build-Codesign-Capability.pdf

Office of Disease Prevention and Health Promotion. (n.d.). Social determinants of health. *Healthy
People 2030.* U.S. Department of Health and Human Services. https://health.gov/healthypeople
/objectives-and-data/social-determinants-health

Office of Homeland Security, Federal Emergency Management (2019). National response framework,
4th edition. https://www.fema.gov/sites/default/files/2020-04/NRF_FINALApproved_20110
28.pdf

Pickover, A. M., Allbaugh, L. J., Sun, S., Casimir, M. T., Graves, C. C., Wood, K. A., Ammirati, R.,
Cattie, J. E., Lamis, D. A., & Kaslow, N. J. (2020). Ecological framework for social justice advocacy by behavioral health professionals in public healthcare. *Psychological Services, 17*(S1),
5–11. https://doi.org/10.1037/ser0000388

Pittman, P. (2019). Rising to the challenge: Re-embracing the Wald Model of Nursing. *The American
Journal of Nursing, 119*(7), 46–52.

Positive Deviance Collaborative. (n.d.). *What is positive deviance?* https://positivedeviance.org/

Puddifoot, K. (2019). Stereotyping patients. *Journal of Social Philosophy, 50*(1), 1–126. https://doi
.org/10.1111/josp.12269

Rajput, V., Mookerjee, A., & Cagande, C. (2017). The contemporary hidden curriculum in medical
education. *MedEdPublish, 6,* 155. https://doi.org/10.15694/mep.2017.000155

Ramaswamy, V., & Ozcan, K. (2014). *The co-creation paradigm.* Stanford University Press.

Robert Wood Johnson Foundation. (2022). Visualizing health equity: One size does not fit all
infographic. https://www.rwjf.org/en/insights/our-research/infographics/visualizing-health-equity
.html?cid=xsh_rwjf_ec_00053819

Rothberg, E. (n.d.). Lillian Wald. National Women's History Museum. https://www.womenshistory
.org/education-resources/biographies/lillian-wald

Roux, A. V. (2016). On the distinction—or lack of distinction—between population health and
public health. *American Journal of Public Health, 106*(4), 619–620. https://doi.org/10.2105
/AJPH.2016.303097

Rural Health Information Hub. (2022). *New Mexico mobile screening program for miners.* https://
www.ruralhealthinfo.org/project-examples/939

Sánchez de la Guía, L., Puyuelo Cazorla, M., & de-Miguel Molina, B. (2017). Terms and meanings
of "participation" in product design: From "user involvement" to "co-design." *The Design Journal, 20*(Sup 1), S4539–S4551. https://doi.org/10.1080/14606925.2017.1352951

Sanders, E. B-N., & Stappers, P. J. (2008). Co-creation and the new landscapes of design.
International Journal of CoCreation in Design and the Arts, 4(1), 5–18. https://doi.org/10.1080
/15710880701875068

Schneider, E. C., Shah, A., Doty, M. M., Tikkanen, R., Fields, K., & Williams, R. D. (2021). *Mirror,
mirror 2021—reflecting poorly: Health care in the U.S. compared to other high-income countries.* The
Commonwealth Fund. https://www.commonwealthfund.org/publications/fund-reports/2021
/aug/mirror-mirror-2021-reflecting-poorly

Soni, A., Wherry, L., & Somin, K. (2020). How have ACA insurance expansions affected health
outcomes? Findings from the literature. *Health Affairs, 39*(3), 371–378. https://doi.org/10.1377
/hlthaff.2019.01436

Staats, C., Capatosto, K., Wright, R., & Contractor, D. (2015). *State of the science: Implicit bias review
2015.* Kirwan Institute, The Ohio State University. https://kirwaninstitute.osu.edu/sites/default
/files/pdf/2015-implicit-bias-review.pdf

Stanhope, M., & Lancaster, J. (2016). *Public health nursing: Population-centered health care in the community* (9th ed.). Mosby Elsevier.

Stobierski, T. (2019). *How to do a cost-benefit analysis and why it's important.* Harvard Business School Online. https://online.hbs.edu/blog/post/cost-benefit-analysis

The Commonwealth Fund. (2023). *Improving population health through communitywide partnerships.* https://www.commonwealthfund.org/publications/newsletter-article/improving-population-health-through-communitywide-partnerships

Theprimes.com. (n.d.). *The Primes: Stake.* https://theprimes.com/stake/

The University of Kansas. (n.d.). *Center for community health and development.* https://communityhealth.ku.edu/

Trasande, L. (2014). Further limiting Bisphenol A in food uses could provide health and economic benefits. *Health Affairs, 33*(2), 316–323.

UNISDR. 2017. *Terminology.* https://www.undrr.org/terminology/disaster (accessed February 26, 2023).

United Nations Sustainable Development Goals. (2015). Sustainable development goals. https://www.undp.org/sustainable-development-goals

United Nations. (n.d.a). *The 17 goals: History.* https://sdgs.un.org/goals

United Nations. (n.d.b). *Goal 2: End hunger.* https://sdgs.un.org/goals/goal2

United Nations. (n.d.c). *Goal 3: Ensure healthy lives and promote well-being for all at all ages.* https://sdgs.un.org/goals/goal3

University of North Carolina, Wilmington. (2021). *How nurses can shape health policy.* https://onlinedegree.uncw.edu/articles/nursing/how-nurses-shape-health-policy.aspx

Vargas, C., Whelan, J., Brimblecombe, J., & Allender, S. (2022). Co-creation, co-design and co-production for public health: A perspective on definitions and distinctions. *Public Health Research and Practice, 32*(2), e3222211. https://www.phrp.com.au/wp-content/uploads/2022/06/PHRP3222211.pdf

Vela, M. B., Erondu, A. I., Smith, N. A., Peek, M. E., Woodruff, J. N., & Chin, M. H. (2022). Eliminating explicit and implicit biases in health care: Evidence and research needs. *Annual Review of Public Health, 43*, 477–501. doi: 10.1146/annurev-publhealth-052620-103528

Ward, M., Schulz, A. J., Israel, B. A., Rice, K., Martenies, S. E., & Markarian, E. (2018). A conceptual framework for evaluating health equity promotion within community-based participatory research partnerships. *Evaluation and Program Planning, 70*, 25–34. https://doi.org/10.1016/j.evalprogplan.2018.04.014

Whitmee, S., Haines, A., Beyer, C., Boltz, F, Capon, A. G., de Souza Dias, B. F, Ezeh, A., Frumkin, H., Gong, Pl. Head, P., Horton, R. Mace, G. M., Marten, R., Myers, S. S., Nishtar, S., Osofsky, S. A., Pattanayak, S. K., Pongsiri, M. J., Romanelli, C., Soucat, A., Vega, J., & Yach, D. (2015). Safeguarding human health in the Anthropocene epoch: report of The Rockefeller Foundation-*Lancet* Commission on planetary health, *The Lancet, 386*, 1973–2028.

Williams, D. R. (1997). Race and health: Basic questions, emerging directions. *Ann. Epidemiology, 7*, 322–333. doi: 10.1016/s1047-2797(97)00051-3

Williams, D. R., Lawrence J. A., & Davis, B. A. (2019). Racism and health: Evidence and needed research. *Annual Review of Public Health, 40*, 105–125. doi: 10.1146/annurev-publhealth-040218-043750

World Health Organization. (2010). *Framework for action on interprofessional education and collaborative practice.* WHO Department of Human Resources for Health. WHO Press. https://www.who.int/publications/i/item/framework-for-action-on-interprofessional-education-collaborative-practice

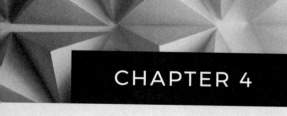

CHAPTER 4

Scholarship for the Nursing Discipline

Catherine Tymkow, DNP, MS, APN, WHNP-BC

True scholarship consists in knowing not what things exist, but what they mean; it is not memory but judgment.

—James Russell Lowell

Any discussion of scholarship and evidence-based practice (EBP) and the Doctor of Nursing practice (DNP) degree must first begin with some essential questions. These include questions as basic as the following: What is scholarship? Are EBP and clinical scholarship the same thing? How does clinical scholarship differ from the traditional definition of scholarship? Why do we need nursing scholars and advanced practice nurses (APNs) in practice settings? What is the role of the DNP-prepared nurse in clinical scholarship? What are the knowledge resources, tools, methods, and competencies necessary to implement and support clinical scholarship and EBP?

These questions are important ones to consider as healthcare organizations and schools of nursing redefine and expand nurses' roles. The merging of nursing leadership skills, evidence-based decision making, and expert clinical care will ensure that nursing has a strong and credible presence in an ever-changing and complex healthcare system. In a presentation by former president Faye Raines to the American Association of Colleges of Nursing (AACN), the leader noted that "the DNP degree more accurately reflects current clinical competencies and includes preparation for the changing healthcare system" (Raines, 2010, p. 5). The DNP's academic preparation—with a strong curricular base in advanced practice principles, experiential learning, intra- and interprofessional collaboration, and application of the best clinical research evidence—as illustrated by growth in numbers over the past decade, is positioned to fulfill nursing's goals for leadership in practice and clinical education. In addition, clinical scholarship, including critical inquiry, analysis, synthesis, creativity, and translational research coupled with implementation science, must be a distinguishing feature of the DNP's role and expertise. The development of these competencies and skills through education and experience will ensure the need for, and the sustainability of, the DNP role in scholarship and practice.

The purpose of this chapter is to define and explore the meaning of clinical scholarship; to distinguish EBP from other forms of scholarly activity; to describe the unique role of the DNP in scholarship; and to provide an overview of the language, methodological tools, strategies, thought processes and competencies that are necessary to ensure that nursing's scholarship is useful, significant, and of the highest quality.

Selected Concepts for Nursing Practice Represented in the Domain

The concepts to be specifically highlighted in this chapter will include evidence-based practice (EBP), policy, ethics, and communication as they relate to advanced level practice in the domain of scholarship as identified in the revised AACN Essentials, *The Essentials: Core Competencies for Professional Nursing Education* (AACN, 2021). The defining feature of EBP is a problem-solving approach that links current research findings with patients' conditions, values, and circumstances. In addition, "it is the generation, synthesis, translation, application, and dissemination of nursing knowledge to improve health and transform healthcare" (AACN, 2021, p. 10). It is through the incorporation of intuition, observation, theory, research, intelligent analysis, and judgment based on the data that nurses provide care that is truly individualized, reflective, and evidence based. With an increased knowledge of the theory and the tools necessary to critique and translate research into practice, the DNP-educated nurse is in a prime position to affect the delivery of care and disseminate the evidence to improve overall care and outcomes in a myriad of clinical areas.

Policy and evidence-based practice based on scholarship are linked because policy frequently delineates the boundaries of practice. Knowledge of policy processes is an important component of interpreting and gaining support for policy for practice change.

Ethical research is a core component of clinical scholarship as the incorporation of the bioethical principles of autonomy, beneficence, nonmaleficence, and justice safeguard patients. Institutional Review Board (IRB) processes ensure a systematic application and review of these principles in research involving human participants and an IRB determination about whether a project is human subjects research is recommended for any DNP project.

Communication facilitates the dissemination of research and other scholarly endeavors in a variety of ways. Clear, effective communication promotes understanding for patients and families, the delivery of quality care, and the advancement of the profession of nursing. The translation and dissemination of clinical knowledge constitute the core of clinical scholarship.

Each section that follows will include a discussion of the components of the selected competencies and subcompetencies, elaborate on the meaning of the competencies and how the DNP manifests these competencies as essential components of scholarship in practice. Where appropriate, specific examples of the Level II competencies and the assessment(s) that are appropriate for advanced nursing practice related to scholarship will be incorporated.

Level II Competencies of the Domain

Advance the Scholarship of Nursing

In order to advance nursing scholarship, its meaning must be contextualized for its application in nursing practice. The AACN's Position Statement on *Defining Scholarship for the Discipline of Nursing* (1999) defined scholarship as "those activities that systematically advance the teaching, research, and practice of nursing through rigorous inquiry that: 1) is significant to the profession, 2) is creative, 3) can be documented, 4) can be replicated or elaborated, and 5) can be peer-reviewed through various methods" (p. 1). According to the National Organization of Nurse Practitioner Faculties (NONPF), scholarly projects can be varied but should meet the needs of a group, community, or population versus an individual. Examples include, but are not limited to, translating research in practice, quality improvement (QI), implementing and evaluating EBP guidelines, and collaborating on legislative change using evidence (NONPF, 2007).

These definitions and examples of scholarly activities remain congruent with the evolving definition of scholarship in academia since Boyer's (1990, 1997) groundbreaking work, *Scholarship Reconsidered: Priorities of the Professoriate*. Ernest L. Boyer was an American educator, chancellor, and president of the Carnegie Foundation for the Advancement of Teaching (Carnegie Foundation for the Advancement of Teaching, 1996). Since the publication of *Scholarship Reconsidered* (1990), a new and expanded role for scholarship has emerged in academia that makes the previously mentioned definitions of scholarship more compatible with the goals and processes of practice disciplines. The traditional definition of scholarship in academia did not account for the nuances and rigors of clinical practice knowledge and its application for problem solving and interactive, human engagement (AACN, 2006). Boyer's model (1990, 1997), however, is well suited to scholarship in nursing practice. In Boyer's view, scholarship is not linear; rather, there is a constant, reciprocal, iterative relationship between each of its four aspects. It embraces the concepts of discovery (building new knowledge through research and careful inquiry to refine existing knowledge); integration (interpreting knowledge through dissemination in various forms); application (using knowledge for problem solving, service, and growth); and teaching (developing and testing instructional materials to advance learning, including the formation and sustaining of an engaging environment for learning between teacher and student) (Boyer, 1990, 1997; Stull & Lanz, 2005). The discussion of the subcompetencies which follows further exemplifies the concept of advancing scholarship in nursing.

Apply and Critically Evaluate Advanced Knowledge in a Defined Area

The dynamic nature of health care requires that DNPs be up to date on current information and that they be able to discern nuances in research findings and to translate those findings in understandable ways that improve care and practice. When data from practice has been generated and analyzed, areas of gaps and/or problems can be discerned. Identifying problems in defined areas of practice is one of the most critical steps in the design of evidence-based interventions.

Table 4-1 Hierarchy for Evaluating Evidence for Practice

Level 1 (strongest)	Systematic reviews/meta-analysis of all randomized controlled trials (RCTs); clinical practice guidelines based on RCT data
Level 2	Evidence from one or more RCTs
Level 3	Evidence from a controlled trial; no randomization
Level 4	Case control or cohort studies
Level 5	Systematic reviews of descriptive/qualitative studies
Level 6	Single descriptive or qualitative study
Level 7 (weakest)	Opinions of authorities/experts

Note: All levels assume a well-designed study.
Data from Grove, S. K., et al., (2013). *The practice of nursing research: Appraisal, synthesis, and generation of evidence* (7th ed., p. 30). St. Louis, MO: Elsevier Saunders

The problem statement provides the direction for the design of an intervention and is usually stated at the beginning of any proposal or evaluation. Essential to good design is adequate background information that includes a rationale for pursuing an intervention, evidence from research that has already been done on the topic, and the goals to be achieved (Fain, 2013). Depending on the problem to be addressed, evidence-based interventions for practice change may be generated from quantitative research, qualitative research, outcome studies, patient concerns and choices, or clinical judgment. The next step is to conduct a literature review of the current and background evidence related to the problem and potential solutions. An analysis, based on the hierarchy of evidence (**Table 4-1**) and a search of all relevant databases (e.g., Cochrane, CINAHL, PubMed), is essential.

Engage in Scholarship to Advance Health

Advancing health through scholarship requires conscious commitment to sustained, purposeful inquiry, engagement in the process, translation of evidence, and dissemination of new knowledge and findings. Scholarship in practice is often related to an incident, uncommon finding, or phenomenon that is observed but not easily explained. More commonly, there has been an identified need for practice change. Once a triggering event or issue has been established, and the clinical practice issue has been clearly defined, there should be a review of best evidence for practice change. Critical questions include the following: What patients will be affected? What treatment or intervention or practice change is involved? What old practice would need to be discontinued? What outcomes are expected? (Collins et al., 2008). A framework, map, or theoretical base made up of concepts provides structure for the review, project design and dissemination of findings. Several models, such as, but not limited to, the Stetler Model (Stetler et al., 2014), the Johns Hopkins Model (Newhouse, et al., 2008), the Advancing Research and Clinical Practice

Through Collaboration (ARCC) model (Melnyk & Fineholt-Overholt, 2002), and the Iowa Model (Titler et al., 2001; Titler, 2002), have been used to implement practice change.

Discern Appropriate Applications of QI, Research, and Evaluation

The translation and application of research and evaluation are an important part of the scholarly process to improve quality of care. Application involves the use of qualitative and quantitative methods to support use of the acquired evidence for practice.

Qualitative Research Evidence. Qualitative research questions and methods provide an avenue for truly knowing patients and practicing both the "art" and "science" of nursing. These are the hallmarks of nursing that nurses at every level must retain, and that DNPs must foster as role models to ensure that "best practice" does not exclude the best of nursing's perspective. The following are guidelines for evaluating qualitative research evidence:

1. *Question, purpose, and context:* Is the research question clear, the primary purpose and the focus of the study stated, and the context described?
2. *Design:* Was the design appropriate; were the units of analysis and sampling strategy described, and the sampling criteria clear?
3. *Data collection:* What types of data were collected? Were data collection processes systematic and adequately described? How were logistical issues addressed?
4. *Data analysis:* Was data analysis systematic and rigorous? What controls were in place? What analytical approach or approaches were used? How were validity and confidence in the findings established?
5. *Results:* Were results surprising, interesting, or suspect? Were conclusions supported by data and explanation (theory)? Were the authors' positions clearly stated?
6. *Ethical issues:* How were ethical issues and confidentiality addressed?
7. *Implications:* What is the worth/relevance to knowledge and practice? (Gifford et al., 2007; Grove et al., 2013; M. Patton, 1990; Russell & Gregory, 2003)

The results of qualitative research to inform practice may be used singly or coupled with quantitative evidence.

Quantitative Research Evidence. The *research problem* is often derived because there is a gap in knowledge that needs to be addressed or described. Research problems or questions often arise from direct observations made in practice. The *purpose* of the study should address the problem. The *literature review* provides for understanding the nature and scope of the problem and determining if or how the research done fits the problem to be addressed. A framework, map, or theoretical base made up of concepts provides structure and helps the project leader discern applicability of the findings to practice. The *research objectives, questions,* or *hypotheses* set the study limits in terms of who was studied, what question(s) were addressed, and what relationships among variables exist in theoretical and operational terms and how they were measured.

Once the applicability of the evidence has been established, the selection of the project design, including the population to be included, the methods of measurement, the plan for data collection, and data analysis are determined. Implementing the plan follows, including piloting the project, collecting and analyzing the data, and evaluating and interpreting the outcomes, including identifying limitations (any issue within the project that serves to limit its generalizability beyond the population or sample where the project is conducted). The last step is to communicate the project findings. A brief description of research process steps and methodological considerations follows. The reader is directed to a research book for a complete description of each of the steps in this process.

When a quantitative study is appraised for use in practice, three questions are generally considered: Is the study valid? Is the study reliable? Is the study applicable in the identified case?

Is the Study Valid? Specifically, were the methods used scientifically sound? Are the independent (manipulated variable) and dependent variables (observed result) clearly identified? Was the study free from bias or confounding variables? In research, bias (sometimes called systematic variation) may occur when participants' characteristics specifically differ from those of the population (Grove et al., 2013). It is less likely to occur, however, if the sampling strategy is well planned and followed. Bias may also occur if the instruments or measurement tools are faulty or if the data or statistics are inaccurate. An example of one type of bias, *selection bias*, may occur if in a study where two types of instruction are compared, students are allowed to choose the group they enter. Random assignment to the groups minimizes the risk of selection bias. Another form of bias is *gender bias*. Gender bias occurs in research when one gender is used more than the other to study research interventions, thus impacting generalizability of results (Polit & Beck, 2013). Since Polit and Beck's study, there remains a problem with gender bias in nursing studies and medical studies and this may impact the way diseases are managed. While nurses are predominantly female and focus on female participants, medical research is predominantly focused on male participants (Merone et al., 2022). A balance in the genders of healthcare providers and study participants, and an intentional focus on gender perspectives is essential to prevent bias in research, scholarship, and quality of care.

Is the Study Free of Confounding Variables? *Confounding* may occur when comparing two groups that may be different in additional ways from the treatment being studied (Leedy & Ormrod, 2010). Randomizing participants to either the intervention or study group helps to eliminate the possibility of confusion because there is an equal chance that extraneous variables will appear equally in both groups, thus minimizing the confounding effect.

In one example of confounding, a researcher was interested in comparing lung cancer and smoking incidence in various regions of the country. In this study, a region was seen to have a significantly higher rate of lung cancer death among smokers (15 times higher) than other regions of the country. The confounding factor was that these smokers had also worked in asbestos coal mines for many years. When the researchers controlled for the variable of working with asbestos by removing the confounder, the rate of cancer due to smoking was nearly the same as that in other regions of the country. **Figure 4-1** shows the relationship among the independent variable (smoking) and confounding variable (working in an asbestos coal mine) in relationship to the dependent variable (lung cancer).

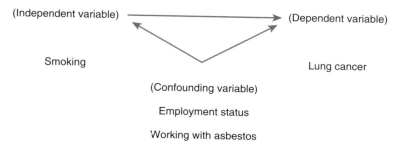

Figure 4-1 Interrelationships Among Smoking, Working in an Asbestos Coal Mine, and Risk for Lung Cancer in a Cohort/Case Control Study

Used with permission of IDRC Canada, www.idrc.ca.

Is the Study Reliable? The *reliability* of a study is based on questions such as the following: Does the instrument or test measure what it is supposed to measure? Does it do this consistently? Do the items on the instrument consistently measure the same characteristic? Is there consistency between raters? (Fain, 2013; Grove et al., 2013). Reliability is measured using a reliability coefficient (*r*) and ranges from 00.0 (lowest) to 1.00 (highest). Therefore, the closer a reliability score is to 1.00, the higher the reliability. In most cases, a coefficient of 0.80 or higher is considered acceptable if the instrument has already been tested and has been used frequently. If an instrument is new, a reliability coefficient of 0.70 may be acceptable depending on the purpose of the study (Griffin-Sobel, 2003). Reliability also focuses on stability (test–retest reliability—whether an instrument yields the same results for the same two people on two different occasions); homogeneity (internal consistency—the extent to which all the items within a single instrument yield similar results); and equivalence (interrater reliability—the extent to which two or more individuals evaluating the same product or performance give identical judgments) (Fain, 2013; Leedy & Ormrod, 2010).

A simple example of reliability is seen in the selection of timing devices used in sports events. Timing devices must work consistently every time so that competitors are ensured an equal chance of winning. An example of interrater reliability is that of a classroom situation in which two evaluators are trained to use the same tool with a Likert scale to measure student performance on oral presentations.

Are the Results of the Study Applicable in the Identified Case? Once the science of a study has been appraised and the reliability of results assessed, the next important questions are: Do the results apply to the case of interest? Are the populations in the study and in the proposed population for application similar? If the populations studied are not similar, the significance of results in the study has little value for real-life implementation in a given clinical situation.

Is the effect size sufficient so that application of the study intervention makes a significant difference? The *effect size* is calculated by determining the mean difference between two groups (intervention and control) and dividing by the standard deviation. It is not the same as the statistical significance but rather is the size of the difference between two groups. The effect size is often used in meta-analysis for combining and comparing estimates from different studies to determine the effectiveness of an intervention. "An effect size is exactly equivalent to the Z-score of a normal standard deviation. For example, an effect size of 0.8 means that the score of the average person in the experimental group is 0.8 standard deviations above the average person in the control group, and hence exceeds the scores of 79% of the control group" (Coe, 2002, p. 2). Thus,

$$\text{Effect size} = \frac{\text{Mean size of experimental group} - \text{Mean of control group}}{\text{Standard deviation}}$$

Generally, in evaluating any quantitative study, additional questions include the following: Why was the study done? How was the sample size decided? How were the data analyzed? Were there any surprises or unexpected events that occurred during the study? How do the results of this study compare with others? (Melnyk & Fineout-Overholt, 2019). The standard of care for practice is increasingly based on scientific evidence. Finding the most current research based on well-conducted clinical trials is an important first step. What happens if the evidence conflicts with patients' values and preferences, or our own experiences? The key is that the evidence must be relevant to the problem and tested through application. In addition, once evidence used for making changes in practice is implemented, the results must be evaluated. Did the evidence support better decision making? Was the patient's care improved? In what ways were care or outcomes improved? If they were not improved, why not? (Melnyk & Fineout-Overholt, 2019). Outcomes may be classified according to population served (e.g., pediatric, adult, geriatric); time (long term, medium term, or short term); or type (care related, patient related, or performance related) (Rich, 2015, 2022).

Using Benchmarks to Evaluate Clinical Outcomes and Trends. One method of evaluating practice is to evaluate practice patterns against national benchmarks to determine variances in clinical outcomes and population trends. Benchmarking is the process of comparing performance with an external standard to motivate improvement (AHRQ, 2013). Organizations that regularly collect data on outcomes in health care are state boards of health and the Centers for Medicare and Medicaid Services (CMS). The Joint Commission and the Magnet Recognition Program (American Nurses Credentialing Center, 2018) also have performance measurement standards that are based on quality indicators. Benchmarking is especially important since the passage of the Patient Protection and Affordable Care Act (2010). One interesting example was a study that compared NP and PA practices and productivity in outpatient oncology clinics at national comprehensive cancer network institutions. NPs were seen to be marginally more productive in seeing follow-up patients, whereas PAs conducted slightly more procedures. Both providers were a useful addition to oncology practices in these centers (Hinkel et al., 2010).

Nursing services are an important aspect of outcome evaluation and reporting at any healthcare institution because nurses make up such a large part of the healthcare workforce. Effectiveness of nursing care is determined by nurse-sensitive indicators. As leaders in clinical care and outcome evaluation, DNPs must be at the forefront of designing outcome evaluation plans for advanced practice. As the number of DNP programs has increased so have the studies that benchmark the trends in curriculum, program outcomes, and DNP impact on practice.

According to Gallagher (2009), the general approach to measurement includes six steps: "1) identifying the opportunities for improvement, 2) involving

Table 4-2 Websites for Healthcare Outcome Information

Organization	Website
Academy Health	www.academyhealth.org
Agency for Healthcare Research and Quality	www.ahrq.gov
Centers for Medicare and Medicaid Services	www.cms.gov
Institute for Healthcare Improvement	www.ihi.org
International Society for Pharmacoeconomics and Outcomes Research	www.ispor.org
The Joint Commission	www.jointcommission.org
National Cancer Institute	www.cancer.gov/
National Committee for Quality Assurance	www.ncqa.org
National Quality Forum	www.qualityforum.org/Home.aspx

Data from Rich, K. A. (2015). Evaluating outcomes of innovations. In N. A. Schmidt & J. M. Brown (Eds.), *Evidence-based practice for nurses: Appraisal and application of research* (3rd ed., pp. 487–504). Burlington, MA: Jones & Bartlett Learning.

representation from medical specialties and other care disciplines, 3) linking measures to an evidence base, 4) supporting clinical judgment and patient preferences, 5) testing measures, and 6) promoting a single set of measures for widespread use and multiple purpose" (p. 185). **Table 4-2** contains a brief listing of websites for healthcare outcomes and data.

Collaborate to Advance Scholarship

Participating in collaborative research is an excellent way for APNs/DNPs to resolve clinical dilemmas and highlight their expertise through well-constructed questions that interest scientists and engage professional peers within and outside nursing. The dynamic nature of scientific evidence and the speed with which it is now possible to generate new knowledge using technology demand that all care providers combine their expertise to interpret, plan, and evaluate the outcomes of interventions based on these new discoveries. Collaboration "implies collective action toward a common goal in a spirit of trust and harmony" (D'Amour et al., 2005, p. 116). Examples of interprofessional education programs to better integrate teaching, research, and professional activities among the healthcare and related disciplines are increasing. Some best practice models are those of the University of Washington School of Medicine (Seattle), Rosalind Franklin University of Medicine (North Chicago, Illinois), and the University of Florida (Gainesville) (Bridges et al., 2011). Others include Thomas Jefferson University, (Philadelphia); University of California (San Francisco), University of Minnesota (Minneapolis), and the IPEC Collaborative, 2022 (Washington, DC). The models incorporate didactic, community-based, and simulation experiences with interprofessional team building and service learning in a variety of ways. Specialization in nursing, medicine, and other healthcare disciplines demands collaboration between peers and patients to resolve complex clinical dilemmas if patients are to be treated holistically.

In addition to the models presented above, nursing has a body of knowledge, separate and unique from that of medicine, that provides the basis for unique, yet collaborative, contributions to science and to the care of individuals. According to Fairman (2008), "nursing scholarship remains contextual and contingently situated" (p. 10). Nurses have shown in practice that they are creative and capable of managing changing circumstances and dynamic cultural milieus, thus ensuring that APNs with both research and clinical skills are in a prime position to function as practice consultants in collaborative knowledge-generating research (AACN, 2006). However, nursing's collaboration across organizational and academic sites and across disciplines is underutilized but shows signs of increasing. In one example, Albert et al. (2020) at the Cleveland Clinic conducted a cross-sectional research study of academic–clinical collaborations through the Office of Nursing Research and Innovation. The researchers "compared characteristics, resources, benefits and outcomes of academic-clinical collaboration of nursing research leaders from academia, clinical and joint-employer sites." The study method included sending validated questionnaires to members of the Midwest Nursing Research Society (MNRS). While it was expected that participants from academic–clinical research collaboratives would publish more research outcomes than those from single institutions, "the results were that the outcomes were similar." The authors concluded that "nurse researchers who really want to conduct research will find a way" but that "more research on academic-research collaboratives is needed to foster, facilitate multidisciplinary, interdisciplinary and multisite collaboration in order to advance nursing science" (pp. 435–444). In order to further collaboration between degree holders, MNRS has reached out to DNP APNs to foster collaboration between DNPs and PhDs. The name of the MNRS research interest groups (RIG) has recently been changed to research interest and implementation groups (RIIGs) (MNRS, 2023). In a recent study about hospitals' collaboration, Lombardo et al. (2022) found that "collaborative research across multiple hospitals, provided efficiencies and expertise not otherwise available in every organization" (p. 1162). In this study, "an infrastructure of leadership, regular meetings, formal presentations, and facilitation of the IRB application process, and coordinated site leader functions" (p. 1162) were the instrumental processes. Other studies on collaboration efforts include those by McConkey et al. (2022) and Allen et al. (2023).

Disseminate Scholarship to Diverse Audiences

A primary reason for disseminating research is to use the findings to improve practice and health outcomes. Communicating the results of research and EBP trials is the culminating step of the research and research utilization processes. It is one of *the* most important steps in research and the application of research in practice because it is the communication of research findings that provides the basis for meaningful critique, development of new questions, and testing of research evidence in practice (Lyder & Fain, 2009).

The methods used to communicate evidence from practice trials are similar to those used for communicating research findings: journal publications, podium or poster presentations, internet webinar sessions, podcasts and other media communications, journal clubs, and community presentations. However, the forums for dissemination may be broader because the audience of interest may be more diverse, including those with practice, research, and community development interests. In addition, the choice of method for communicating information depends on several factors. For example, a journal publication may be personally advantageous to the author, but the time from submission to actual publication and dissemination may delay utilization of important evidence-based treatments in practice. Oral reports at national conferences may facilitate timelier dissemination. Webinars may be the fastest way to disseminate information but may not reach all the desired audiences. Journal clubs are useful forums for discussions of research findings in academic settings. Reports of community-based studies to advisory boards or media venues may also become the basis for further research and political support that help nonprofit and other community organizations. Nevertheless, because theory, research, and practice must be constantly intertwined, the circular and reciprocal relationship among these elements must be apparent regardless of where the research is presented (McEwen & Wills, 2014) or project results/outcomes shared.

Preparing a Journal Publication. Preparing a journal article for publication is time consuming and at times tedious, but the rewards of feeling that you have contributed and seeing your work in print are worth the effort. Once the topic for an article has been established, the next step is selecting the journal. Peer-reviewed journals have the most rigorous review criteria. Therefore, publication in one of these journals is more credible. The actual content will be determined by the editorial guidelines of the journal, which may be found in the "Information for Authors" section of the journal or from the journal website. It is especially important to follow the submission requirements because many journals will not review articles that are not submitted in the correct format.

It is not uncommon for the review process to last several weeks or months; articles may be rejected, accepted with revisions, or accepted. The key to success is to be persistent, correct those things that can be corrected, explain those that cannot, and return the submission in the agreed-on time frame.

Preparing a DNP Scholarly Project Presentation. Regardless of where or how evidence is reported, the essential element is that it combines the knowledge and values of the project population with practitioner expertise and the best in available and current research evidence. Specifically, the presenter must ask the following questions: What is the specific content to be addressed? How will the audience use the information? What is the knowledge level of those who are to receive the information? What is the time allowed for the presentation? What audiovisual resources are available for the presentation? Once these questions have been answered, specific learning objectives should be developed to guide and organize the presentation.

An outline for presentation of scholarly project findings is shown in **Table 4-3**. Important points of each aspect of the scholarly project can be displayed in a PowerPoint presentation or podcast to help keep the presentation within the designated time frame and allow the audience to stay focused on the essential elements. Some useful websites for building PowerPoint presentations are listed in **Table 4-4**.

Table 4-3 Outline for Scholarly Presentation

I. Introduction
II. Purpose of the project
III. Theoretical framework
IV. Design
    A. What kind of project
    B. Intervention
    C. Sample
        1. Population
        2. Inclusion/exclusion criteria
    D. Instruments
V. Analysis
    A. Method
    B. Types of statistical tests used
VI. Findings
VII. Discussion
VIII. Implications
    A. Research
    B. Clinical practice

Table 4-4 Resources and Websites for Developing Multimedia and PowerPoint Presentations

PosterPresentations.com (Scientific Template)	www.posterpresentations.com
Villanova University, Instructional Technology Resources	https://www1.villanova.edu/villanova/unit/instructionaltech/blackboard/bbtraining/multimedia_tools.html; https://www1.villanova.edu/villanova/unit/instructionaltech/audiovideo/ppodcasting/createpodcast.html
Audacity, a free, open-source, easy-to-use, multi-track audio editor and recorder for Windows, Mac OS X, GNU/Linux, and other operating systems.	http://www.audacityteam.org/download/
University of North Carolina, Academic Poster Presentations	http://gradschool.unc.edu/academics/resources/postertips.html
Synergis Education	https://www.synergiseducation.com/podcasting-best-practices-for-preparation-of-engaging-podcasts/

Preparing a Poster Presentation. Disseminating information from scholarship—original research, practice innovations, clinical projects—through poster presentations has become an accepted medium for the exchange of ideas in a more personal and less formal environment than the podium presentation.

It is both efficient and effective. Presenters and participants have the freedom to engage in a dialogue that allows for education, clarification, and networking. Posters also allow for the formatting of data in creative ways. Like any presentation, posters require preparation. The following steps are essential.

Plan Ahead. A good poster presentation requires considerable planning. In this stage, ample thought should be given to the message you are trying to convey. What is the purpose? Is the conference only for nurses, only for APNs, or for a multidisciplinary audience? How much background information or detail do you need to include? Is the audience familiar with the topic? If they are, do not include familiar details, but if they are not, do not make the information so specific that those who are not familiar with the topic will be put off. Avoid using abbreviations that only a select audience will understand (Berg, 2005; Hardicre et al., 2007).

Decide on Layout and Format. A good poster presentation is focused on a single message, uses graphics to tell the story, and is orderly with an obvious sequence (Hess et al., 2013). Most people read top to bottom, left to right. This is the usual sequence for poster layout. The layout for a research poster presentation is as follows: title, abstract, introduction, methods, results, discussion, and acknowledgments. If the presentation is a practice innovation, the layout will be different. The innovation is usually in the center, with explanatory text at the periphery or below the diagram or explanation of the protocol or change (Hardicre et al., 2007). References are also included. The poster should be easy to read from 4 to 6 feet (Halligan, 2005; Hess et al., 2013). Section heads should be at least 40 points and supporting text 32 points (Halligan, 2005, p. 49). Titles should be short, with letters 2 to 3 inches high (Berg, 2005).

Determine the Content. The content of the poster should follow the format established by the conference guidelines. If the study or project is funded by an outside or government agency, some grant-funded projects or studies require specific wording of the acknowledgment. If an abstract is required, it should include the main purpose of the study, be clearly worded, and be succinct. A key component is to keep it simple because posters "show," they do not "tell" (Miracle, 2008). Schmidt and Brown (2022) provide a chart of typical poster content and a depiction of a logical layout for EBP posters (pp. 546–547).

Clinical project content will vary according to the specific topic and scope. The title for either a research study or clinical innovation should be creative, but, most important, it should accurately reflect the content of the project and "highlight the project's take-home message" (Christenbery & Latham, 2013). The title banner should also include authors and affiliations in order of authorship and/or contribution to the effort (Hardicre et al., 2007).

Prepare a Brief Presentation. "The poster is a story board of information" (Jackson & Sheldon, 1998; Hardicre et al., 2007, p. 398). Preparing a short script or handouts allows you to organize your thoughts and prepare for questions from participants. Be sure to include your name and contact number or attach a business card so that participants may contact you with questions. This is an effective networking tool (Miracle, 2008).

Preparing a Podcast. Podcasts are another effective way to supplement educational content and vary the delivery modality. With the increase in online learning, this form of delivery has proliferated. Some questions to ask before preparing a podcast are: Will a podcast help to improve course content delivery, and understanding of the material? Will it help to engage learners with different learning styles? Podcasts, like other presentations, require time and organization. Some essential first steps are: (1) Knowing what and why you are presenting the information; (2) preparing an outline for the presentation; (3) adding value to the information—for example, don't repeat what can be read; (4) do repeat what is important; (5) rehearse; (6) take your time and resist the urge to rush through the content; and (7) listen to what you record (Synergis Education, 2012–2023).

Media Communications. This kind of communication is essential when there is a major event or change, such as a policy to be initiated. It is usually best to engage the resources of a professional organization to make the preliminary contact and to aid in constructing the message.

Journal Club Presentations. Another way to facilitate the communication of evidence-based research is through journal club presentations. Journal clubs can be used to facilitate EBP development and as a forum for clinical guideline development (Kirchoff & Beck, 1995; McQueen et al., 2006).

Additionally, with the aid of the Internet, evidence-based articles or studies can be posted in advance and facilitated online, thus increasing the possibility of wider participation. This technique may be especially helpful in garnering increased participation through social media forums such as Twitter and may be an avenue for further research to assess its effectiveness (Lachance, 2014; Wray, Auerbach, & Arora, 2018). **Box 4-1** presents an outline of a journal club.

Box 4-1 Online Journal Club

Outline of the Journal Club

1. A specific clinical question is chosen.
2. All evidence-based literature related to the question is derived from online databases.
3. A reference list of all literature for review is generated.
4. High-level evidence, randomized controlled trials, and systematic reviews are critiqued and given more weight than quasi-experimental case studies and opinions.
5. Participants critically appraise the relevant literature before attending the journal club.
6. Journal club discussions center on the critical appraisal of evidence found for clinical interventions.
7. Implications for practice and further research are discussed, with key findings recorded in minutes.
8. A resource folder that includes a reference list, guidelines for practice, treatment resources, standardized assessments, disease management strategies, and gaps in evidence is created.
9. A system for ongoing evaluation of outcomes and changes in practice is communicated.

Data from McQueen, J., Miller, C., Nivison, C., & Husband, V. (2006). An investigation into the use of a journal club for evidence-based practice. *International Journal of Therapy and Rehabilitation, 13*(7), 313.

Whether live or Internet-based, journal clubs provide a mechanism for promoting professional debate, increasing confidence, and, most important, improving practice and quality care (Sheratt, 2005; McQueen et al., 2006). With their educational background and advanced skills, DNPs are in an excellent position to implement this kind of strategy in a collaborative, interdisciplinary format.

Advocate Within the Interprofessional Team and Other Stakeholders for the Contributions of Nursing Scholarship

To identify gaps in care that are of concern to APNs/DNPs, nurses must have representatives from their ranks on research and quality improvement decision-making bodies. To have their voices heard and their studies funded and disseminated, DNPs must use the power of their professional organizations and garner positions on national and international research and EBP collaboratives. The AHRQ is positioned to take the lead in outcomes research, whereas the NIH focuses on biomedical aspects of disease management (O'Grady, 2008). Nurses with doctorates have collaborated on studies funded by these organizations. In addition, the Robert Wood Johnson Foundation (RWJF) and AARP are other prominent organizations that have supported nurses educational progress for the purpose of increasing the number of nurses with doctorates to translate research into practice and advance the science of nursing. A number of university nursing programs have joined the RWJF campaign to promote the Institute of Medicine (IOM) recommendation of expanding nursing's opportunities for leading and disseminating collaborative health improvement efforts through collaboration with other health providers including the National Academy of Medicine to establish a *Culture of Health* and health equity for the next decade (RWJF, 2017, 2023). The four components of this initiative are evidence for action, health data for action, policy for action, and systems for action. Nursing's involvement in the scholarship of action and the dissemination of these initiatives will ensure their place as a key stakeholder in scholarship to advance health.

Integrate Best Evidence Into Nursing Practice

As electronic access to sources of data has increased, the amount of evidence now available as a basis for clinical practice has become overwhelming. In addition, the use of translational science has increased and includes several processes, including knowledge translation, quality improvement, adoption of innovation, implementation science (applied research) for quality, and safety improvement (May, 2013; Newhouse et al., 2013). The key to making best practice decisions is using the best quality evidence—evidence that is scientifically based and that has been replicated with success in repeated research and application.

Use Diverse Sources of Evidence to Inform Practice

According to the Agency for Healthcare Research and Quality (West et al., 2002), three benchmark domains must be considered when evaluating evidence: quality, quantity, and consistency. *Quality* refers to the absence of biases due to errors in selection, measurement, and confounding biases (internal validity). *Quantity* refers to the number of relevant, related studies; total sample size across studies; size of the treatment effect; and relative risk or odds ratio strength (causality). *Consistency* refers to the similarity of findings across multiple studies (or statistical power), regardless of differences in study design. These considerations make it essential that all types of evidence be considered when delivering individual care and implementing systems of care. Based on these domains of evidence, a critical appraisal of types of studies can be facilitated and evaluated to determine the best approach for practice (Melnyk & Fineout-Overholt, 2019; West et al., 2002). A distinguishing feature of EBP is that nurses treat and work *with* patients rather than "work on them" (McSherry, 2002). In addition, nursing's approach is more holistic, so that "effectiveness of treatment" is but one indicator; cost-effectiveness and patient acceptability also matter (McSherry, 2002).

While the AHRQ domains identified here remain relevant, other researchers have noted the shift toward more population-based research, risk and disease assessment, prevention, health promotion, and the need for inclusion of all "stakeholders value assumptions" (Fernandez et al., 2015). Of note, the Robert Wood Johnson Foundation has engaged in support for "actionable research" with community leaders in housing, transportation, and other environmental agencies outside of healthcare to inform policy makers and impact population health and health equity (Titler & Shuman, 2017). DNPs are in an excellent position to engage with other stakeholders in population-based and environmental health promotion and disease prevention efforts.

Lead Translation of Evidence Into Practice

Because of their education, APNs, particularly DNPs, are expected to have proficiency in essential information so that the teaching of staff, patients, and communities becomes a key function of the role. Although most practicing nurses are exposed to "research" and "evidence" in practice, the DNP must not only embrace the process but also implement the findings in ways that change or improve practice and outcomes. Translating evidence into practice is facilitated by the use of models and frameworks that show the relationships between concepts and make the path toward implementation for practice flow logically and systematically.

Conceptual Frameworks for Evidence and Practice Change. Several models that were originally designed for research utilization were the historical precursors to EBP. Four well-known models for research utilization and EBP are the Conduct and Utilization of Research in Nursing (CURN) model (Horsely et al., 1978), the Kitson model (Kitson et al., 1998), the Stetler/Marram model (Stetler, 1994; Stetler & Marram, 1976; Stetler et al., 2014), and the Iowa Model of Research Utilization (Titler et al., 1994). As EBP has evolved, some of these models have been adapted and/or revised with emphasis on EBP use in organizational settings. Other models have also been developed. Some later models include the Advancing Research and Clinical Practice Through Close Collaboration (ARCC) model (Melnyk & Fineout-Overholt, 2002), the revised Iowa Model of Evidence-Based Practice to Promote Quality Care (Titler et al., 2001; Titler, 2002), the Johns Hopkins model (Newhouse, et al., 2008), the PARiHS framework (Rycroft-Malone et al., 2002, 2004, 2013), and the AGREE model (2001). Each of these models has been successful in disseminating research and/or facilitating the implementation of change toward EBP. The ARCC model is one model that is useful for implementing

EBP in community and hospital settings. As noted by Schaffer, Sandau, and Diedrick (2013), it is primarily used for implementation of EBP and helps to assess an organization's culture and readiness for change. In their text and companion website, *thePoint* (http://the point.lww.com/Melnyk 4e), Melnyk and Fineout-Overholt (2019) provide examples of EBP in practice and tools to assess feasibility of implementation and evaluate outcomes.

The revised Iowa model (Titler et al., 2001; Titler, 2002) has been used extensively in designing organizational practice change. As shown in **Figure 4-2**, the model shows a number of algorithmic steps and decision points that include determining whether a problem is an organization priority, searching for evidence and deciding adequacy of the evidence, piloting a change if evidence affirms adequacy, deciding on a practice change based on the outcome of the pilot, and ongoing evaluation and dissemination of the results (Schaffer et al., 2013).

Another conceptual framework that helps in the promotion and translation of evidence into practice is the PARiHS (promoting action on research implementation in health services) model (Rycroft-Malone et al., 2013). The PARiHS model, which is based on the work of Kitson et al. (1998, 2008), suggests that the integration of evidence is based on three factors: the nature of the evidence, the context of the desired change, and the mechanism of facilitating change. This evidence, and its translation for practice, includes practice guidelines and other forms of evidence specific to patient outcomes. The use of randomized controlled trials was central to implementation of this model. The model was revised by Rycroft-Malone et al. (2002, 2004) to include research information, clinical experience, and patient choice.

Further work by Doran and Sidani (2007) identified gaps in the PARiHS model that led to an intervention framework that specifically addressed indicators for evaluating nursing services, systems, performance measures, and feedback to design and evaluate practice change. The framework included "clinical (e.g., signs and symptoms), functional (e.g., activities of daily living), satisfaction (e.g., perceived benefit of care) and cost (i.e., both direct and indirect cost to the health care system and the patient)" (Doran & Sidani, 2007, p. 5). **Figure 4-3** depicts Doran and Sidani's (2007) outcomes-focused knowledge translation intervention framework.

The PARiHS model has continued to be used and referenced extensively and was revised again in 2013; it continues to be refined to include more deliberative processes for implementation of the framework in practice including greater emphasis on the role of individuals and the evaluation of outcomes (Rycroft-Malone et al., 2013).

The Johns Hopkins Nursing Evidence-Based Practice Model (JHNEBP), another evidence-based model, was developed as a collaborative effort between Johns Hopkins Hospital and the Johns Hopkins School of Nursing (Johns Hopkins Center for Health Services and Outcomes Research, 2012). The model is explained in six sections. Section I introduces the concept, the evolution of EBP, and the role of critical thinking in EBP. Section II describes the components of the model, which uses the PET process—practice question, evidence, and translation. Section III further explores the PET process in developing EBP projects. Section IV describes the environment necessary for the success of EBP. Section V provides examples of EBP projects. Section VI contains tools used for EBP at Johns Hopkins. The model was revised in 2017 and again in 2022. The 2022 version "highlights EPB as an interprofessional activity to enhance team collaboration and

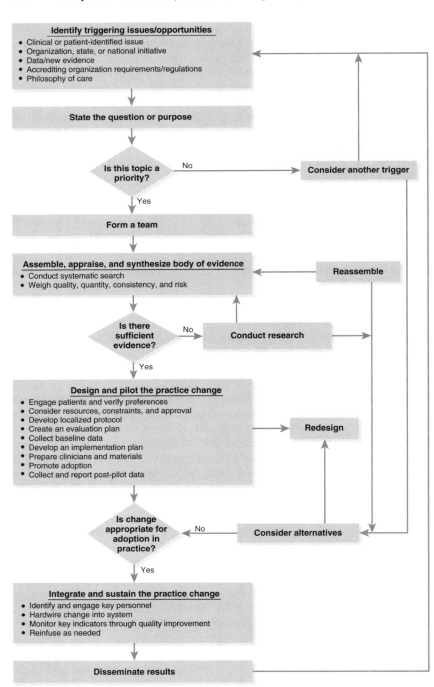

Figure 4-2 The Iowa Model Revised: Evidence-Based Practice to Promote Excellence in Health Care

Reproduced from Iowa Model Collaboration. (2017). Iowa Model of evidence-based practice: Revisions and validation. *Worldviews on Evidence-Based Nursing, 14*(3), 175–182. doi: 10.1111/wvn.12223

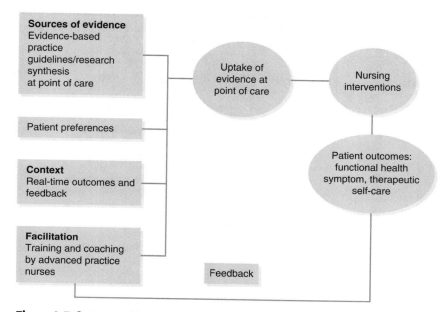

Figure 4-3 Outcomes-Focused Knowledge Translation Intervention Framework

Reproduced from Doran, D. M., & Sidani, S. (2007). Outcomes-focused knowledge translation: A framework for knowledge translation and patient outcomes improvement. *Worldviews on Evidence-Based Nursing,* 4(1), 3–13.

patient care coordination" (Dang et al., 2022). A copyright permission form for use of the tools is available online as a zipped file. An overview and comparison of the uses and features of some of the EBP models discussed here as well as other models can be found in a discussion paper by Schaffer et al. (2013) in the *Journal of Advanced Nursing.*

Once the evidence has been verified, assessing applicability to the population and environment is crucial. Questions to be considered may include the following: Will implementing this practice increase patient safety? Are there ethical or legal considerations? Will other departments or providers be affected? How will the change affect practitioner time? How will patients react to the change? The next step is to develop a plan for the change. Who are the key stakeholders? How will they be apprised and included? Who has final sign-off authority? Is a pilot study indicated before full-scale implementation? Finally, determine the methods of education and communication. How much time, money, and personnel resources will be needed?

When implementing the plan, the following questions should be considered: Who is responsible for coordinating the effort? What contingency plans are in place if a change must be made? Who is managing issues that may arise? Will evaluation of implementation be ongoing? How will feedback be generated? Who will conduct the evaluation? What is the method of analysis? What are the measurement tools? How will results of the evaluation be presented? (Collins et al., 2008). The answers to some of these questions can be found through clinical practice guideline implementation. Carey et al. (2009) in **Table 4-5** summarize their use of theoretical constructs and specific strategies based on evidence to promote use of guidelines and improve the care of cardiac patients. Although the examples reference general

Table 4-5 Strategies to Promote Guideline Implementation: Theoretical Constructs and Examples of Application

Strategy	Relevant Constructs	Key Illustrative Examples
Concrete and specific recommendations	Knowledge, executability, decidability	Concrete and specific recommendations were more likely to be adopted by general practitioners (GPs) than vague, nonspecific recommendations. Observational study (Grol et al., 1998).
Identify priorities Set targets for implementation	Goal setting, action planning	Of 228 primary care patients with cardiovascular disease risk factors who made an action plan to identify behavioral change goals, 53% also reported making behavioral change related to their action plan. Descriptive study (Handley et al., 2006).
Present a rationale	Beliefs, attitudes, perceived relative advantage	Recommendations compatible with current values were more likely to be adopted by GPs than those perceived as controversial or incompatible with values. Observational study (Grol et al., 1998).
highlight clinical norms	Normative beliefs, attitudes, modeling/verbal persuasion	An intervention to improve myocardial infarction care that involved using local medical opinion leaders to influence peers through small-group discussions, informal consultation, and revisions of clinical protocols was compared with performance feedback alone. Hospitals in both groups improved from baseline to follow up on indicators of quality; however, the improvement was greatest for those allocated to the peer intervention. Randomized controlled trial (Soumerai et al., 1998).
Orient to the need of the end user	Complexity	Among the guideline characteristics most commonly endorsed to promote use by GPs was "clarity, simplicity and availability of a short format." Descriptive study of 391 GPs (Watkins et al., 1999).
Skills training	Skills, knowledge, self-efficacy	Continuing medical education (CME) improves knowledge, skills, attitudes, and patient outcomes. CME that is interactive, uses multimedia, uses live media, and involves multiple exposures is more effective than other types. Systematic review (Marinopoulos et al., 2007).

Strategy	Relevant Constructs	Key Illustrative Examples
Social influences	Normative beliefs, attitudes, modeling, verbal persuasion	The use of local opinion leaders in hospital settings can be effective in promoting evidence-based practice. Systematic review of 12 studies (Doumitt et al., 2007).
Environmental influences	Cues to action, environmental triggers	Guideline adherence improved due to the implementation of a computerized clinical decision aid that gave clinicians real-time recommendations for venous thromboembolism prophylaxis. Time series study (Durieux et al., 2000).
Patient mediated	Knowledge, skills, and attitudes of patients	Patient request for a new drug and patient acceptability were cited as contributing to decisions to prescribe a new drug in approximately 20% of cases. Descriptive study (Prosser et al., 2003).
Feedback	Positive/negative reinforcement, goal setting, skill development	Audit and feedback are effective strategies for improving care, particularly when baseline adherence to the recommended practice is low. Systematic review of 118 studies (Jamtvedt et al., 2006).
Incentives	Positive/negative reinforcement	Five of six studies examining physician-level incentives and seven of nine studies examining provider-group-level incentives demonstrated partial or positive effects on quality indicators. Systematic review (Peterson et al., 2006).
Pilot testing with iterative refinement of implementation strategies	Perceived advantages, beliefs, trialability	Breakthrough collaborative model intervention that involved a series of iterative plan-do-study-act cycles was found to be effective in improving care for chronic heart failure. Quasi-experimental, controlled study (Asch et al., 2005).

Reproduced from Carey, M., Buchan, H., & Sanson-Fisher, R. (2009). The cycle of change: Implementing the best-evidence clinical practice. *International Journal for Quality in Health Care, 21*(1), 37–43. Reproduced with permission.

practitioner (GP) practice and earlier research outcomes, the strategies and constructs are applicable to APN/DNP practice. In her study of ($n = 712$) patients with atrial fibrillation, a DNP noted the increased use of CPGs by advanced practice nurses. "Patients were randomized to a systematic approach using guidelines software. [This] nurse led clinic had significantly reduced composite outcomes, death, cardiovascular events, and hospitalizations compared to patients randomized to standard cardiology care" (Deaton, 2012, p. 263).

Implementation science provides the tools—methods, interventions, and variables—that facilitate decision making toward practice change (May, 2013; Newhouse et al., 2013). These tools include "theories, measures of implementation process and outcomes, and research" (frontiersin.org). Table 4-5 is an example of many of these tools and strategies.

Another tool, the AGREE instrument, as defined by the collaborators, "is to provide a framework for assessing the quality of clinical practice guidelines" (AGREE Collaboration, 2001, p. 2). As further described, quality means that potential biases are addressed and that the recommendations are valid and feasible for practice. In addition, as described in AGREE, "this process involves [considering] the benefits, harms, and costs of the recommendations, as well as the practical issues attached to them. Therefore, the assessment includes the judgments about the methods used for developing the guidelines, the content of the final recommendations, and the factors linked to their uptake" (AGREE Collaboration, 2001, p. 2). The AGREE instrument consists of 23 items organized into six domains: scope and purpose (items 1–3), stakeholder involvement (items 4–7), rigor of development (items 8–14), clarity of presentation (items 15–17), applicability (items 18–21), and editorial independence (items 22–23). The complete instrument and user guide are available for download from the internet.

In another application of the AGREE instrument, Zadvinskis and Grudell (2010) used the guideline to appraise the National Kidney Foundation Kidney Disease Outcomes Quality Initiative Clinical Practice, Guideline for Chronic Kidney Disease. Since its original publication in 2003, AGREE was revised as AGREE II. The 4-point Likert-type scale has been replaced with a 7-point scale. The domains and item numbers remain essentially the same in the two versions except that in the AGREE II version, the term *patient* has been replaced by *target population* to account for a broader focus, including nonclinical guideline evaluation (e.g., public health policy). The updated AGREE II scale and the process of guideline evaluation can be conducted online. A user's manual and online tutorial is available from the AGREE Trust website, www.agreetrust.org. Practice exercises allow users to rate a sample guideline and compare their scores with that of the experts (Levin & Ferrara, 2011). Since its revision, the use of AGREE has expanded internationally and continues to afford improvements in the "quality of patient care and system performance through the differentiation and reporting of clinical practice guidelines [CPGs]" (Makarski & Brouwers, 2014, p. 103).

Further research in implementation science was proposed to update implementation strategies for greater consensus and uptake of clinical practice guidelines and strategic change toward EBP at institutional levels (Gagliardi & Alhabib, 2015; Liang et al., 2017; Stetler et al., 2014; Purtle, Peters, & Brownson, 2016; Nilsen et al., 2013). DNPs as practice experts and health leaders in community settings need to play a part in these processes.

Address Opportunities for Innovation and Practice Changes

In patient care, a process that facilitates continuous improvement is central to an environment that produces changes in practice, is patient centered and focused on care, and is both evidence based and of high quality. The process must be based on a commitment by all those involved to change practice, and this commitment must be made in advance so that the research findings are applied early in the process (French, 1999). As changes are made, they must be continuously evaluated for their impact on care and care systems. The EBP process is consistent with total quality improvement, and often the same resources can be used for both processes.

DNPs, in whatever role they assume, must be constantly attuned to and knowledgeable about changes in practice to ensure that current best practice is maintained, considering the context of empirical evidence and patients' preferences and using processes and frameworks that aid translation evaluation help to ensure quality. In their presentation at the 2019 DNP National conference in Washington, D.C., four DNP-educated leaders in distinct roles described how DNPs can impact healthcare policy on the local, regional, and national levels and how the DNP-educated nurse engages in interprofessional teams to improve health outcomes. The presentation, *The expert role of the DNP prepared nursing impacting healthcare system: Bench to bedside, classroom to boardroom*, included several examples of changes in practice (Tenhunen et al., 2019).

Collaborate in the Development of New/Revised Policy Regulation Based on New Evidence

As nurses collaborate in EBP and other research activities, they must be cognizant of the policies that affect health and healthcare delivery. Often innovations in science and technology move ahead of the policy that is needed to either embrace or regulate change. Curriculum that includes health policy as a core part of DNP education can facilitate advanced practice nurses' collaboration with health providers in various disciplines to inform legislators of new research and evidence to support changes in policy that impact health. Course content that includes the "how to's" of legislation and legislative processes and resources is key to successful participation. A review of legislative websites provides nurses with the knowledge and tools to determine what policy or bills currently exist or are in process on the issue. Searching state or federal websites such as Congress.gov or the state government website are good places to begin, followed by analyzing the content from news sources, professional organization websites, and peer- reviewed publications to provide the evidence for engaging with legislators in an informed way. Since coalitions of communities of interest have more sway than single individuals, garnering support for a policy change is easier when there is a collaborative initiative among stakeholders, such as that seen in the passage of recent legislation in Illinois on regulating the manufacture and sale of assault weapons (Protect Illinois Communities Act Public Act 102-1116, (HB 5471), 2023).

Articulate Inconsistencies Between Practice Policies and Best Evidence

Since the impetus to improve patient safety generated by the IOM reports *To Err Is Human* (Kohn et al., 2000), *Crossing the Quality Chasm* (IOM, 2001), *Health Professions Education: A Bridge to Quality* (IOM, 2003), and *The Future of Nursing* (IOM, 2011, 2016), significant gains have been made in the availability of support for

EBP through educational restructuring and systems support. However, inconsistencies between best practice and policy continue to exist. In this regard, collaborative engagement and priority setting needs to be broader and more systematic to reduce the practice-translational-dissemination gap (Brown & Crabtree, 2013; Cooke et al., 2015; RWJF Culture of Health, 2017, 2023). DNPs are in an excellent position to initiate this kind of practice-based dialogue in community-based practice settings.

The AMA, the AACN, ANA, NONPF, and other professional nursing organizations in each specialty all have agendas for advancing research and evidence for practice in their respective areas. These and other nursing specialty organizations provide excellent forums for proposing practice change based on the outcomes and translation of current research into practice. Using and articulating these evidenced-based outcomes in a common voice is essential to make the case for policy change at organizational and legislative levels.

The Joint Commission, the National Database of Nursing Quality Indicators, and individual hospital report cards may be used as sources of research or outcome analysis to identify gaps in care delivery or in patient or staff education institutions or practice groups. Examples include adverse events, smoking cessation, rates of adherence to best practice, blood glucose control, patient satisfaction rates, time spent with patients, tests ordered, and number of consultations (care related); knowledge, functional status, and access to care (patient related); and collaboration, technical quality, exam comprehensiveness, and adherence to guidelines (performance related) (Kleinpell, 2021). Within these and other categories, the gaps may be identified through the development of a specific plan based on target areas of APN practice.

Evaluate Outcomes and Impact of New Practices Based on Evidence

As nursing moves practice decisions from those based on tradition to those based on empirical evidence, the APN, particularly the DNP, is in the best position to affect and assess change within the clinical setting. Why? EBP and quality management are both practice-driven processes (French, 1999). Each is informed by experience and outcomes that can be directly seen and measured. In most cases, the observations that arise during daily practice provide the basis for questions, which can be empirically tested, and their results implemented and evaluated. The findings of previous research studies can be replicated in a variety of settings with resources that are already in place. Listed in **Table 4-6** are some recent examples of clinical studies concerning advanced practice nursing interventions and outcomes designed by DNPs.

Promote Ethical Conduct of Scholarly Activities

The promotion and maintenance of ethical conduct in the range of scholarly activities in advanced practice nursing is of major concern to the profession, schools of nursing and health-related institutions. In the following subsections, the scholars' role(s) in ethical concerns, historical background and ethical initiatives, federal regulations and guidelines, and institutional requirements for

Table 4-6 Selected DNP Scholarly Publications: Evidence-Based Research Interventions and Outcomes

Author/Year	Design, Sample, Setting	Framework/Intervention/Measures	Goal/Aim	Outcomes/Findings
Anderson J. (2022)	Q.I.: 60 staff in a rural Missouri Level II Trauma hospital. Patients in mass casualty	Kurt Lewin's Change Theory; Pre-test, Net Learning Module; post-test; Mock scenario participation usimg AHRQ tool kit.	QI.: Update current hospital policy based on AHRQ mass casualty preparation guidelines; improve employee compliance with current national statutes regarding mass casualty readiness	Education and mock trials resulted in improved staff knowledge; current policy was changed using information from AHRQ, CDC and FEMA.
Falk (2017)	QI: Development and evaluation of an evidence-based Organizational Improvement Readiness Assessment (OIRA) tool.	Delphi-Based System Architecting Framework with modified Delphi method, and Rogers Diffusion of Innovation Model. Collected data at item and scale level of content to confirm validity of the tool employing 13 subject matter improvement experts in 3 review rounds of evaluation at item and scale levels.	Assist healthcare institutions to assess readiness for implementing and sustaining improvement initiatives	Tool effective; made improvement and modifications for usability; established foundation for future studies to test theory and advance outcome improvement.

(continues)

Table 4-6 Selected DNP Scholarly Publications: Evidence-Based Research Interventions and Outcomes *(continued)*

Author/Year	Design, Sample, Setting	Framework/Intervention/Measures	Goal/Aim	Outcomes/Findings
Koman (2018)	Utilized video education program to decrease HCV transmission rates in a public health STD clinic; $n = 26$.	Pre-/post-test design of educational video intervention. Measures included the Brief Hepatitis C Knowledge Scale (Balfour et al., 2009).	Increase in HCV knowledge; knowledge retention; decrease in HCV transmission.	Increase in post-test knowledge scores by 9% at 3-week follow up; brief intervention was effective in increasing HCV knowledge.
Patton, Lim, Ramlow, and White (2015)	QI; institution of a collaborative multidisciplinary approach to increase efficiency of evaluating patients presenting with chronic cough; retrospective sample of 165 medical records divided into two groups: current practice and intervention group.	Institute for Healthcare Improvement Collaborative Model with focus on Lean/Six Sigma and Awareness, Desire, Knowledge, Ability, Reinforcement (ADKAR) change management; interventions included education of referring providers, software changes, collaborative interdepartmental scheduling, inter-clinic communication, and decision support dashboard.	Quality; decrease utilization and unnecessary referrals; decrease length of time to complete evaluation.	Multidisciplinary collaboration; communication associated with decreased costs and utilization of resources. Reduced number of referrals per patient from $M = 3.33$ to 1.22; reduced length of itinerary from $M = 126.93$ to 12.9 days.

ethical role responsibility in scholarship, legal mandates, ethical best practice and application in research, scholarship, and healthcare problem-solving practices are discussed.

Identify and Mitigate Potential Risks and Areas of Ethical Concern in Conducting Scholarly Activities

Scholarly activities that include or impact human beings have potential risks, whether original research, or evidence-based synthesis and translation interventions for implementation in practice. These risks require consideration and must be factored into decisions about the process and progress of any study or practice intervention. A risk–benefit analysis which predicts outcomes of a study or practice change is an essential first step in designing a study, practice change, or intervention. The benefits may be direct or indirect, and the risks to patients may be known or unknown. However, in all cases they must be proactively assessed.

As "there is time for everything and a season for everything under heaven," there is a time and place for policy development, modification, and implementation. Sometimes it is a triggering event, at others the dawning of a new discovery, an off-the-cuff conversation that spawns new thinking, or an idea generated by a policy think-tank. This is often the case when research and new evidence sparks the need for new policy. This is most evident in terms of research in the events in history (Tuskegee, Nuremberg) that led to many of the changes that now frame our current Institutional Review Board processes.

Apply IRB Guidelines Throughout the Scholarship Process

An institutional review board (IRB) is a committee that is charged with reviewing and ensuring that any research activity is safe and ethically conducted (Grove, et al., 2013). There are three levels of review: exempt (no apparent risks); expedited (only minimal risks may be present); full review (there is greater than minimal risk). The key features of review that the IRB conducts are that (1) subjects' rights and welfare are protected during the study; (2) there is appropriate informed consent; and (3) that potential benefits outweigh the risks. Institutions have specific rules, guidelines, and procedures that all investigators, including students, must follow to have a study or quality improvement project approved. While not every project or study needs a full review, projects must be submitted to the assigned review board for a determination of review status.

Ensure Protection of Participants in the Conduct of Scholarship

The guidelines designed to protect participants in scholarly endeavors are based on historical events that necessitated subsequent codes for ensuring ethical research conduct and protection of research participants. They include, but are not limited to the Nuremberg Code, the Declaration of Helsinki, the Belmont Report, and federal regulations promulgated by the U.S. Department of Health and Human Services (U.S. DHHS). The most current regulations were approved in 2009 as part of the U.S. code of Federal Regulations (CFR), Title 45, Part 46, Protection of Human Subjects. The regulations can be accessed online as cited in the reference list (Grove et al., 2013). Another department within DHHS, the Office of Human Resource Protection (OHRP) is charged with clarifying the regulations, developing educational programs, overseeing research regulations and maintenance, and providing ethical advice related to biomedical and social-behavioral research (Grove et al., 2013).

Implement Processes to Support Ethical Conduct in Practice as Well as Scholarship

Ethical conduct in scholarship and practice means that scholars are required to protect human rights. The processes that support ethical practice and scholarship endeavors are based on Nursing's Code of Ethics (American Nurses Association [ANA], 2015). The guidelines for ethical conduct include protection of patient and research participant rights for self-determination, privacy, anonymity and confidentiality, fair treatment, and protection from harm (Grove et al., 2013). In terms of implementation of these codes, colleges and universities, and institutions that conduct research (e.g., teaching hospitals, magnet hospitals) require that researchers and those involved with any interventions/projects complete a course or online certificate of completion that details these guidelines before conducting any study or project. Such courses are available from the Collaborative, Institutional Training Initiative Program (CITI) and the U.S. DHHS (n.d.). Concepts included in required education include discussions of assuring that studies have social or scientific validity, that subject selection is fair, that benefits of the study or intervention outweigh risks, that there is independent review by peers (IRB review), that there is informed consent of participants which includes participant's right to withdraw at any point during a trial, and that respect for potential and enrolled participants is maintained during and after the completion of the research or project (Emanuel, Wendle, & Grady, 2000). In addition, the Code of Federal Regulations (FR) Title 45, Part 46 (2009) provides additional special protective rules for pregnant women, fetuses, neonates, children, and prisoners involved in research. A sample informed consent template is included in **Table 4-7**. Depending on the type of project, not all sections may be needed, but need would be determined by the agency and/or school IRB.

Apply Ethical Principles to the Dissemination of Nursing Scholarship

Just as the conduct of research must follow guidelines previously identified, all scholarly endeavors must be disseminated with integrity. That means that in all forms of dissemination, written or oral, the data and recommendations presented must be truly based solely on the findings, even those contradicting one's own views/beliefs. They must include appropriate attribution of the ideas of others and show permission for the use of data, tables, and artifacts obtained from other researchers or scholars. The discussion of the design and methodology of the study or project must be the same as that approved by the IRB. The results must be reported free of bias or interpretation not consistent with the actual results (Martinson, Anderson, & DeVries, 2005).

Table 4-7 Sample Informed Consent Template

NOTE: Depending on the nature of your research or project, additional language (for example, a statement about mandatory reporting or FERPA statement) may be required. Consult the IRB for additional required language. Some Quality Improvement initiatives may not require this level of detail. Consult your IRB for required language.

[Insert College here]
[Insert Division/Department here]

Title of Research/Project Study: [insert title of research study here]

Principal Investigator: [insert name of principal investigator/faculty sponsor]

Key Information:

The following is a short summary of this study or project to help you decide whether to participate or not. More detailed information is listed later in this consent form. [For the section below, include items in a bulleted format.]

- I am inviting you to participate in a research study or project about [insert brief purpose of the study/project].
- Participation in this study is <u>voluntary</u> and you can choose not to participate or withdraw at any time without penalty.
- I am asking you to [insert brief statement of the procedures including everything that participants will be asked to do].
- I expect that your participation in this study or project will take [insert expected duration of the study, and if applicable, the number of times the participant will be asked to participate].
- The risks of participating are [briefly summarize nature of risks or say that risks are no greater than those experienced in daily life].

The benefits of the study/project include [describe benefits. NOTE: Most social behavioral studies do not benefit participants directly. You may say: Participation in the study will not benefit you directly, but it may help the researchers better understand [purpose of the study].

- As a token of appreciation, we are offering participants [include information about compensation. For a lottery or raffle, state the odds of winning a prize and how it will be delivered to participants].

Why am I being asked to participate in this research study or project?
I am asking you to participate in this research study or project because [fill in the reason/eligibility for recruiting these participants].

What should I know about participating in a research or project study?
- Whether or not you participate is up to you. You can choose not to participate.
- You can agree to participate and then later change your mind.
- Your decision will not be held against you or result in penalty.
- You can ask all the questions that you want before you decide.

(continues)

Table 4-7 Sample Informed Consent Template *(continued)*

What happens if I agree to participate in the research study or project?
[Tell the participant what to expect using lay language and simple terms.
Whenever appropriate include the following items]:

- A description of the research/project activities and procedures, including when and where the research/project will be done
- How often study/project activities and procedures will be performed
- What is being performed as part of the research/project study and what is being performed as part of standard or customary practice (i.e., if the study/project takes place in the classroom, describe what is the customary educational activity and what is part of the research or project). If the study/project involves any type of clinical care (e.g., mental health care), describe what is standard care/procedure and what is part of the research/project.
- Describe if you are audio or video recording any research/project activities. Include if agreement to be recorded is required for participation or if it is optional.

Will being in this study or project help me in any way?
[Include if there are direct benefits to participation. For example, subjects may benefit from a study/project that includes a therapeutic or behavioral intervention. Otherwise, delete.]

Is there any way being in this study or project could be bad for me?
[Include if there are risks. Otherwise, delete.]

[Describe each of the following risks, if appropriate. If known, describe the probability and magnitude of the risk, and how it will be minimized.]

- Physical risks
- Psychological/emotional risks
- Privacy risks
- Legal risks
- Social risks
- Economic risks
- Group or community harms

What happens if I do not want to be in this research or project?
Participation in research/project is voluntary. You can decide to participate or not to participate.

[Include if there are alternatives other than participating. Otherwise, delete.]
Instead of being in this research study/project, your choices may include: [List alternatives procedures/options. For example, for student participant pools, describe alternatives for course credit.]

What happens if I say "Yes," but I change my mind later?
You can leave the research/project at any time, and it will not be held against you.

[Describe what will happen to data collected to the point of withdrawal. You may say: If you decide to leave the study/project, your information will not be used.]

What happens to the information collected for the research?
[Describe how data will be protected. Specifically, address the confidentiality of data: will the data be anonymous or confidential (coded), what information will be kept, where, for how long, and who will have access to it]

Data Sharing
[If you plan to share the de-identified data from the study/project with other investigators]: De-identified data from the study could be used for future research studies or shared with other investigators without your additional informed consent.

[If you do not plan to share the data]: Data from this study/project will not be used for future research studies/projects or shared with other investigators, even if all your identifiers are removed.

What else do I need to know?
[Include for research where this is a possibility. Otherwise, delete.] We will tell you about any new information that may affect your health, welfare, or choice to stay in the research/project.

Who can I talk to?
If you have questions, concerns, or complaints, talk to the Principal Investigator [Name and contact phone or email] and [You can list another investigator such as a student if appropriate].

This research/project has been reviewed and approved by an Institutional Review Board ("IRB"). You may contact the IRB at irb@____.edu if you have questions or concerns regarding your rights as a research/project participant. You may also contact_____(role, phone).

Signature for Adult 18 or older

Signing here means that you are agreeing (consenting) to participate in this research and that you are giving the researchers permission to use the information that they collect from your participation.

_____   _____
Signature of participant   Date

Printed name of participant

_____   _____
Signature of person obtaining consent   Date

_____
Printed name of person obtaining consent

Provided by Informaticist: Jane Matejcek, DNP, RN

Summary

Scholarship and EBP are not the same, but each has elements that support the other. Scholarship involves research and application, as does EBP. Whereas scholarship may be a joint or singular effort, EBP requires teamwork and collaboration. The outcome of scholarship is a scholarly product, a new way of thinking, or a change in awareness about a subject or phenomenon—an end in itself. EBP is based on the scholarship of research and evidence gathering and synthesis. It is a means for improving care for patients or effecting a change in a system that results in better care for patients, providers, and communities. It is a transformation of knowledge to new levels of understanding and integration. Changing to a model of EBP does not just happen; it requires the integration of skills, such as the use of good research and the synthesis of best information and other "evidences," including patient choice and professional expertise. Dissemination of information gleaned from synthesis and translation in practice is essential for successful change. Using the knowledge of research methods to discover and interpret the best evidence for practice gives the DNP the tools to transform care.

References

Agency for Healthcare Research and Quality (AHRQ). (2013). *Module 7. Measuring and benchmarking clinical performance.* http://www.ahrq.gov/professionals/prevention-chronic-care/improve /system/pfhandbook/mod7.html

AGREE Collaboration. (2001). *AGREE instrument.* http://www.agreetrust.org/?o=1085

Albert, N. M., Chipps, E., Klein, C. J., Briskin, I., Olson, A. C. F., Hand, L. L., Harmon, M. M., Heitschmidt, M., & Talsma, A. (2020). A cross-sectional study of United States academic-clinical research collaborations: Characteristics, resources, benefits, and outcomes. *Journal of Clinical Nursing, 31*(3–4), 435–444. https://doi.org/10.1111/jocn.15597

Allen, D. H., Arthur, E. K., Blazey, M., Brassil, K, Cahill, J. E., Cooley, M. E., Fadol, A. P., Hammer, M. J., Hartranft, S., Murphy, B., Nolan, T., Sun, V, Whisenant, M. & Yoder, L. (2023). A scoping review on the nurse scientist role with health systems. *Worldviews on Evidence-Based Nursing, 20*(1) 47–55.

American Association of Colleges of Nursing (AACN). (1999). *Defining scholarship for the discipline of nursing.* https://www.aacnnursing.org/News-Information/Position-Statements-White-Papers /Defining-Scholarship-Nursing

American Association of Colleges of Nursing (AACN). (2006). *The essentials of doctoral education for advanced nursing practice.* https://www.aacnnursing.org/DNP/DNP-Essentials http://www.aacn .nche.edu/news/articles/2015/enrollment

American Association of Colleges of Nursing (AACN). (2021). *The essentials: Core competencies for professional nursing education.* Author

American Nurses Credentialing Center. (2018). *Magnet Recognition Program overview.* http://nursing world.org/organization-program/magnet

American Nurses Association. (2015). *Code of Ethics with Interpretive Statements.*

Anderson, J. (2022). *Improving mass casualty in the emergency department: A quality improvement project.* Doctor of Nursing Practice Repository. https://www.doctorsofnursingpractice.org/wp-content /uploads/project_form/complete_271022124653.pdf

Asch, S. M., Baker, D. W., Keesey, J., Broder, M., Schonlau, M., Rosen, M., & Keeler, E. B. (2005). Does the collaborative model improve care for chronic heart failure? *Medical Care, 43*(7), 667–675.

Audacity. http://www.audacityteam.org/download/

Balfour, L., Kowal, J., Corace, K. M., Tasca, G. A., Krysanski, V., Cooper, C. L., & Garber, G. (2009). Increasing public awareness about hepatitis C: Development and validation of the brief hepatitis C knowledge scale. *Scandinavian Journal of Caring Sciences, 23*(4), 801–808.

Berg, J. A. (2005). Creating a professional poster presentation: Focus on nurse practitioners. *Journal of the American Academy of Nurse Practitioners, 17*(7), 245–248.

Boyer, E. L. (1990). *Scholarship reconsidered: Priorities of the professoriate.* The Carnegie Foundation for the Advancement of Teaching. Jossey-Bass.

Boyer, E. L. (1997). *Scholarship reconsidered: Priorities of the professoriate* (Rev. ed.). The Carnegie Foundation for the Advancement of Teaching. Jossey-Bass.

Bridges, D. R., Davidson, R. A., Odegard, P. S., Maki, I. V., & Tomkowiak, J. (2011). Interprofessional collaboration: Three best practice models of interprofessional education. *Medical Education Online, 16.* https://doi.org/10.3402/meo.v16i0.6035

Brown, M. A., & Crabtree, K. (2013). The development of practice scholarship in DNP programs: A paradigm shift. *Journal of Professional Nursing, 29,* 330–337.

Carey, M., Buchan, H., & Sanson-Fisher, R. (2009). The cycle of change: Implementing the best-evidence clinical practice. *International Journal for Quality in Health Care, 21*(1), 37–43.

Carnegie Foundation for the Advancement of Teaching. (1996). *Ernest L. Boyer.* 91st annual report of the Carnegie Foundation for the Advancement of Teaching. Princeton, NJ: Author.

Christenbery, T. L., & Latham, T. G. (2013). Creating effective scholarly posters: A guide for DNP students. *Journal of the American Association of Nurse Practitioners, 25,* 16–23.

Coe, R. (2002, September). *It's the effect size, stupid: What effect size is and why it is so important.* Paper presented at the annual conference of the British Educational Research Association, University of Exeter, England.

Collaborative Institutional Training Initiative (CITI). Human Subjects Research (HSR) https://about.citiprogram.org/course/biomedical-biomed-basic/

Collins, P. M., Golembeski, S. M., Selgas, M., Sparger, K., Burke, N., & Vaughn, B. B. (2008, January 25). Clinical excellence through evidence-based practice: A model to guide practice changes. *Topics in Advanced Practice E-Journal.* https://pdfs.semanticscholar.org/29e9/eae052beb4d3cb6301edb238fa000e5444a6.pdf

Cooke, J., Ariss, S., Smith, C., & Read, J. (2015). Ongoing collaboration priority-setting for research activity: A method of capacity building to reduce the research-practice translational gap. *BMC Health Research Policy and Systems, 13*(25). https://doi.org/10.1186/s12961-015-0014-y

D'Amour, D., Ferrada-Videla, M., San Martin-Rodriguez, L., & Beaulieu, M. D. (2005). The conceptual basis for interprofessional collaboration: Core concepts and theoretical frameworks. *Journal of Interprofessional Care, 19*(Suppl. 1), 116–131.

Dang, D., Dearholt, S., Bissett, K., Ascenzi, J., & Whalen, M. (2022). *Johns Hopkins Nursing evidence-based practice for nurses and health professionals: Model and guidelines* (4th ed.). Sigma Theta Tau International.

Deaton, C. (2012). Implementing clinical practice guidelines: A responsibility for nurses and allied health professionals? *European Journal of Cardiovascular Nursing, 11*(3), 263–264. https://doi.org/10.1177/1474515112438294

Doran, D. M., & Sidani, S. (2007). Outcomes-focused knowledge translation: A framework for knowledge translation and patient outcomes improvement. *Worldviews on Evidence-Based Nursing, 4*(1), 3–13.

Doumitt, G., Gattelliari, M., Grimshaw, J., & O'Brien, M. A. (2007). Local opinion leaders: Effects on professional practice and healthcare outcomes. *Cochrane Database Systematic Review, 4,* Art. No. CD000125. https://doi.org/10.1002/14651858.CD000125.pub3

Durieux, P., Nizard, R., Ravaud, P., Mounier, N., & Lepage, E. (2000). A clinical decision support system for prevention of venous thromboembolism: Effect on physician behavior. *Journal of the American Medical Association, 283*(21), 2816–2821.

Emanuel, E.J., Wendler, D., & Grady, C., (2000), What makes clinical research ethical? *Journal of American Medical Association* (JAMA), 283(20) 2701–2711, doi.10.1001/jama 283.20.2701

Fain, J. A. (2013). *Reading, understanding, and applying nursing research* (4th ed.). F. A. Davis.

Fairman, J. (2008). Context and contingency in the history of post-World War II scholarship in the United States. *Journal of Nursing Scholarship, 40*(1), 4–11.

Falk, L. H. (2017). *Organizational Improvement Readiness Assessment (OIRA) Tool Evaluation.* A Scholarly Project Presented to the Faculty of the School of Nursing Boise State University In partial fulfillment of the requirements for the Degree of Doctor of Nursing Practice.

Fernandez, A. Sturmberg, J., Lukersmith, S., Madden, R., Torkfar, G., Colaguiri, R., Salvador-Carulla, L. (2015). Evidence-based medicine: Is it a bridge too far? *Health Research and Policy Systems, 13*(66). https://doi.org/10.1186/s12961-015-0057-0

French, P. (1999). The development of evidence-based nursing. *Journal of Advanced Nursing, 29*(1), 72–78.

Frontiersin.org. *Going beyond the traditional tools of implementation science.*

Gagliardi, A. R., Alhabib, S., & members of the Guidelines International Network Implementation Working Group. (2015). Trends in guideline implementation: A scoping systematic review. *Implementation Science, 10*(54), 1–11. https://doi.org/10.1186/s13012-015-0247-8

Gallagher, R. M. (2009). Participation of the advanced practice nurse in managed care and quality initiatives. In L. A. Joel (Ed.), *Advanced practice nursing: Essentials of role development* (2nd ed., pp. 172–190). F. A. Davis.

Gifford, W., Davies, B., Edwards, N., Griffin, P., & Lybanon, V. (2007). Managerial leadership for nurses' use of research evidence: An integrative review of the literature. *Worldviews on Evidence-Based Practice, 4*(3), 126–145.

Governors State University. (2022). Informed Consent Template.

Griffin-Sobel, J. P. (2003). Evaluating an instrument for research. *Gastroenterology Nursing, 26*(3), 135–136.

Grol, R., Dalhuijsen, J., Thomas, S., Veld, C., Rutten, G., & Mokkink, H. (1998). Attributes of clinical guidelines that influence use of guidelines in general practice: Observational study. *British Medical Journal, 317*(7162), 858–861.

Grove, S. K., Burns, N., & Gray, J. R. (2013). *The practice of nursing research: Appraisal, synthesis, and generation of evidence* (7th ed.). Elsevier Saunders.

Halligan, P. (2005). Poster perfect. *World of Irish Nursing and Midwifery, 13*(8), 49.

Handley, M., MacGregor, K., Schillinger, D., Sharifi, C., Wong, S., & Bodenheimer, T. (2006). Using action plans to help primary care patients adopt healthy behaviors: A descriptive study. *Journal of the American Board of Family Medicine, 19*(3), 224–231.

Hardicre, J., Devitt, P., & Coad, J. (2007). Ten steps to successful poster presentation. *British Journal of Nursing, 16*(7), 398–401.

Hess, G., Tosney, K., & Liegel, L. (2013). *Creating effective poster presentations.* https://www.tandfonline.com/doi/abs/10.1080/01421590902825131?casa_token=szqxM_J7AooAAAAA%3AQbFXqfoy95Lb8x38ztfAxforDAZEVX0JMaG0RIi0MnL5b9muLYAhbVE7doKkI-cZ1cdj6aGmjTDT&/

Hinkel, J. M., Vandergift, J. L., Perkel, S. J., Waldinger, M. B., Levy, W., & Stewart, F. M. (2010). Practices and productivity of physician assistants and nurse practitioners in outpatient oncology clinics at national comprehensive cancer network institutions. *Journal of Oncology Practice, 6*(4), 182–187.

Horsely, J. A., Crane, J., & Bingle, J. D. (1978). Research utilization as an organizational process. *Journal of Nursing Administration, 8*(7), 4–6.

Institute of Medicine (IOM). (2001). *Crossing the quality chasm: A new health system for the 21st century.* National Academies Press.

Institute of Medicine (IOM). (2003). *Health professions education: A bridge to quality.* National Academies Press.

Institute of Medicine (IOM). (2011).The future of nursing; Leading change, advancing health. National Academies Press.

Institute of Medicine (IOM). (2016). Assessing progress on the Institute of Medicine Report: The future of nursing. National Academies Press.

Jackson, K. I., & Sheldon, J. M. (1998). Poster presentation: How to tell a story. *Pediatric Nurse, 10*(9), 36–37.

Jamtvedt, G., Young, J. M., Kristofferson, D. T., O'Brien, M. A., & Oxman, A. D. (2006). Audit and feedback: Effects on professional practice and healthcare outcomes. *Cochrane Database of Systematic Reviews, 2*, CD000259.

Johns Hopkins Center for Health Services and Outcomes Research. (2012). Homepage. http://www.jhsph.edu

Kirchoff, K., & Beck, S. (1995). Using the journal club as a component of the research utilization process. *Heart and Lung: The Journal of Acute and Critical Care, 24*(3), 246–250.

Kitson, A., Harvey, G., & McCormack, B. (1998). Enabling the implementation of evidence-based practice: A conceptual framework. *Quality in Healthcare, 7*(3), 149–158.

Kitson, A., Rycroft-Malone, T., Harvey, G., McCormack, B., Seers, K., & Titchen, A. (2008). Evaluating the successful implementation of evidence into practice using the PARiHS framework: Theoretical and practical challenges. *Implementation Science, 3*(1), 1–21.

Kleinpell, R. M. (2021). *Outcomes assessment in advanced practice nursing* (5th ed.). Springer.

Kohn, L. T., Corrigan, J. M., & Donaldson, M. S. (2000). *To err is human: Building a safer health system.* A report of the Committee on Quality of Health Care in America, Institute of Medicine. National Academies Press.

Koman, D. (2018). Increasing hepatitis C virus knowledge through evidence-based educational intervention. *Gastroenterology Nursing, 41*(2), 95–102.

Lachance, C. (2014). Nursing journal clubs: A literature review on the effective strategy for continuing education and evidence-based practice. *Journal of Continuing Education in Nursing, 45*(12), 559–565.

Leedy, P. D., & Ormrod, J. E. (2010). *Practical research: Planning and design.* Pearson.

Levin, R. F., & Ferrara, L. (2011). Evidence-based practice: Using the Appraisal Guidelines for Research Evaluation II to assess clinical practice. *Guideline Research and Theory for Nursing Practice: An International Journal, 25*(3), 160–162. https://doi.org/10.1891/0541-6577.25.3.160

Liang, L., Safi, J. A., & Gagliardi, A. R. (2017). Number and type of guideline implementation tools varies by guideline, clinical condition, country of origin, and type of developer organization: Content analysis of guidelines. *Implementation Science, 12*(136), 1–12. https://doi.org/10.1186/s13012-017-0668-7

Lombardo, M. C., Mackay, P., Stavarksky, D. H., Alderfer, M. E., Dutton, S., Scala, E., & Gerstenhober, M. (2022). An academic and regional nurse research collaborative: Implications for nursing research. *Nursing Forum, 57*(6), 1162–1168.

Lyder, C., & Fain, J. A. (2009). Interpreting and reporting research findings. In J. A. Fain (Ed.), *Reading, understanding, and applying research* (3rd ed., pp. 233–250). F. A. Davis.

Makarski, J., & Brouwers, M. C. (2014). The AGREE Enterprise: A decade of advancing clinical practice guidelines. *Implementation Science, 9*(1), 103.

Marinopoulos, S. S., Dorman, T., Ratanawongsa, N., Wilson, L. M., Ashar, B. H., Magaziner, J. L., . . . Bass, E. B. (2007). Effectiveness of continuing medical education. *Evidence Reports in Technology Assessment, 14*, 1–69.

Martinson, B.C., Anderson, M.S., & DeVries, R., (2005). Scientists behaving badly. *Nature, 435* (7043) 737–738. https://doi.org/10.1038/435737a

May, C. (2013). Towards a general theory of implementation. *Implementation Science, 8*, 18.

McConkey, R.W., Kelly, T., Dalton, R., Rooney, G. Healy, M., Murphy, L., & Dowling, M. (2022). Developing a culture of nursing research through clinical-academic partnership. *International Journal of Urological Nursing.* https://doi.org/10.1111/ijun.12339

McEwen, M., & Wills, E. M. (2014). *Theoretical basis for nursing* (4th ed.). Wolters Kluwer Health Lippincott Williams & Wilkins.

McQueen, J., Miller, C., Nivison, C., & Husband, V. (2006). An investigation into the use of a journal club for evidence-based practice. *International Journal of Therapy and Rehabilitation, 13*(7), 311–316.

McSherry, R. (2002). *Evidence informed nursing: A guide for clinical nurses.* Routledge.

Melnyk, B., & Fineout-Overholt, E. (2002). Putting research into practice. Rochester ARCC. *Reflections on Nursing Leadership, 28*(2), 22–25.

Melnyk, B., & Fineout-Overholt, E. (2019). *Evidence-based practice in nursing and healthcare: A guide to best practice* (4th ed.). Lippincott Williams & Williams, Wolters Kluwer Health. Companion website thePoint: http://thepoint.lww.com/Melnyk4e

Merone, L., Komka, T., Russell, D., & Nagle, C. (2022). Sex inequalities in medical research: A systematic scoping review of the literature. *Women's Health Rep* (New Rochelle), *3*(1), 49–59. https://doi.org/10.1089/whr.2021.0083

Midwest Nursing Research Society (MNRS). (2023). https://mnrs.org/members-center/research-implementation-interest-groups/

Miracle, V. (2008). Effective poster presentations. *Dimensions of Critical Care Nursing, 27*(3), 122–124.

National Organization of Nurse Practitioner Faculties (NONPF). (2007). *NONPF recommended criteria for NP scholarly projects in the practice doctorate program.* www.nonpf.org/associations/10789 /files/ScholarlyProjectCriteria.pdf

Newhouse, R., Bobay, K., Dykes, P. C., Stevens, K. R., & Titler, M. (2013). Methodology issues in implementation science. *Medical Care, 51,* 532–540.

Newhouse, R. P., Dearholt, S. L., Poe, S. S., Pugh, L., & White, K. M. (2008). *Johns Hopkins nursing evidence-based practice model and guidelines: Instructor's guide.* Sigma Theta Tau International.

Nilsen, P., Stahl, C., Roback, K., & Cairney, P. (2013). Never the twain shall meet? A comparison of implementation science and policy implementation research. *Implementation Science, 8,* 63–75.

O'Grady, E. T. (2008). Advanced practice registered nurses: The impact on patient safety and quality. In *Patient safety and quality: An evidence-based handbook for nurses.* http://www.ahrq.gov /qual/nurseshdbk/

Patient Protection and Affordable Care Act. (2010). http://www.dpc.senate.gov/healthreformbill /healthbill04.pdf

Patton, C. M., Lim, K. G., Ramlow, L. W., & White, K. M. (2015). Increasing efficiency in evaluation of chronic cough: A multidisciplinary, collaborative approach. *Quality Management in Health Care, 24*(4), 177–182.

Patton, M. Q. (1990). *Qualitative evaluation and research methods* (2nd ed.). Sage.

Peterson, L. A., Woodward, L. D., Urech, T., Daw, C., & Sookanan, S. (2006). Does pay-for-performance improve the quality of health care? *Annals of Internal Medicine, 145*(4), 265–272.

Polit, D. F., & Beck, C. T. (2013). Is there still gender bias in nursing research? An update. *Research in Nursing and Health, 36,* 75–83.

PosterPresentation.com.

Prosser, H., Almond, S., & Walley, T. (2003). Influences on GP's decision to prescribe new drugs: The importance of who says what. *Family Practice, 20*(1), 61–68.

Protect Illinois Communities Act (2023), Public Act 102-1116, Sec.702 ILCS 5/24-1.9(a)(1). il.ga.gov./legislation/

Purtle, J., Peters, R., & Brownson, R. C.,(2016). A review of policy dissemination and implementation research funded by the National Institutes of Health, 2007-2014, *Implementation Science, 11,* 1–8.

Raines, C. F. (2010, March). *The doctor of nursing practice: A report on progress.* Presentation at the annual meeting of the American Association of Colleges of Nursing. https://www .aacnnursing.org/Search-Results?sb-search=Raines%2c+C.+F.+(2010%2c+March).+The +doctor+of+nursing+practice%3a+A+report+on+progress&sb-inst=42_dnn_avtSearch_pnl Input&sb-logid=345628-ak5n4tg7beetd7id

Rich, K. A. (2015). Evaluating outcomes of innovations. In N. A. Schmidt & J. M. Brown (Eds.), *Evidence-based practice for nurses: Appraisal and application of research* (3rd ed., pp. 487–504). Jones & Bartlett Learning.

Rich, K.A. (2022). Evaluating outcomes of innovations, In N. A. Schmidt & J. M. Brown (Eds.), *Evidence-based practice for nurses: Appraisal and application of research* (5th ed., pp. 519–537). Burlington, MA: Jones & Bartlett Learning

Robert Wood Johnson Foundation (RWJF). (2017). *What is health equity?* https://www.rwjf.org/en /insights/our-research/2017/05/what-is-health-equity-.html

Robert Wood Johnson Foundation (RWJF). (2023). *Building a Culture of Health.* https://www.rwjf .org/en/building-a-culture-of-health.html

Russell, C., & Gregory, D. (2003). Evaluation of qualitative research studies. *Evidence-Based Nursing, 6*(2), 36–40.

Rycroft-Malone, J., Kitson, A., Harvey, G., McCormack, B., Seers, K., Titchen, A., & Estabrooks, C. (2002). Ingredients for change: Revisiting a conceptual framework. *Quality and Safety in Health Care, 11*(2), 174–180.

Rycroft-Malone, J., Sears, K., Chandler, J., Hawkes, C. A., Crichton, N., Allen, C., . . . Strunin, L. (2013). The role of evidence context and facilitation in an implementation trial: Implications for the development of the PARIHS framework. *Implementation Science, 8,* (28). https://doi .org/10.1186/1748-5908-8-28

Rycroft-Malone, J., Sears, K., Titchen, A., Harvey, G., Kitson, A., & McCormack, B. (2004). What counts as evidence in evidence-based practice? *Journal of Advanced Nursing, 47*(1), 81–90.

Schaffer, M. A., Sandau, K. E., & Diedrick, L. (2013). Evidence-based practice models for organizational change: Overview and practical applications. *Journal of Advanced Nursing, 69*(5), 1197–1209.

Schmidt, N., & Brown, J. M. (2015). Sharing the insights with others. In N. A. Schmidt & J. M. Brown (Eds.), *Evidence-based practice for nurses: Appraisal and application of research* (3rd ed., pp. 539–566). Jones & Bartlett Learning.

Sheratt, C. (2005). The journal club: A method for occupational therapists to bridge the theory-practice gap. *British Journal of Occupational Therapy, 68*(7), 301–306.

Soumerai, S. B., McLaughlin, T. J., Gurwitz, J. H., Guadagnoli, E., Hauptman, P. J., Borbas, C., . . . Gobel, F. (1998). Effect of local medical opinion leaders on quality of care for acute myocardial infarction. *Journal of the American Medical Association, 279*(17), 1358–1363.

Stetler, C. B. (1994). Refinement of the Stetler/Marram model for application of research findings to practice. *Nursing Outlook, 42*(1), 15–25.

Stetler, C. B., & Marram, G. (1976). Evaluating research findings for applicability in practice. *Nursing Outlook, 24*(9), 559–563.

Stetler, C. B., Ritchie, J. A., Rycroft-Malone, J., & Charns, M. P. (2014). Leadership for evidence-based practice: Strategic and functional behaviors for institutionalizing EBP. *Worldviews on Evidence-Based Nursing, 11*(4), 219–226.

Stull, A., & Lanz, C. (2005). An innovative model for nursing scholarship. *Journal of Nursing Education, 44*(11), 493–497.

Synergis Education. (2012–2023). https://www.synergiseducation.com/podcasting-best-practices-for-preparation-of-engaging-podcasts/

Tenhunen, M. L., Heinonen, S., Buchko, B. L., & Frumenti, J. (2019). *The expert role of the DNP prepared nurse impacting healthcare systems: Bench to bedside, classroom to boardroom*. Presentation at the 2019 DNP National Conference, Washington, D.C. August 8, 2029. http://hdl.handle.net/10755/21142. Sigma Repository.

Titler, M. G. (2002). Use of research in practice. In G. LoBiondo & J. Haber (Eds.), *Nursing research methods: Critical appraisal and utilization* (5th ed., pp. 410–431). Mosby.

Titler, M. G., Kleiber, C., Steelman, V., Goode, C., Rakel, B., Barry-Walker, J., . . . Buckwalter, K. (1994). Infusing research into practice to promote quality care. *Nursing Research, 43*(5), 307–313.

Titler, M. G., Kleiber, C., Steelman, V. J., Rakel, B. A., Budreau, G., Everett, L. Q., . . . Goode, C. J. (2001). The Iowa model of evidence-based practice to promote quality care. *Critical Care Nursing Clinics of North America, 13*(4), 497–509.

Titler, M. G., & Shuman, C. S. (2017). *Implementation science*. In P.A. Grady & A.S. Hinshaw, Eds. Using research to shape health policy, pp. 33-54. Springer Publishing.

University of North Carolina. *Academic Poster Presentations*. http://gradschool.unc.edu/academics/resources/postertips.html

U.S. Department of Health and Human Services (DHHS, n.d.). *Human research protection training*. https://www.hhs.gov/ohrp/education-and-outreach/human-research-protection-training/index.html

Villanova University. *Multimedia tools*. https://www1.villanova.edu/villanova/unit/instructionaltech/blackboard/bbtraining/multimedia_tools.html

Villanova University. *Podcasting*. https://www1.villanova.edu/villanova/unit/instructionaltech/audiovideo/podcasting.html

Watkins, C., Harvey, I., Langley, C., Gray, S., & Faulkner, A. (1999). General practitioners' use of guidelines in the consultation and their attitudes to them. *British Journal of General Practice, 49*(438), 11–15.

West, S., King, V. Carey, T. S., Lohr, K. N., McKoy, N., Sutton, S. F., & Lux, L. (2002). *Systems to rate the strength of scientific evidence* (Evidence Report/Technology Assessment No. 47). Agency for Healthcare Research and Quality.

Wray, C. M., Auerbach, A. D., & Arora, V. M. (2018). The adoption of an online journal club to improve research dissemination and social media engagement among hospitalists. *Journal of Hospital Medicine, 13*(11), 764–769. https://doi.org/10.12788/jhm.2987

Zadvinskis, I. M., & Grudell, B. A. (2010). Clinical practice guideline appraisal using the AGREE instrument: Renal screening. *Clinical Nurse Specialist, 24*(4), 209–214.

CHAPTER 5

Quality and Safety

Carol G. Klingbeil, DNP, RN, APNP, CPNP-PC, CNE
Carolyn Ziebert, DNP, RN, PCNS-BC

*He who every morning plans the transaction of the day and follows out that
plan, carries a thread that will guide him through the maze of the most busy
life. But where no plan is laid, where the disposal of time is surrendered merely
to the chance of incidence, chaos will soon reign.*

—**Victor Hugo**

Background

Quality and safety in health care are intertwined and impacted by just about every
domain of *The Essentials: Core Competencies for Professional Nursing Education* of the
American Association of Colleges of Nursing (AACN) (2021). Competency in all
domains will impact and enable quality and safety transformation in health care as
well as assist in elevating the general health of the populations cared for and the
professionals designing and delivering care. In the early 2000s, the first few land-
mark reports on quality and safety emerged, addressing the challenges of providing
high-quality and safe care to citizens. The first Institute of Medicine (IOM) report in
2000, *To Err Is Human: Building a Safer Health System*, followed by the 2001 report,
Crossing the Quality Chasm: A New Health System for the 21st Century, catapulted organizations and healthcare professionals into a new awareness of issues with quality
and safety in health care. These reports and others will continue to drive the daily
practices of health care forever. There has been an explosion in the complexity of
health care that is not only fueled by medical specialization but also by advances
in technology. Challenges with healthcare funding and access issues as well as consumer advocacy, chronic care demands, globalization, and supply chain issues that
emerged during the COVID-19 pandemic continue to add complexity to health
care as well. Overwhelming evidence of healthcare disparities, healthcare burnout,
and staffing issues have all emerged as central problems that impact the quality and
safety of health care and became magnified during COVID-19.

APN/DNP nurses are prepared with leadership, EBP, and knowledge and skills
in quality improvement methods throughout their education in order to transform health care (Bowie et al., 2019). Evidence supports that they can identify

opportunities for change and lead teams of stakeholders to improve care and identify innovative solutions. APN/DNP-prepared nurses can also move further to impact and anchor improvements into organizational and even governmental policy solutions. Through reflective practice, systematic approaches, and interprofessional collaboration, recognition of problems can move forward to potential solutions (Flynn et al., 2017).

The purpose of this chapter is to address advanced level quality and safety competencies for the APN/DNP nurse (AACN, 2021). Integrated concepts and resources that will enable leading the advancement of care and assuring safety in a variety of settings will be discussed and explored. The APN/DNP nurse will need to envision innovative solutions and use appropriate methodologies, tools, and engagement of appropriate stakeholders in improvement processes and safety approaches in healthcare settings. The competencies and subcompetencies in the quality and safety domain, as outlined by the AACN, offer guidance for APN/DNP students to receive educational training and gain experiences during practicums to address changes needed to support a culture of patient safety.

Selected Concepts for Nursing Practice Represented in the Domain

Concepts of clinical judgment, evidence-based practice (EBP), communication, health policy, and ethics are most relevant in the discussion of this domain and will be addressed when appropriate. This brief discussion highlights some of the aspects of these concepts' relevance to quality and safety. Nursing clinical judgment is primary when identifying problems in the clinical arena that impact the delivery of high-quality and safe care. Clinical judgment must be anchored on the six aims of quality care established by the IOM in 2001: safe, timely, efficient, effective, equitable, and patient-centered. Clinical judgment is also a part of the trifecta of EBP: best research evidence, clinical experience, and patient preference (Cronenwett et al., 2007). Communication is central to quality and safety in foundational ways such as talking with patients and families, speaking up when concerns or ethical issues arise, practicing interprofessional and intraprofessional collaboration and teamwork to address problems, and systematically carrying out quality improvement. The APN/DNP nurse must also continually ask about the evidence base for care decisions and the delivery of care in multiple settings. Engaging with patients and families to illicit their preferences in care decisions is an important aspect of EBP. Ease of searching, accessing, and evaluating the relevance and quality of evidence is essential in advanced nursing practice in order to lead improvement efforts and enact safety approaches in healthcare settings. The potential to address policy issues that are out of date, need to be incorporated into practice, or need to be initiated due to new evidence or regulations will also be integral to high-quality care. Lastly, ethical considerations must be integrated into the care of a variety of populations, especially when addressing health equity issues that have not been focused on for far too long. Recognition that addressing health disparities and considering the presence of social determinants of health will impact attaining high-quality outcomes for patients, clients, and their families.

Three competencies will be addressed in detail in this section focusing on quality and safety in health care. Subcompetencies identified for each competency will be discussed and explored in their relevance to the advanced level of practice for the DNP-prepared nurse, focusing on knowledge, skills, attitudes, and resources. It is important to note that data-driven decisions for quality and safety rely on informatics competencies involving the design of systems and analysis of data. It is assumed that entry-level competencies are foundational for the advanced competencies, and they are not consistently included in the discussion of the advanced competencies for the APN/DNP.

Level II Competencies of the Domain

Apply Quality Improvement Principles in Care Delivery

It is helpful to start with a brief discussion of several frameworks that commonly organize overall quality improvement efforts and measures. An overall broadly adopted policy framework to improve healthcare quality emerged from a well-established organization, the *Institute for Healthcare Improvement (IHI)* (IHI, 2023), and provides four broad goals for the focus of health-focused improvement efforts titled the *Quadruple Aim* (Bodenheimer, & Sinsky, 2014). The four pillars include goals to: (1) improve health of populations; (2) control costs; (3) improve the experience of care; and (4) address the healthcare providers' experience. More specifically, each outcome must have quality measures, which are often organized under six aims of high-quality health care and originally were set forth in a seminal report on quality, *Crossing the Quality Chasm* (IOM, 2001). The six aims are focused on the essentials of care: safe, timely, efficient, effective, equitable, and patient-centered.

The Donabedian (1966) quality improvement framework is often used to develop and monitor measures with a longstanding approach to organizing and measuring outcomes with structure, process, and outcomes. The underlying foundation for the framework is that the right structure upholds and supports the right processes, and in turn will result in the desired outcomes.

Fundamental to the competencies in this chapter are basic quality improvement methods, tools, and benchmarking measures for processes and outcomes. The IHI is a key organization to use as a resource for understanding the processes and tools used for quality improvement. The IHI has many education modules, courses, and credentials that can be useful for a successful quality improvement project (IHI, 2023). The IHI QI Toolkit includes tools, templates, and examples for professionals to access and use. Collaboration with QI staff within organizations is also an important resource for the APN/DNP nurse.

The Quality and Safety Education for Nurses (QSEN) Project (2007, 2009) emerged as a national initiative and partnership of nurses to advance the priority of patient care quality and safety by establishing competencies at the undergraduate and graduate levels (Cronenwett et al., 2007, 2009). This incredible body of work was organized with knowledge, skills, and attitude competencies under patient-centered care, teamwork and collaboration, evidence-based practice, quality improvement, safety, and informatics. While the work has now transitioned into the AACN 2021 *The Essentials: Core Competencies for Professional Nursing Education*, the products of this work remain accessible and intact under the QSEN website, www.qsen.org.

Nurses' reflection of their experience in daily practice with patients and families, and awareness of outcome measures and guidelines for care offer a myriad of opportunities for inquiry and improvement (Horton-Deutsch & Sherwood, 2017). Nurses continually observe and ask questions stimulated by their clinical practice, providing the source for clinical inquiry. Another very useful model is the *I3 Model for Advancing Quality Patient Centered Care,* that provides nurses with an algorithmic guide to understand how inquiry (research and EBP), improvement (QI), and innovation are all important processes that must be considered when approaching clinical questions (Hagle et al., 2020). The visual model in **Figure 5-1** is very useful to see the flow of processes and decisions that need to be made when addressing clinical practice issues. It is common for nursing students at all levels to struggle with how these processes are intertwined and delineated while also remaining curious and open to opportunities that need new and innovative approaches to improve care.

Establish and Incorporate Data-Driven Benchmarks to Monitor System Performance

Data-driven quality improvement is essential to monitor care outcomes in organizations. Quality measures are determined, and in many cases required, to be used by different government agencies, insurance companies, and credentialing and accrediting bodies in addition to internally identified measures (Anderson et al., 2022). Measures in all settings need to be useful and actionable when used to compare performance against a set standard with the intent to improve care through benchmarking (Willmington et al., 2022). Benchmarking is used either internally to improve care, or externally for comparison to report quality care for the public to use when deciding where to seek care (Anderson et al., 2022). Measures that are both useful as important to consumers, providers, and agencies and actionable so that when used they can reflect a change and improved care are important when benchmarking (Sherwood & Barnsteiner, 2021). Quality measures have characteristics such as reliability, validity, variation, and practicality. Measures also may need to be risk adjusted based on the populations that different institutions serve in order to be fair to those organizations seeing higher-risk populations. Risk adjustment is important so that severity of illness and patient characteristics of populations are accounted for when comparing measures (Sherwood & Barnsteiner, 2021).

A number of different organizations provide specific measures and benchmarking resources. Key examples of benchmarking and quality outcome organizations and resources for the APN/DNP nurse to be aware of are listed in **Table 5-1**. Nurses practicing at the advanced level must be competent to identify and understand appropriate measures for different spheres of care and settings such as The Joint Commission, service lines such as the Quality Oncology Practice Initiative (QOPI), and populations such as Centers for Medicare and Medicaid Services (CMS). Identifying and understanding these different spheres and settings is also needed to attain certain credentials signaling excellence and quality of nursing care such as the Magnet Recognition Program (ANCC, 2023) and the National Database of Nursing Quality Indicators' (NDNQI) nurse-sensitive indicators (now managed by Press Ganey).

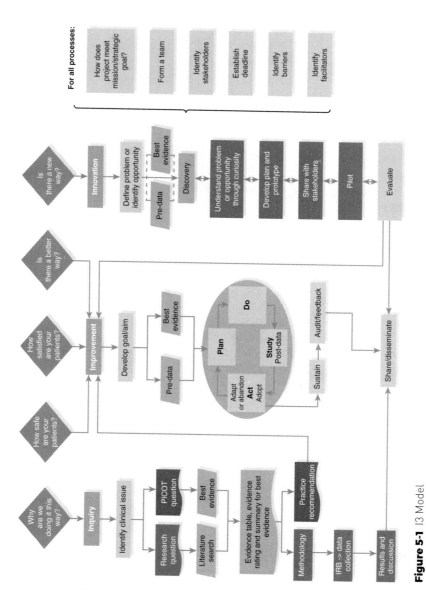

Figure 5-1 I3 Model

© Clement J. Zablocki VA Medical Center

Table 5-1 Healthcare Benchmarking and Quality Outcomes Organizations and Websites

Organization	Website
Agency for Healthcare Research and Quality (AHRQ) Quality Indicators (prevention, in-patient, patient safety, and pediatric)	www.quality indicators.ahrq.gov
Agency for Healthcare Research and Quality (AHRQ) National Healthcare Quality and Disparities Report (NHQDR)	www.ahrq.gov
Centers for Medicare and Medicaid Services (hospitals, nursing homes, home care)	www.cms.gov
Hospital Consumer Assessment of Healthcare Providers and Systems (HCAHPS) (consumer measures of in-patient and out-patient care)	www.hcahpso nline.org
Institute for Healthcare Improvement (in-patient, out-patient, rapid response, adverse events, primary care access)	www.ihi.org
The Joint Commission (in-patient, out-patient, surgical, emergency care, in-patient psych and substance use, staffing)	www.joint commission.org
Leapfrog (healthcare associated infections, medication safety, maternity, pediatric, surgical)	www.hospitalsafety grade.org
National Database of Nursing Quality Indicators (NDNQI) now under Press Ganey since 2014 (nurse-sensitive indicators)	https://www .pressganey.com /platform/ndnqi/
National Committee for Quality Assurance (HEDIS measures focused on effectiveness, access, utilization, and EHR data, patient-centered medical home)	www.ncqa.org
National Quality Forum (adult immunization, Alzheimer's and dementias, care coordination, health workforce and person-centered care)	www.qualityforum.org
Quality Oncology Practice Initiative (QOPI®) (out-patient focused)	https://practice .asco.org/quality -improvement /quality-programs /quality-oncology -practice-initiative

Carol G. Klingbeil and Carolyn Ziebert

Use National Safety Resources to Lead Team-Based Change Initiatives

Many of the organizations that provide benchmarking and outcomes measures are also a source of national safety and quality improvement resources. The APN/DNP must be aware of and use a multitude of resources, some of which are broad based in scope and others that are focused on sectors of healthcare professionals, inter-professional work, or consumers of health care. Given that quality and safety are so intertwined and central to the work of all healthcare organizations, many organizations leverage or create focused resources for their organization. Central to all improvement efforts is establishing a solid team that is inclusive of key stakeholders representing those involved or impacted by the change or targeted improvement. Membership in organizations can be at the organization or individual level and some resources that are sponsored by the government or self-sustaining are free to use. Each organization has certain target groups they are designed to assist and provide resources in the form of toolkits, models, and educational resources such as webinars, podcasts, articles, or guidelines. Detailing each safety resource is beyond the scope of this chapter; however, a list of commonly cited national resources are listed in **Table 5-2**.

Integrate Outcome Metrics to Inform Change and Policy Recommendations

APN/DNP-prepared nurses must be prepared to use outcome metrics to advocate for important institutional, regional, state, and even national change in practice guidelines and policies. Creating a data-driven approach to one's practice is a central theme and competency for the APN/DNP. Without outcome metrics of care, you have no gauge for improvement work or safe care. Making meaningful and lasting change will only be sustained through creating informed data-driven change and then anchoring the changes in policy. Organizations with a solid system for policy and procedure review that is evidence based and built on results from quality improvement efforts will most likely be top performers. The consumer/patient and family partnership lens is also an important vantage point that can inform policy recommendations. One example of this, from an institutional policy, is that at a local Children's Hospital it is recommended to engage a parent as a stakeholder for every quality improvement project impacting patients and families. Another example from the same organization is that the patient education committee must also have several parent representatives. APN/DNP nurses often lead policy and procedure committees within organizations.

At the federal level, there has been a National Quality Strategy to guide governmental programming and strategic planning for the past decade. In 2015, six evolving priorities emerged and included:

- Making care safer by reducing harm caused in the delivery of care.
- Ensuring that each person and family members are engaged as partners in their care.
- Promoting effective communication and coordination of care.
- Promoting the most effective prevention and treatment practices for the leading causes of mortality, starting with cardiovascular disease.
- Working with communities to promote wide use of best practices to enable healthy living.
- Making quality care more affordable for individuals, families, employers, and governments by developing and spreading new healthcare delivery models. (AHRQ, 2015)

Since 2015, this quality report has been integrated with the National Healthcare Quality and Disparities Report in response to policy from the Affordable Care

Table 5-2 National Safety and Quality Improvement Resources from Organizations

Organization	Key Resources	Website
American Association of Critical-Care Nurses (AACN)	Healthy work environments focusing on teamwork and collaboration	www.aacn.org
American Nurses Credentialing Center (ANCC) Magnet® recognition program	Standards for nursing excellence, nursing leadership, quality improvement, and organizational culture	www.nursingworld .org/organizational -programs/magnet
Agency for Healthcare Research and Quality (AHRQ)	QI toolkit and resources	https://www.ahrq.gov /prevention/resources /index.html
	Surveys on Patient Safety Culture (SOPS)	https://www.ahrq.gov /sops/index.html
	Patient Safety Organizations (PSOs) that voluntarily collect/analyze safety data.	https://pso.ahrq.gov/
	TeamSTEPPS® is an evidence-based collection of tools focused on effective teamwork.	https://www.ahrq.gov /teamstepps-program /index.html
Institute for Healthcare Improvement (IHI)	QI Toolkit QI Modules and Credentialing	www.ihi.org
Interprofessional Education Collaborative (IPEC)	Interprofessional competency domains for education and practice and teamwork	www.ipecollaborative
The Joint Commission (TJC)	Institutional Accreditation and annual list of National Patient Safety Goals (NPSG) with resources for improvement	www.jointcommission .org
National Academy of Medicine (NAM), previously Institute of Medicine (IOM)	Landmark reports on quality, safety, nursing, and health equity	www.nam.edu
Nursing Alliance for Quality Care (NAQC) (under the ANA)	Organized voice for nursing quality, safety, patient advocacy, and policy makers	www.nursingworld .org/practice-policy /naqc
Solutions for Patient Safety/Children's Hospitals	150+ children's hospitals working together on patient safety to prevent harm. Tools and resources	www.solutionsfor patientsafety.org

Carol G. Klingbeil and Carolyn Ziebert

Act (ACA) calling for the establishment of an Interagency Working Group on Health Care Quality (IWG). The group has leaders from 24 federal agencies responsible for quality and safety improvement for the nation. Each year, over 440 quality metrics and benchmarking opportunities are published in an effort to advocate for measuring the quality of the nation's health by state (AHRQ *National Healthcare Quality and Disparities Report*, 2022). This population health report focuses on health disparities across the nation, is an important source for data, and serves as a report card for making progress with closing the gap on healthcare disparities.

Collaborate in Analyzing Organizational Process Improvement Initiatives

Many organizations have systems-level process improvement departments with teams that organize education, projects, and interprofessional systems-level initiatives. The APN/DNP nurse would be a very valuable asset to these teams and could in fact cultivate a future role within a process improvement department once expertise and competency is established. Personnel in these departments are often accessible or a part of QI initiatives within organizations, especially those that are systems-wide projects. These QI personnel can facilitate access to data, complete data analytics, prepare data visualization tools, and assist or collaborate with presentations at organization, regional, state, or national levels. It is common to find APN/DNP-prepared nurses leading process or outcomes improvement teams with the support of institutional staff focused on QI. As a working example, in one hospital the Clinical Nurse Specialist team initiated how chlorhexidine gluconate (CHG) baths were done. The measures were monitored and documented and then the team analyzed the data to determine the next steps (G. Altmiller, personal communication, February 14, 2023).

De-implementation science is a new emerging focus in the EBP and quality improvement arena and, interestingly, a new area of change management (Ingvarsson et al., 2022; Rietbergen et al, 2020; Walsh-Bailey et al., 2021). Certainly, there have been discussions related to "sacred cows" in the nursing literature for a number of years and identification of interventions and practices that we should consider doing away with (de-implementing) due to limited evidence showing efficacy have surfaced (Hanrahan et al., 2015). *Choosing Wisely* is a campaign started in 2012 by the American Board of Internal Medicine (ABIM) to help inform the public about practices, tests, and procedures that are low-value care provided by or ordered by doctors or nurses that waste resources or time and can even be harmful to patients (Rietbergen et al., 2020). Overall, knowledge of these low-value practices is central to leading an evidence-based practice approach to quality improvement and focusing not only on implementation science but also on de-implementation science when practices are ineffective or even harmful. APN/DNP nurses must recognize that certain evidence-based practices need to be initiated while others may need to be stopped. Evidence on how to de-implement practices is limited but evolving (Grimshaw et al., 2020).

Lead the Development of a Business Plan for Quality Improvement Initiatives

Leadership of quality improvement initiatives is a competency that is expected in advanced nursing practice. Moving teams forward takes clear and effective

---

Box 5-1 Outline of a Business Case Plan

Executive Summary (1–2 pages)

Analysis of the Problem, Associated Needs, and Alignment with Strategic Plan

Proposed Solutions with Options

Goals for Success

Implementation Plans

Evaluation Plans with Cost Analysis

Risk-Adjusted Cost–Benefit Analysis

Data from Bartlett Ellis, R. J., Embree, J. L., & Ellis, K. G. (2015). A Business Case Framework for Planning Clinical Nurse Specialist–Led Interventions. *Clinical Nurse Specialist, 29*(6), 338-347. doi:10.1097/NUR.0000000000000162 Welch, T. D., & Smith, T. B. (2022). Anatomy of a business case. *Nursing Administration Quarterly, 46*(1), 88-95. doi:10.1097/NAQ.0000000000000498

communication, knowledge, and skills in EBP, reflective practice, and planning. Health care has been shifting from a fee for service model to a value-based model in the past few decades and the APN/DNP nurse needs to be prepared to drive improvements not only with quality and safety goals, but also considering the cost and revenue aspects involved (Bartlett Ellis et al., 2015). Engaging a set of stakeholders and setting initial expectations is the first step in the process, but making sure that early on you have the right stakeholders at the table is a task for the entire team. Planning and evaluating progress will be greatly facilitated by creating a business plan for the project and help decision makers in the organization allocate resources as well as justify the business case to stakeholders and eventually the governing board of the organization. A business case plan (BCP) is "a structured framework for evidence-based, transparent business decisions" (Welch & Smith, 2021, p. 88). The outline for a BCP is included in **Box 5-1**. Depending upon the scope and focus of the project, it is important to make the case for the return on investment (ROI) for the proposed project. A cost analysis is a standard part of any BCP but is often a missed element of DNP Projects. There is a current gap in knowledge around the language of business practices for many nurses in advanced practice. Welch and Smith (2022) outline the details and definitions of the BCP to address the need-to-know elements.

Advocate for Change Related to Financial Policies That Impact the Relationship Between Economics and Quality Care Delivery

Data from quality initiatives can inform institutional and government agencies to make changes in covered services, medications, and policies. One of the most important changes to scholarly and improvement projects that could make a large impact on decision makers is to include a cost analysis whenever possible in the planning of projects. Cost savings speak loudly to leaders in organizations and call stakeholders' attention to the importance of making change in the clinical arena on behalf of patients and families. Cost analysis is an area that needs much more attention in the initial education of students, and the continuing education of staff and providers in organizations.

Another example that greatly impacts the financial health of organizations is related to the Hospital-Acquired Condition (HAC) Reduction Program established within health systems to monitor a number of reportable conditions and infections to CMS (CMS, 2022). There are financial implications with lower reimbursement from CMS for hospitals performing in the lowest quartile of institutions as measured by a Total HAC Score for six quality measures of adverse events and certain identified conditions. These quality measures have implications for patient care overall as well as for consumers who are making decisions about where to seek care from reportable data on websites such as Leapfrog or institutional websites. Stakeholders from a variety of units and centralized improvement team staff regularly meet to determine focal areas, monitoring issues and rates for these reportable conditions. The APN/DNP both leads and advocates for addressing safety issues impacting the quality of care or experience of patients and families. Advocating for change and improvements that impact the financial health of the organization and the health of patients and families seeking care in the organization are central to the role of APN/DNP nurses.

Advance Quality Improvement Practices Through Dissemination of Outcomes

Dissemination of quality improvement projects is an important competency for the APN/DNP prepared nurse. Publication knowledge and skills are areas of improvement for many advanced practice nurses and leaders as well as for DNP programs. Learning how to move a project from poster to publication is a unique skillset that requires mentorship, leadership, and teamwork. A focus of DNP programs is to be sure that QI projects are designed with publication in mind so that rigor and a systematic approach will provide a project that is publishable. Standards for Quality Improvement Reporting Excellence (SQUIRE) guidelines were first developed in 2008 to provide a standardized approach to both planning and publishing quality improvement projects. Davies and colleagues (2015) published results identifying challenges with following and understanding the guidelines. In 2016, the SQUIRE 2.0 guidelines were launched and published, after several improvement revisions in the guidelines through consensus building conferences, interviewing editor journals, and pilot testing of the revised guidelines (Ogrinc et al., 2016). SQUIRE friendly journals are listed on their website, www.squire-statement.org. The SQUIRE 2.0 publication guidelines and access to a reviewer checklist for the guidelines can be found at the following website: http://www.squire-statement.org/index.cfm?fuseaction=Page.ViewPage&PageID=471.

Dissemination of quality improvement efforts through scholarly presentations and posters are also avenues that are available and important to reach a variety of audiences. One unique aspect of QI projects is that they are overall not generalizable due to the complex context and unique nature of each setting. This lack of being generalizable is a determining factor that must be recognized when planning and evaluating each published project and something students need to understand when they are submitting to an IRB for determination of the project status as research versus quality improvement. A common issue with DNP projects is that they do not have enough data, cycles of improvement, and data that shows sustainability over time to make the projects publishable.

Contribute to a Culture of Patient Safety

Primum non nocere. (First, do no harm.)

— **Thomas Sydenham**, MD

In 1999, the Institute of Medicine (IOM) published its groundbreaking report *To Err Is Human: Building a Safer Health System*. This report indicated there are approximately 44,000 to 98,000 deaths experienced per year in healthcare systems as a result of medical errors. In 2013, James reported this number was approaching 400,000 people dying each year. More recently it has been reported that medical errors may have contributed to over 250,000 deaths per year, becoming the third leading cause of death (Boussat et al., 2021). These errors are the result of a combination of human errors and deficiencies in system structures, policies, and processes. The complexity of health care requires healthcare professionals and organizations to contribute to a culture of patient safety and find ways to improve the care provided to those using these healthcare systems.

Culture has been described as key to patient safety. It can be defined as "The product of individual and group values, attitudes, perceptions, competencies and patterns of behavior that determine the commitment to, and the style and proficiency of, an organization's health and safety management" (Churucca et al., 2021, p. 2). This definition speaks to these shared traits being applicable to individual healthcare professionals, units or departments, and organizations overall. Therefore, it is essential that patient safety is addressed from multiple perspectives.

Many national organizations and regulatory agencies have now instituted requirements for organizations to focus on a culture of safety. Two to note are The Joint Commission (TJC) and Centers for Medicare & Medicaid Services (CMS). TJC establishes yearly national patient safety goals for healthcare systems to focus on. These are developed for healthcare systems across the continuum of care, including hospitals as well as long-term care and ambulatory centers (TJC, 2023). CMS (2017) has also implemented patient safety standards. With the passage of the Affordable Care Act, CMS now has requirements for hospitals to use patient safety evaluation systems and work with a Patient Safety Organization (PSO). The intent is for hospitals to collect, manage, and analyze patient safety events to reduce preventable harm.

Evaluate the Alignment of System Data and Comparative Patient Safety Benchmarks

Available Tools and Resources. Because a culture of patient safety is key to providing safe, quality care, a number of organizations now require healthcare systems to regularly assess their safety culture. These include the National Quality Forum's Safe Practices for Healthcare and the Leapfrog Group (Yount et al., 2022). Table 5-1, presented earlier in this chapter, lists other resources for the APN/DNP to use.

A widely used validated tool to align a healthcare system's data and compare not only perceptions on the culture of patient safety, but patient safety outcomes as well, is the AHRQ's *Surveys on Patient Safety Culture*™ (SOPS). Similar to TJC national patient safety goals, the AHRQ offers surveys to be used across the continuum of care to enable hospitals, medical offices, nursing homes, ambulatory centers, and even community pharmacies to assess how their staff perceives various aspects of their patient safety culture. Organizations typically use this survey on a yearly basis in order to track progress over time. User guides are available to organizations to implement these surveys. The AHRQ also offers a database for organizations to compare their results on the SOPS to other similar types of organizations for benchmarking purposes. Additionally, the AHRQ offers a toolkit for developing and implementing action plans for the unit/department or systems level. See **Figure 5-2**.

Another opportunity for aligning and comparing data exists through patient safety collaboratives. Patient safety collaboratives have been developed by capitalizing on cooperation among healthcare systems readily sharing best practices. These collaboratives are often referred to as hospitals engagement networks (HENS). Member facilities share their own quality improvement and patient safety initiatives with each other. HENS also direct training programs to teach hospitals and systems how to improve patient safety. Work to standardize how outcomes are analyzed within these HENS continues to ensure reported improvements and initiatives are effective (Pronovost & Jha, 2014).

Ways to examine your survey data	Questions to ask
Look at your lowest-scoring results	**Do your survey scores highlight areas for improvement?** ■ What are the lowest scoring composite measures? ■ What are the lowest scoring items?
Compare your survey scores to other facilities or to your prior scores	**How do your scores compare with:** ■ SOPS Database results? ■ Other facilities like yours? You can examine SOPS Database results by bed size, geographic region, number of operating/procedure rooms, ownership, single specialty vs. multispecialty, teaching status, and other characteristics. ■ Your facility's scores from a previous survey administration (if applicable)? Have your scores improved over time?
Investigate whether any areas within your facility contribute to lower scores	**Do your survey scores vary based on respondent characteristics or work areas? For example, look for high- or low-performing groups based on:** ■ Job title. ■ Staff position. ■ Tenure. ■ Hours worked per week. ■ Interaction with patients/residents. ■ Work areas, units, departments.

Figure 5-2 Examining Your Survey Data to Identify Areas to Improve

Reproduced from Yount N, Edelman S, Sorra J, Gray L. *Action Planning Tool for the AHRQ Surveys on Patient Safety Culture™ (SOPS®)*. (Prepared by Westat, Rockville, MD, under Contract No. HHSP233201500026I/ HHSP23337004T). Rockville, MD: Agency for Healthcare Research and Quality; November 2022. AHRQ Publication No. 23-0011.

The pediatric population is as vulnerable to adverse events as the adult population. It has been estimated that almost 50% of adverse events in hospitalized children are preventable (Lyren et al., 2017). The Ohio Children's Hospitals' Solutions for Patient Safety (SPS) network was established among eight children's hospitals to measure and share patient safety initiatives among member hospitals to reduce preventable harm and sustain results. This structured collaborative has since spread and includes more than 150 children's hospitals across the nation. Much of the success of SPS is due to the rapid sharing of evidence-based practices and tools to help reduce harm and also sharing interventions aimed at improving the culture of patient safety in hospitals. Four domains are used to help focus the work of SPS, including error-prevention methods, leadership methods, cause analysis, and patient–family engagement. Member hospitals adhere to the philosophies of "all teach, all learn" and "we will not compete on safety" (Lyren et al., 2017). These philosophies are unique to safety as the member hospitals most likely compete on hiring professionals, market share of patients, and other business aspects of health care. Through measurement of hospital-acquired conditions and serious safety events, member hospitals are able to compare their own data to the benchmarks achieved through the collaborative.

Challenges in Assessing Safety Culture. Although much attention has been paid and work has been accomplished in creating and sustaining a culture of patient safety, ongoing work is needed. Understanding safety culture and the elements contributing to safe patient care is challenged by differences in definitions and methods of assessment. The terms *safety culture* and *safety climate* are often used interchangeably in the literature. Often safety climate is described as individuals' perceptions of their organization, while safety culture, as defined earlier in this section, is aimed more at how multileveled perceptions and behaviors reflect the organization's health and management of safety (Churruca et al., 2021). **Box 5-2** is reflective of the many tools and surveys available for organizations to use.

In terms of measurement, a systematic review by Churruca et al. (2021) examined which elements of safety culture have been studied and what type of quantitative and qualitative methods were used to assess safety culture. This review found the vast majority of studies used surveys; very few studies used qualitative methods or mixed methods combining qualitative methods with surveys. Eleven themes related to safety culture were identified across all studies but no one method of study or tool captured all eleven themes. Over a decade ago, Halligan and Zecevic (2011)

Box 5-2 Staff Patient Safety Surveys

Hospital Survey on Patient Safety Culture
Safety Attitudes Questionnaire
Patient Safety Climate in Healthcare Organizations
Safety Climate Survey
Hospital Safety Climate Scale
Teamwork and Safety Climate Survey
Operating Room Management Attitudes Questionnaire

called for a move to develop more common definitions and measurement of the dimensions important to safety culture. The work by Churruca et al. (2021) confirmed the need for more standardization in this area. In addition, more qualitative and mixed methods studies are recommended to help provide more detail and insight into the quantitative surveys. Organizations need to decide how to balance the resources needed to gather and evaluate data, as well as which methods will support the development of meaningful action plans aimed at improving safety culture and ANPs/DNPs can assist in this work.

Lead Analysis of Actual Errors, Near Misses, and Potential Situations That Would Impact Safety

Another step to improve safety culture and safety outcomes is for organizations to analyze events and near misses which have occurred within their institutions. Safety events are typically categorized as actual errors or near misses. Actual errors reach the patient, resulting in some type of harm. Harm can range from mild effects to the death of the patient. Near misses can be defined as variations in normal processes that, if left to continue, have the potential to negatively impact patients. Near misses may not result in full-scale harm but by investigating these events, important information can be discovered and evaluated to avoid these situations in the future (Marra et al., 2020). This potential for some level of harm is why analyses of both these categories of errors are necessary. The TJC has also defined sentinel events. Sentinel events are not related to the normal course of a patient's illness and result in death, severe harm, or temporary harm. Organizations accredited by the TJC are required to perform a systematic review of sentinel events (Oster & Braaten, 2016, Chapter 7). After the review is complete, the organization can voluntarily submit the review to the TJC for feedback.

Another important consideration when evaluating the risks posed to patient safety from actual errors or near misses is to consider both individual and organizational factors which played into the events. Common individual factors found to play a role in safety events are not following policy, inappropriate decision making/critical thinking, or not stopping next actions in the face of uncertainty. Top organizational factors playing a role in errors have been found to include interruptions/disruptions in workflows, poor communication among the healthcare team, and/or complete lack of policies and procedures to guide individuals' actions (Speroni et al., 2014). Evidence shows that individual factors do play a role in the cause of events, but system or organizational factors are the root cause of most events (Hughes, 2008). APNs/DNPs can be leaders in the analysis of errors as their practice is aimed at many levels of the organization, from patient care to systems-level projects focusing on improvements.

One of the most common methods used to investigate errors and near misses is the root cause analysis (RCA). An RCA is a reactive assessment that begins after an event, retrospectively outlining the sequence of events leading to that identified event. RCAs are conducted in a systematic manner using standardized tools to guide the analysis involving a team. The goal is to identify system issues which led to the event occurring. This analysis is done by asking what happened, how did it happen, and why did it happen (Oster & Braaten, 2016, Chapter 7). RCAs began in the engineering and aviation industries and migrated to health care partly due to the IOM reports (2000; 2001) published regarding patient safety. Although

RCAs can be carried out in a number of ways, a systematic approach involving the following steps is often cited in the literature: (a) gathering information and mapping out the event timeline if applicable; (b) assembling a team; (c) identifying root causes—most events have multiple root causes; (d) developing an action plan; (e) ensuring the action steps are measurable; and (f) disseminating findings. Action planning is one of the most important steps in an RCA. The action steps need to be specific, identify who is responsible for carrying the steps out and how success will be measured, and set a time frame for making necessary changes. If the action steps are not prioritized in an RCA, the ability to drive change or improvement is lost. As discussed in the quality section of this domain, under the first competency, the Donabedian (1966) framework can be used to identify structural, process, and outcome action steps. Again, the TJC not only requires some type of RCA for sentinel events, but also development of robust action plans which are monitored for effectiveness and can lead to improvements (Hughes, 2008). There is little evidence that conducting an RCA alone can improve patient safety. Finally, in order for both individuals and organizations to learn from errors and hopefully prevent them from happening again, the results of the RCA, including the action plan, should be shared widely. Specific details can be de-identified to protect those involved. It is important for the APN/DNP to understand that often the same type of events cross professions and departments with an organization.

Design Evidence-Based Interventions to Mitigate Risk

Accidents do not occur because people gamble and lose, they occur because people do not believe that the accident that is about to occur is at all possible.

— **James Reason**

In addition to analysis of actual events and near misses, it is important to identify potential risks and design interventions to mitigate the risks. In recent years, it has been recommended to take a more proactive approach to patient safety. Although a reactive approach, through conducting an RCA, for example, is needed to evaluate actual events or near misses, the use of proactive strategies and tools might mitigate potential risks. These may include failure modes and effects analysis (FMEA), standardized handoffs, improving usability of the electronic health record (EHR) systems, huddles, bundles/checklists, education, and personal reflection.

Failure Modes and Effects Analysis (FMEA). FMEAs can be used proactively to identify potential areas of failure which could lead to safety events. This process can help identify all ways in which a process could fail. FMEAs can also estimate the probability of failures happening, as well as what consequences may ensue. Alternative processes, once identified, can be trialed and monitored. By focusing on the systems of care, structures can be put in place to support healthcare professionals in knowing and doing the right thing to avoid errors in the first place. Through proactive improvement in processes, it makes it obvious for the healthcare professional to do the right thing, and improbable for them to choose to do the wrong thing. Since 2001, TJC has mandated accredited organizations to conduct proactive risk assessments on a yearly basis focusing on one or two high-priority areas. The benchmarking data discussed earlier can help to identify these high-priority areas. Again, the goal is to predict system weaknesses and adopt changes to minimize patient harm (Hughes, 2008).

Standardized Tools. Several tools are available for healthcare professionals to use to help mitigate risks. A few of them will be discussed here. Patient handoffs used during transfers to other units/facilities, shift change reports, and other instances when the transfer of responsibility and accountability will occur during the care of patients are key to avoiding adverse events and minimizing safety risks to the patient. Ineffective communication among members of the healthcare team has been identified as a main risk factor for adverse events and patient harm (Graan et al., 2016; Padgett, 2018). For handoffs to be effective, they not only need to contain pertinent assessment data related to the patient, but also a plan of care and escalation plan if patients' responses to the plan of care don't proceed as expected (Graan et al., 2016). To ensure complete information, another standardized tool which can be embedded into handoffs is to present patient data using the SBAR (situation, background, assessment, and recommendations) format. A systematic review conducted by Segall et al. (2012), determined several recommendations for handoffs, including using a standardized process (SBAR, checklist, etc.), completing urgent clinical tasks prior to information transfer so these tasks aren't missed, allowing only patient-centered discussions during handoffs, requiring all relevant team members to be present, and providing training in team communication. Because missing vital information when transferring responsibility and accountability to another member of the team can be detrimental to the patient, the TJC has made handoff standardization a national patient safety goal for the past several years.

Huddles among members of the healthcare team are another strategy to mitigate risks. Patient safety huddles are brief, multidisciplinary daily meetings where information is shared for healthcare team members to stay informed and review events and/or unit QI data (Lamming et al, 2021). The goal is to coordinate care and to discuss who on the unit may be at risk for harm or decompensation as well. Lamming et al. (2021) discovered the defining criteria of what to include in these daily huddles may change to ensure what is presented is most useful to the staff at the huddle and found huddles to be an important influence on outcomes for different groups of staff. Some of the more common tenets of daily huddles include conducting the daily huddle at the same time and place every day, reviewing the number of days since the last harm event, sharing QI data, debriefing on any harm events since the last huddle, keeping it short (less than 15 minutes), and providing a nonjudgmental and fear-free space to ask questions and discuss any other concerns.

Larson et al. (2022) described the use of a daily reflection assessment tool in the intensive care unit (ICU). This tool offered staff the opportunity to assess patient safety, workload, and work environment on a daily basis over time. Shifts were rated using a green, yellow, red rating. Free text could be added if the shift was rated yellow or red. Communication and collaboration were key to affecting the perception of all three areas when using the daily reflection tool. Data from using the tool can be used by staff and leadership to drive necessary changes and to develop interventions for moving yellow and red ratings to green ratings.

Yang et al. (2021) investigated how second-order problem solving can offer nurses the opportunity to learn from near misses in order to improve outcomes. Nurses often "fix and forget" or temporarily "patch up" the problem when encountering near misses or actual errors instead of taking action to solve problems or get at the root cause. Second-order problem solving involves taking further actions to investigate the root causes and attempting to identify preventative countermeasures (Yang et al., 2021). This approach requires education regarding second-order problem solving, having a supportive environment for frontline staff to take the lead on pursuing solutions, and encouraging learning from near misses to promote patient safety. Nurses can feel empowered if encouraged to use second-order problem solving when facing potential safety risks.

Work-related interruptions and distractions have been found to be a major organizational factor contributing to safety events. Because of this, it is important to have mitigating strategies to overcome these interruptions and distractions. One method is through the use of the acronym STAR (Speroni et al., 2014). STAR involves (1) stopping to concentrate on the task; (2) thinking further about the task and what needs to be done; (3) acting to complete the task; and (4) reviewing how well the task was accomplished. Many organizations have implemented "no talking zones" in medication rooms where focus is needed to avoid interruptions and distractions. Staff can also be empowered to not answer phone calls or pages when critical thinking is required. If interrupted, refocusing using STAR can occur before proceeding with a critical task.

One final strategy to help mitigate safety risks involves patient participation to help prevent adverse errors. When patients and families are given the opportunity to offer input into their care and are kept informed as to the plan of care, communication is enhanced between themselves and healthcare professionals. This trust promotes two-way communication and allows patients and families to question the care they are receiving and speak up if care doesn't appear to be following the plan of care as discussed, thus potentially avoiding safety events or near misses (Andersson et al., 2015).

Evaluate Emergency Preparedness Systems-Level Plans to Protect Safety

APNs/DNPs have the proper educational preparation to examine issues from a practice based on evidence, systems-level thinking, and policy development, all of which are needed to deal with crisis management. Their expertise can be used to focus on prevention and preparedness, response, and recovery and rehabilitation when facing disasters or major public health crises, such as COVID-19 (Ladak et al., 2021). APNs/DNPs can provide support to nursing staff, medical colleagues, and leadership within an organization and can be leaders in implementing crisis management policies.

APNs/DNPs need to share responsibility with the nursing profession and nursing professional organizations to ensure healthcare delivery is available to communities as a whole, especially at-risk populations, to protect safety during disasters and public health crises. Their leadership skills are needed to remain involved at every level of government and within community organizations to be able to prevent, prepare, respond, and recover from these events (Couig et al., 2021). Advocacy in terms of emergency preparedness by APNs/DNPs can help reduce morbidity and mortality for communities and at-risk populations.

The recent COVID-19 pandemic has shed light on deficiencies in how public health crises are managed. Professional nursing organizations can serve as expert resources when designing and evaluating disaster plans. The Association of Community Health Nurse Educators, the Association of Public Health Nursing, and the

Emergency Nurses Association have all published position statements regarding nurses' role in public health preparedness that include mention of at-risk populations. These position statements can be used to further develop organizational policies and procedures. The Association of Healthcare Emergency Preparedness Professionals also has open-source materials available to the APN/DNP regarding lessons learned from the COVID-19 pandemic (https://www.ahepp.org/page /COVIDLessonsLearned).

Universities offering DNP programs can encourage students to focus projects on emergency preparedness to ensure the latest evidence is incorporated into policies and procedures, educational training, and responses to crises. Projects have been completed in the hospital environment in terms of how best to respond to patient emergencies (Hart & Braband, 2015); projects could be expanded beyond direct patient care by using simulation for response to community responses and preparedness. This project focus becomes more important as it has been noted in the literature that nurses lack competencies in emergency preparedness (McNeill et al., 2020). Competencies noted to be lacking were in terms of professional emergency preparedness knowledge (e.g., triage, incident command systems, isolation and quarantine practices) and personal preparedness. It was also noted that intention to return to work after a mass casualty disaster or natural disaster was higher than if the event was related to an infectious disease pandemic or biologic disaster. Administrators should consider increasing education, use of simulation scenarios, and participation in disaster drills to improve nurses' competencies (McNeill et al., 2020; Park & Kim, 2017). APNs/DNPs could partner with administrators to develop, carry out, and evaluate the different methods chosen to increase competencies.

Contribute to a Culture of Provider and Work Environment Safety

Progress on safety comes from going behind the label "human error" where you discover how workers and managers create safety, and where you find opportunities for them to do it even better.

— **David Woods, Sidney Dekker, Richard Cook, Leila Johannesen, and Nadine Sarter**

In the literature, the evidence is quite compelling regarding the need for strong leadership to set the stage for an organization's culture. Leaders do this by establishing missions and visions, setting strategic goals, and providing the necessary resources for carrying out safe, quality care. Safety issues should be on the agendas of meetings held at all levels of the organization to keep safety front and center. Leaders can also role model their responses to errors, asking what happened instead of who made the error. Providing support to staff and patients involved in errors and harm is also key to a work environment which is safe not only for patients, but staff as well (Botwinick et al., 2006).

Another approach to focusing on patient safety is using the framework of high reliability organizations (HROs). Principles of high reliability have commonly been used in industries such as commercial aviation and nuclear energy. Many healthcare organizations have now adopted this framework to improve patient safety and strive to become HROs (Basson et al., 2021; Oster & Braaten, 2016, Chapter 2). Specific principles will be discussed in a below subcompetency.

Advocate for Structures, Policies, and Processes That Promote a Culture of Safety and Prevent Workplace Risks and Injury

As mentioned above, HROs use a framework based on two major categories: (1) anticipation (attempting proactivity in preventing errors) and (2) containment (bouncing back from errors when they do occur). Five principles fall under these two categories. See **Table 5-3**. In HROs, reliability is a top priority. Putting the five principles into practice can make a high-risk environment safer through embedding anticipation and containment strategies into the organization's structure, policies, and processes (Oster & Braaten, 2016, Chapter 2). Proactivity is important to avoid errors and harm if possible; reactivity is also necessary, recognizing it may not be possible to eliminate all harm in the high-risk healthcare environment. The key to improved outcomes is how the organization reacts to and learns from errors and harm.

Another focus needed to promote a culture of safety and prevent workplace risks and injuries is the establishment of a healthy work environment. The status of work environments has been shown to affect both patient and staff outcomes. The American Association of Critical Care Nurses has published ongoing reports of nurse work environments in 2006, 2008, 2013, 2018, and most recently in 2021 (Ulrich et al., 2021). Items measured in the work environment reports include

Table 5-3 **Principles of High Reliability Organizations**

Anticipation	Preoccupation with failure	Heightened awareness of potential risks and near misses in workflows, procedures, and so on. Problems belong to employee until fixed or finds someone to fix.
	Reluctance to simplify	Deliberately questions assumptions. Knowledge/fixes can lie beyond one individual and require multiple perspectives.
	Sensitivity to operations	Ongoing sharing of information and communicating risks across the organization. Allowing small adjustments to prevent errors from accumulating.
Containment	Commitment to resilience	Developing ability to cope with errors and bounce back from events. Hoping to contain event before situation worsens or causes more harm.
	Deference to expertise	Decision making should lie with those with the most expertise with the problem at hand, regardless of role or title. Increase ability to respond quickly.

Data from Oster, C. A., & Braaten, J. S. (2016). *High reliability organizations: A healthcare handbook for patient safety & quality*, Chapter 2. Sigma Theta Tau International.

factors which have been found to contribute to healthy work environments: skilled communication, true collaboration, effective decision making, appropriate staffing, meaningful recognition, and authentic leadership. In the most recent report, a decline in all items measured was evident from 2018 to 2021, with the largest decline in perceptions of appropriate staffing (Ulrich et al., 2021). APNs/DNPs need to play a role in creating and sustaining healthy work environments to support a culture of safety (Ulit et al., 2020).

Nurses, including the APN/DNP, not only provide direct patient care, but often are involved at the organizational level. This places the APN/DNP in a position to advocate for structures, policies, and processes which promote a culture of safety and prevent workplace risks and injuries. Bowie et al. (2019) found recent graduates of DNP programs can identify the importance of their roles at the systems level upon completing the degree. DNP graduates were able to re-envision themselves as agents of change. APNs/DNPs believe they belong at the table where change can happen and decisions are made as they see themselves as equals to other leaders and have confidence in their ability to contribute. Being a change agent at the systems level requires seeing issues, including safety, as complex systems issues. Having the ability to interpret data and apply evidence to practice makes APNs/DNPs valuable members in promoting safety and reducing harm. Ability to lead others was a final subtheme identified. APNs/DNPs have acquired leadership skills through their coursework and their DNP projects. Future research is needed to focus on quantifying the impact APNs/DNPs can have on healthcare outcomes, including cost effectiveness, contributing to the culture of an organization, and decreasing patient morbidity and mortality through patient safety initiatives (Bowie et al., 2019).

Foster a Just Culture Reflecting Civility and Respect

It is known that disruptive behaviors can lead to errors and harm. Because of this, TJC has issued a sentinel event alert regarding behaviors that undermine a culture of safety. This sentinel event alert was originally published in 2008, with the most recent update in 2021. As safety is dependent on teamwork, communication, and collaboration among members of the healthcare team, TJC has stated organizations must address any type of problem behaviors which may threaten the performance of the team (TJC, 2021). These behaviors can be overt actions, such as outbursts, or passive activities, such as exhibiting uncooperative behaviors or refusing to communicate with or help others. This unprofessionalism contributes to unhealthy and potentially hostile work environments. As stated above, skilled communication and true collaboration are necessary for healthy work environments. Incivility and disrespect hinder these activities. As with any discussion related to factors influencing patient safety, disruptive behaviors can have personal and systemic root causes. Health care is a high-stakes, emotional environment in which different personalities and title ranks coexist. The TJC requires accredited organizations to have a code of conduct defining acceptable and disruptive behaviors and a process in place to manage disruptive behaviors. Starting in January 2022, the TJC added a new requirement to address workplace violence, including prevention strategies, reporting systems, and post-incident follow-up (TJC, 2021).

The American Nurses Association (ANA) also has a position statement on civility and respect issued in 2015. The ANA states it is a shared responsibility of both employees and organizations to create and sustain a culture of respect. The ANA calls for evidence-based strategies to be implemented to prevent and mitigate all forms of incivility, bullying, and workplace violence. This position statement offers detailed strategies for both nurses and organizations to address these behaviors at multiple levels. The APN/DNP should utilize these resources to ensure civility and respect are the foundations for healthcare teams (ANA, 2015).

Although there is an abundance of literature regarding the need for education on incivility, bullying, and workplace violence, it is known that education alone cannot change behavior. One primary prevention strategy identified in the literature involves the use of cognitive rehearsal to address disruptive behaviors. This involves the use of learned responses to support healthcare team members in addressing disruptive behaviors in the moment to stop them from proceeding. Scripts and role playing can help reinforce the cognitive rehearsal strategy (Griffin & Clark, 2014). Virtual learning experiences, such as Civility Mentor, have also been designed to educate learners about incivility and its consequences. Civility Mentor also offers opportunities for the learner to interact with on-screen simulations and receive feedback from virtual coaches. This type of intervention addresses all three learning domains of knowledge, skills, and attitudes (Clark & Dunham, 2019). Other interventions include the use of specific scenarios applicable to the unit or department. Once training and completing the practice scenarios, leaders can identify a "re-set" date for behavioral expectations. Individual accountability can come into play once these expectations are set and leaders can address accordingly if the disruptive behaviors continue (Garcia et al., 2021). Carroll (2023) suggests a pneumonic to use in the moment to stop the disrupting behaviors. State the problem, tell the person what is wanted, offer an opportunity to respond, and provide closure (STOP) is an easy framework to remember. It is important for the APN/DNP to search the literature for evidence-based strategies that go beyond education. The APN/DNP has the skillset to modify interventions if necessary and focus on improvements using available quality improvement tools. Measuring and evaluation of strategies by the APN/DNP will also be a key step in eliminating disruptive behaviors from the healthcare setting.

Create a Safe and Transparent Culture for Reporting Incidents

It is often the best people that make the worst mistakes—error is not the monopoly of an unfortunate few. We cannot change the human condition, but we can change the conditions under which humans work.

— James T. Reason

Just Culture. In order to create a safe and transparent culture for reporting incidents, it is important for healthcare organizations to focus on three areas: a just culture, a reporting culture, and a learning culture (TJC, 2017; TJC, 2021). These concepts stem from the extensive research of James Reason, focusing on the psychology of human error. In a just culture, people are encouraged to report safety issues, but there is also a clear distinction between human error (inadvertent actions), at-risk behaviors (deviations or risks which go unrecognized), and reckless behavior (conscious disregard of a substantial and unjustifiable risk). In the early 2000s, David Marx presented a model and algorithm to use to help differentiate among the various types of errors and the approach needed to address them (Oster & Braaten, 2016, Chapter 8). A just culture is not necessarily a blame-free culture; accountability does come into play. Basically, a just culture is a system of shared accountability where organizations are accountable for systems they have designed and responding to staff behaviors in a fair and just manner; staff are accountable for the quality of their choices and reporting both errors and system vulnerabilities. This model is designed to help change an organization's culture by placing less focus on events, errors, and outcomes, and more focus on risk, system design, and the management of behavioral choices. Managing behaviors is different for each type of error: staff are consoled for human errors, coached for at-risk behaviors, and punitive action can come into play for reckless behavior.

The ANA published a position statement in 2010 supporting a just culture within healthcare organizations. Recognizing the importance of nurses speaking up when dealing with errors or safety risks, the ANA endorsed the value of reporting errors and revisiting processes and systems that may leave nurses at risk if not addressed. The ANA's endorsement of reporting errors and an organization's approach via a just culture can help to overcome the fear that reporting errors/risks may result in blame or other negative consequences as well as the doubt that nothing will change if reported (Kennedy, 2016). This fear surrounding consequences of reporting errors is why TJC recognized the importance of focusing on a just culture, a reporting culture, and a learning culture; improvements should be expected to ensure healthcare professionals are supported and the systems in place will support them in making the right decisions.

Unfortunately, there have been instances recently which may exacerbate the barriers to reporting errors and safety risks. The recent conviction of a nurse in Tennessee after a fatal medication error may have unintended consequences in the patient safety movement and stop healthcare professionals from feeling safe to report such issues. The ANA and the Tennessee Nurse Association (TNA) put out a joint statement:

> Health care delivery is highly complex. It is inevitable that mistakes will happen, and systems will fail. It is completely unrealistic to think otherwise. The criminalization of medical errors is unnerving, and this verdict sets into motion a dangerous precedent. There are more effective and just mechanisms to examine errors, establish system improvements and take corrective action. The non-intentional acts of individual nurses like RaDonda Vaught should not be criminalized to ensure patient safety. (ANA & TNA, 2022)

Mark Pelletier, chief operating officer and chief nurse executive with TJC stated, "We not only need more nurses than ever before but need safer systems that provide mechanisms to prevent harm that results in tragic outcomes for both patients and caregivers" (TJC, 2022). Lancaster et al. (2022) encourage leaders and organizations to revisit their focus on their safety culture and the implementation of just culture principles to ensure a safe practice and reporting environment for staff and their overall well-being.

Organizational Reporting. Healthcare organizations also need a safe and transparent culture for reporting incidents. Because the patient safety movement relies on sharing of information and events related to errors and risk, the Patient Safety and Quality Improvement Act (PSQIA) was passed in 2005. This act allowed the creation of patient safety organizations (PSOs). PSOs create a legally secure environment where healthcare professionals and organizations can voluntarily report information on a privileged and confidential basis. Member organizations have data available to them for aggregation and analysis of patient safety events. The goal is to reduce the risks and hazards seen across organizations, thus improving the safety and quality of patient care (*https://www.ahrq.gov/cpi/about/otherwebsites/pso.ahrq.gov/index.html*). PSOs operate in a similar way to the patient safety collaboratives described above, allowing member organizations to "all teach, all learn" from errors. Member organizations can present de-identified cases and discuss the root causes of events using common formats, again without the fear of legal liability or professional sanctions.

Role Model and Lead Well-Being and Resiliency for Self and Team

Individual Resilience. The concept of resilience has received more attention in the past few years. Definitions vary but most have a common thread about the ability to adjust to adversity, maintain equilibrium, retain some sense of control over one's environment, and continue to move on in a positive manner (Oster & Braaten, 2016, Chapter 13). Resilience can be achieved as people confront adversity. This ability to adjust is due to successful coping with challenges. Having to move through adversity, people learn problem-solving skills and gain confidence that they can retain some control and continue to move on as defined above. In the literature, resilience has been measured but it is hard to determine a change in resilience as there are a variety of tools available for measurement. If change is desired, it would be important to use the same tool for measurement over time.

Organizational Resilience. *Resilience* is a term that can be applied to individual healthcare workers or to organizations as a whole. Resilience is seen as a characteristic of HROs. Two types of organizational resilience have been defined: (1) precursor resilience—ability to accommodate change without catastrophic failure or a capacity to absorb shock and (2) recovery resilience—ability to respond to a singular or unique event and bounce back to a state of normalcy. It has been found that HROs are more resilient if they have team training programs in place and engage in process and analysis design on a regular basis (Oster & Braaten, 2016, Chapter 13). Organizational resilience is associated with a strong safety culture, ability to mitigate risks, and encouragement to report safety events and issues.

Relational Resilience. As with many of the concepts discussed under the quality and safety competencies and subcompetencies, resilience is also the result of both individual and organizational factors. Individuals can build resilience through several different strategies. These may include reflective practice, building collegial relationships with others (co-workers or through professional networking), positive thinking and visualization techniques, exercising, and volunteering to name just a few. Each person needs to decide for themselves what works best for them. Leadership is needed to play a key role in providing the necessary policies, support infrastructure, and programs to build resilience. Strategies leaders can use include fostering a healthy work environment so collegial relationships can develop, implementing shared governance structures for individual voices to be heard and be involved with decision making, conducting debriefing sessions if necessary, and offering educational active-learning workshops on the topic of resilience (Barratt, 2018; Hart et al., 2014).

Leaders may need support and training in resilience in order to help others within the organization. One such program involves strength-based coaching. Strength-based coaching allows leaders to create their own competency development plans. Focusing on their strengths helps to maximize effectiveness overall. Further research and program development, such as strength-based coaching, can improve transformational leadership skills and build resilience (Spiva et al., 2021). If leaders are resilient themselves, they will be in a better position to support others on the team. APNs/DNPs could consider participating in or developing programs within their own organizations to benefit themselves and the healthcare team.

Summary

As leaders in the transformation of health care, the APN/DNP is prepared and responsible to embody and advance quality improvement and safety in all spheres of care and settings where health care is delivered. The necessary knowledge, skills, and attitudes to carry out activities to improve health care are outlined and woven throughout every domain of *The Essentials: Core Competencies for Professional Nursing Education* (AACN, 2021). There are many resources focused on quality and safety available for the APN/DNP to leverage and reference in the pursuit of improvement. Dissemination of scholarly work is critical to advance the strategic goals of excellence and safety in care. While learning evolves and new standards emerge, they must be anchored in policy at institutional, regional, state, and national levels. Through innovation, collaboration, and partnership, vision and advocacy, the APN/DNP can lead healthcare initiatives to address challenging and complex issues in health care. High quality and safety will always be the highest of priorities in healthcare settings for patients, families, and healthcare professionals.

References

2022 National Healthcare Quality and Disparities Report. (2022, October). Rockville, MD: Agency for Healthcare Research and Quality. AHRQ Pub. No. 22(23)-0030.

Agency for Healthcare Research and Quality (AHRQ) (2015). *National Strategy for Quality Improvement in Health Care, 2015 Agency-Specific Plans*. https://archive.ahrq.gov/workingforquality/reports/2015-ahrq-agency-specific-plan.pdf

American Association of College of Nursing (AACN). (2021). *The essentials: Core competencies for professional nursing education*. https://www.aacnnursing.org/Essentials

American Nurses Association. (2015). *Incivility, bullying, and workplace violence*. https://www.nursingworld.org/practice-policy/nursing-excellence/official-position-statements/id/incivility-bullying-and-workplace-violence/

American Nurses Association & Tennessee Nurses Association. (2022). *Statement in Response to the Conviction of Nurse RaDonda Vaught*. https://www.nursingworld.org/news/news-releases/2022-news-releases/statement-in-response-to-the-conviction-of-nurse-radonda-vaught/

American Nurses Credentialing Center (ANCC) (2023) Magnet® Recognition Program. www.nursing world.org/organizational-programs/magnet

Anderson, E., Cantlin, D. L., & Watts, S. (2022). Benchmarking: What is it and how can it support the role of nursing in ambulatory care? *AAACN Viewpoint, 44*(4), 1–13.

Andersson, A., Frank, C., William, A. M. L., Sandman, P. O., & Hansebo, G. (2015). Adverse events in nursing: A retrospective study of reports of patient and relative experiences. *International Nursing Review, 62,* 377–385.

Barratt, C. (2018). Developing resilience: The role of nurses, healthcare teams and organisations. *Nursing Standard, 33,* 43–49.

Bartlett Ellis, R. J., Embree, J. L., & Ellis, K. G. (2015). A business case framework for planning clinical nurse specialist–led interventions. *Clinical Nurse Specialist, 29*(6), 338–347. https://doi .org/10.1097/NUR.0000000000000162

Basson, T., Montoya, A., Neily, J., Harmon, L., & Watts, B. V. (2021). Improving patient safety culture: A report of a multifaceted intervention. *Journal of Patient Safety, 17,* e1097–e1104.

Bodenheimer, T., & Sinsky, C. (2014). From triple to quadruple aim: Care of the patient requires care of the provider. *Annals of Family Medicine, 12*(6), 573–576. https://doi.org/10.1370/afm.1713

Boussat, B., Seigneurin, A., Giai, J, Kamalanavin, K., Labarère, J., & François, P. (2021). Involvement in root cause analysis and patient safety culture among hospital care providers. Patient Safety, 17((8): e1194-e1201. doi: 10.1097/PTS.0000000000000456.

Botwinick, L., Bisognano, M., & Haraden, C. (2006). *Leadership Guide to Patient Safety.* IHI Innovation Series white paper. Institute for Healthcare Improvement.

Bowie, B. H., DeSocio, J., & Swanson, K. M. (2019). The DNP degree: Are we producing the graduates we intended? *The Journal of Nursing Administration, 49*(5), 280–285. https://doi.org/10 .1097/nna.0000000000000751

Carroll, K. (2023). Language that respects dignity in nursing practice. *Nursing Science Quarterly, 36,* 21–23.

Centers for Medicare & Medicaid Services (CMS). (2022). Hospital-acquired condition reduction program. https://www.cms.gov/Medicare/Quality-Initiatives-Patient-Assessment-Instruments/Value -Based-Programs/HAC/Hospital-Acquired-Conditions

Centers for Medicare & Medicaid Services (CMS). (2017). *Patient safety standards.* https://www.cms .gov/Medicare/Quality-Initiatives-Patient-Assessment-Instruments/QualityInitiativesGenInfo /ACA-MQI/Patient-Safety/MQI-Patient-Safety

Churucca, K., Ellis, L. A., Pomare, C., Hogden, A., Bierbaum, M., Long, J. C., Olekains, A., & Braithwaite, J. (2021). Dimensions of safety culture: A systematic review of quantitative, qualitative and mixed methods for assessing safety culture in hospitals. *BMJ Open, 11,* e043982. https://doi.org/10.1136/bmjopen-2020-043982.

Clark, C. M., & Dunham, M. (2019). Civility mentor: A virtual learning experience. *Nurse Educator, 45,* 189–192.

Couig, M. P., Travers, J. L., Polivka, B., Castner, J., Veenema, T. G., Stokes, L., & Sattler, B. (2021). At-risk populations and public health emergency preparedness in the United States: Nursing leadership in communities. *Nursing Outlook, 69,* 699–703.

Cronenwett, L., Sherwood, G., Barnsteiner, J., Disch, J., Johnson, J., Mitchell, P., & Warren, J. (2007). Quality and safety education for nurses. *Nursing outlook, 55*(3), 122–131.

Davies, L., Batalden, P., Davidoff, F., et al. (2015). The SQUIRE Guidelines: An evaluation from the field, 5 years post release. *BMJ Quality & Safety, 24,* 769–775.

Donabedian, A. (1966). Evaluating the quality of medical care. *Milbank Memorial Fund Quarterly, 44,* 166–206.

Flynn, R., Scott, S. D., Rotter, T., & Hartfield, D. (2017). The potential for nurses to contribute to and lead improvement science in health care. *Journal of Advanced Nursing, 73*(1), 97–107. https://doi.org/10.1111/jan.13164

Garcia, M. G., Allen, S., Griffis, L., Tidwell, J., & Watt, J. (2021). Incorporating a civility program into a healthcare system: Journey or expedition. *Clinical Nurse Specialist, 35,* 171–179.

Graan, S. M., Botti, M., Wood, B., & Redley, B. (2016). Nursing handover from ICU to cardiac ward: Standardized tools to reduce safety risks. *Australian Critical Care, 29,* 165–171.

Griffin, M., & Clark, C. M. (2014). Revisiting cognitive rehearsal as an intervention against incivility and lateral violence in nursing: 10 years later. *The Journal of Continuing Education in Nursing, 45,* 535–542.

Grimshaw, J. M., Patey, A. M., Kirkham, K. R., Hall, A., Dowling, S. K., Rodondi, N., Ellen, M., Kool, T., Van Dulmen, S. A., Kerr, E. A., Linklater, S., Levinson, W., & Bhatia, R. S. (2020). De-implementing wisely: Developing the evidence base to reduce low-value care. *BMJ Quality & Safety, 29*(5), 409–417. https://doi.org/10.1136/bmjqs-2019-010060

Hagle, M., Dwyer, D., Gettrust, L., Lusk, D., Peterson, K., & Tennies, S. (2020). Development and implementation of a model for research, evidence-based practice, quality improvement, and innovation. *Journal of Nursing Care Quality, 35*(2), 102–107.

Halligan, M., & Zecevic, A. (2011). Safety culture in healthcare: A review of concepts, dimensions, measures and progress. *BMJ Quality & Safety, 20,* 338–343.

Hanrahan, K., Wagner, M., Matthews, G., Stewart, S., Dawson, C., Greiner, J., . . . & Williamson, A. (2015). Sacred cow gone to pasture: A systematic evaluation and integration of evidence-based practice. *Worldviews on Evidence-Based Nursing, 12*(1), 3–11.

Hart, J. L., & Braband, B. (2015). Doctor of Nursing Practice practice improvement project: A simulation-based emergency preparedness program in immediate care. *Clinical Scholars Review, 8,* 201–207.

Hart, P. L., Brannan, J. D., & DeChesnay, M. (2014). Resilience in nurses: An integrative review. *Journal of Nursing Management, 22,* 720–724.

Hogden, A., Bierbaum, M., Long, J. C., Olekains, A., & Braithwaite, J. (2021). Dimensions of safety culture: A systematic review of quantitative, qualitative and mixed methods for assessing safety culture in hospitals. *BMJ Open.11,* e043982.

Horton-Deutsch, S., & Sherwood, G. D. (2017). *Reflective practice: Transforming education and improving outcomes* (Vol. 2). Sigma Theta Tau.

Hughes, R. G. (2008). Tools and strategies for quality improvement and patient safety. *Patient Safety and Quality: An Evidence-Based Handbook for Nurses.* https://www.ncbi.nlm.nih.gov/books/NBK2682/

Ingvarsson, S., Hasson, H., von Thiele Schwarz, U., Nilsen, P., Powell, B. J., Lindberg, C., & Augustsson, H. (2022). Strategies for de-implementation of low-value care—a scoping review. *Implementation Science, 17*(1), 73. https://doi.org/10.1186/s13012-022-01247-y

Institute for Healthcare Improvement (IHI) (2023). *Improving health and health care worldwide.* https://www.ihi.org/

Institute of Medicine. (2000) *To err is human: Building a safer health system.* National Academies Press.

Institute of Medicine. (2001) *Crossing the quality chasm: A new health system for the 21st century.* National Academies Press.

James, J. T. (2013). A new evidence-based estimate of patient harms associated with hospital care. *Journal of Patient Safety, 9,* 122–128.

The Joint Commission (TJC). (2023). *Hospital: 2023 National patient safety goals.* https://www.jointcommission.org/standards/national-patient-safety-goals/hospital-national-patient-safety-goals/

The Joint Commission (TJC). (2022). *Joint Commission response to the recent Tennessee nurse conviction.* https://www.jointcommission.org/resources/news-and-multimedia/news/2022/03/joint-commission-response-to-the-recent-tennessee-nurse-conviction

The Joint Commission (TJC). (2021). *Sentinel event alert 40: Behaviors that undermine a culture of safety.* https://www.jointcommission.org/resources/sentinel-event/sentinel-event-alert-newsletters/sentinel-event-alert-issue-40-behaviors-that-undermine-a-culture-of-safety/#.Y_NpY3bMI2w

The Joint Commission (TJC). (2017). *Sentinel event alert 57: The essential role of leadership in developing a safety culture.* https://www.jointcommission.org/resources/sentinel-event/sentinel-event-alert-newsletters/sentinel-event-alert-57-the-essential-role-of-leadership-in-developing-a-safety-culture/#.Y_Np23bMI2w

Kennedy, B. (2016). Toward a just culture. *Nursing Management, 47,* 13–15.

Ladak, A., Lee, B., & Sasinski, J. (2021). Clinical nurse specialist expands to crisis management role during COVID-19 pandemic. *Clinical Nurse Specialist, 35*(6), 291–299.

Lamming, L., Montague, J., Crosswaite, K., Faisal, M., McDonach, E., Mohammed, M. A., Cracknell, A., Lovatt, A., & Slater, B. (2021). Fidelity and the impact of patient safety huddles on teamwork and safety culture: An evaluation of the Huddle Up for Safer Healthcare (HUSH) project. *BMC Health Services Research, 21,* 1–11.

Lancaster, R. J., Vizgirda, V., Quinlan, S., & Kingston, M. B. (2022). To err is human, just culture, practice, and liability in the face of nursing error. *Nurse Leader, 20,* 517–521.

Larson, I., Aronsson, A., Noren, K., & Walling, E. (2022). Healthcare workers' structured daily reflection on patient safety, workload and work environment in intensive care: A descriptive retrospective study. *Intensive & Critical Care Nursing, 68,* 103–122.

Lyren, A., Brilli, R. J., Zieker, K., Marino, M., Muething, S., & Sharek, P. J. (2017). Children's hospitals' Solutions for Patient Safety Collaborative impact on hospital-acquired harm. *Pediatrics, 140*(3): e20163494. https://doi.org/10.1542/peds.2016-3494

Marra, A. R., Algwizani, A., Alzunitan, M., Brennan, T. M. H., & Edmond, M. B. (2020). Descriptive epidemiology of safety events at an academic medical center. *International Journal of Environmental Research & Public Health, 17,* 1–11.

McNeill, C., Swanson, M., Adams, L., Alfred, D., & Heagele, T. (2020). Emergency preparedness competencies among nurses: Implications for nurse administrators. *Journal of Nursing Administration, 50,* 407–413.

National Quality Strategy Alignment Toolkit. Content last reviewed August 2017. Agency for Healthcare Research and Quality, Rockville, MD. https://www.ahrq.gov/workingforquality/nqs-tools/alignment-toolkit.html

Ogrinc, G., Davies, L., Goodman, D., Batalden, P. B., Davidoff, F., & Stevens, D. (2016). SQUIRE 2.0 (Standards for Quality Improvement Reporting Excellence): Revised publication guidelines from a detailed consensus process. *BMJ Quality and Safety, 25,* 986–992.

Oster, C. A., & Braaten, J. S. (2016). *High reliability organizations: A healthcare handbook for patient safety & quality.* Sigma Theta Tau International.

Padgett, T. M. (2018). Improving nurses' communication during patient transfer: A pilot study. *The Journal of Continuing Education in Nursing, 49,* 378–384.

Park, H.-Y., & Kim, J.-S. (2017). Factors influencing disaster nursing core competencies of emergency nurses. *Applied Nursing Research, 37,* 1–5.

Pronovost, P., & Jha, A. K. (2014). Did hospital engagement networks actually improve care? *New England Journal of Medicine, 371,* 691–693.

Rietbergen, T., Spoon, D., Brunsveld-Reinders, A. H., Schoones, J. W., Huis, A., Heinen, M., Persoon, A., van Dijk, M., Vermeulen, H., Ista, E., & van Bodegom-Vos, L. (2020). Effects of de-implementation strategies aimed at reducing low-value nursing procedures: A systematic review and meta-analysis. *Implementation Science, 15*(1), 38. https://doi.org/10.1186/s13012-020-00995-z

Segall, N., Bonifacio, A. S., Schroeder, R. A., Barbeito, A., Rogers, D., Thornlow, D. K., Emery, J., Kellum, S., Wright, M. C., & Mark, J. B. (2012). Can we make postoperative patient handovers safer? A systematic review of the literature. *Anesthesia and Analgesia, 115,* 102.

Sherwood, G., & Barnsteiner, J. (Eds.). (2021). *Quality and safety in nursing: A competency approach to improving outcomes,* 3rd ed. Wiley.

Sorra, J., Gray, L., Franklin, M., Streagle, S., Tesler, R., & Vithidkul, A. (2016). *Action planning tool for the AHRQ surveys on patient safety culture.* Agency for Healthcare Research and Quality.

Speroni, K. G., Fisher, J., Dennis, M., & Daniel, M. (2014). What causes near-misses and how are they mitigated? *Plastic Surgical Nursing, 34,* 114–119.

Spiva, L., Hedenstrom, L., Ballard, N., Buitrago, P., Davis, S., Hogue, V., Box, M., Taasoobshirazi, G., & Case-Wirth, J. (2021). Nurse leader training and strength-based coaching: Impact on leadership style and resiliency. *Nursing Management, 52*(10), 42–50.

Ulit, M. J., Eriksen, M., Warrier, S., Cardenas-Lopez, K., Cenzon, D., Leon, E., & Miller, J. A. (2020). Role of the clinical nurse specialist in supporting a healthy work environment. *AACN Advanced Critical Care, 31,* 80–85.

Ulrich, B., Cassidy, L., Barden, C., & Delgado, S. (2021). National nurse work environments—October 2021: A status report. *Critical Care Nurse, 42,* 58–70.

Walsh-Bailey, C., Tsai, E., Tabak, R. G., Morshed, A. B., Norton, W. E., McKay, V. R., Brownson, R. C., & Gifford, S. (2021). A scoping review of de-implementation frameworks and models. *Implementation Science, 16*(1), 1–18. https://doi.org/10.1186/s13012-021-01173-5

Welch, T. D., & Smith, T. B. (2022). Anatomy of a business case. *Nursing Administration Quarterly, 46*(1), 88–95. https://doi.org/10.1097/NAQ.0000000000000498

Willmington, C., Belardi, P., Murante, A. M., & Vainieri, M. (2022). The contribution of benchmarking to quality improvement in healthcare: A systematic literature review. *BMC Health Services Research, 22*(1), 1–20. https://doi.org/10.1186/s12913-022-07467-8

Yang, Y., Liu, H., & Sherwood, G. D. (2021). Second-order problem solving: Nurses' perspectives on learning from near misses. *International Journal of Nursing Sciences, 8,* 444–452.

Yount, N., Edelman, S., Sorra, J., & Gray, L. (2022, November). *Action Planning Tool for the AHRQ Surveys on Patient Safety Culture™ (SOPS®).* (Prepared by Westat, Rockville, MD, under Contract No. HHSP233201500026I/ HHSP23337004T.) Rockville, MD: Agency for Healthcare Research and Quality. AHRQ Publication No. 23-0011.

CHAPTER 6

Interprofessional Partnerships

Cheri Friedrich, DNP, RN, CPNP-PC, IBCLC, FNAP, FAAN
Diane M. Schadewald, DNP, MSN, RN, WHNP-BC, FNP-BC, CNE

Great teams consist of individuals who have learned to trust each other. Over time, they have discovered each other's strengths and weaknesses, enabling them to play as a coordinated whole.

—Dr Amy Edmondson

Background

The Institute of Medicine's (IOM) 2001 report, *Crossing the Quality Chasm: A New Health System for the 21st Century*, identified four key issues contributing to poor quality of care and undesirable health outcomes: the complexity of the knowledge, skills, interventions, and treatments required to deliver care; the increase in chronic conditions; inefficient, disorganized delivery systems; and challenges to greater implementation of information technology. The report went on to outline 10 recommendations intended to improve health outcomes, one of which focuses on interprofessional collaboration. It emphasizes the need for providers and institutions to actively collaborate, exchange information, and make provisions for care coordination because the needs of any persons or population are beyond the expertise of any single health profession (IOM, 2001; Yeager, 2005). An earlier IOM report (1999), *To Err Is Human: Building a Safer Health System*, addressed issues related to patient safety and errors in health care. This report articulated interprofessional communication and collaboration as primary measures to improve quality and reduce errors. A more recent IOM report focused on *Measuring the Impact of Interprofessional Education (IPE) on Collaborative Practice and Patient Outcomes* (IOM, 2015).

The professions of nursing and medicine each recognize the need to create organizational environments that promote interprofessional collaboration; however, in many practice arenas, effective collaboration is far from reality. The American Nurses Association (ANA) report *Nursing's Agenda for Health Care Reform* (2008) placed particular emphasis on the role of collaboration in chronic disease management and patient safety. The American College of Physicians (ACP, 2009) also acknowledged that the future of healthcare delivery requires interprofessional teams that are prepared to meet the diverse, multifaceted health issues of the population. Despite this historical emphasis each discipline places on the value of collaborative work, the healthcare delivery system remains hierarchical and siloed, impeding true interprofessional collaboration. To practice in teams learners need to train in teams, and like the practice partners, education continues to be very siloed, with minimal opportunities for collaboration (Bankston & Glazer, 2013). There is a continued call for providers, policy leaders, and health systems to shift mindsets from traditional models of linear, disease-focused care to new delivery approaches. In these new, redesigned healthcare models, it is important to reconsider who should lead the team, and how to shape new relationships and intentionally engage patients in the healthcare team (Brandt, 2015). No one profession owns the process. Each discipline brings specialized skills and abilities, practices at the highest level of the individual provider's scope, assumes new roles, and participates in a shared partnership with other professionals to provide high-quality, safe, cost-effective, patient-focused care. This call to action demands that advanced practice nurses (APNs) and doctor of nursing practice (DNP)–prepared nurses in advanced nursing specialty practice perform at the highest level of clinical expertise and collaborate interprofessionally to improve patient and population health outcomes.

Little agreement exists among healthcare professionals as to the terminology used to describe interprofessional collaboration. Dictionary.com defines *collaborate* as "to work, one with another; cooperate." Leaders in the business world further describe collaboration as a concept involving "strategic alliances" or "interpersonal networks" in an effort to accomplish a project (Ring, 2005). As healthcare professionals, we can learn from successful business and management practices and use the collaborative processes of communicating, cooperating, transferring knowledge, coordinating, problem solving, and negotiating to more effectively reach a healthcare goal or outcome. The ACP (2009) suggests that collaboration involves mutual acknowledgment, understanding, and respect for the complementary roles, skills, and abilities of the interprofessional team. The Robert Wood Johnson Foundation (RWJF, 2015) in its project *Identifying and Spreading Practices to Enable Effective Interprofessional Collaboration* described effective interprofessional collaboration as the active participation of each discipline, where all disciplines work together, disciplinary contributions are respected, the patient and caregivers are engaged in the process, and leadership on the team adapts based on patient needs. Furthermore, the World Health Organization (2010) defines interprofessional collaboration as follows: "collaborative practice happens when multiple health workers from different professional backgrounds work together with patients, families, carers and communities to deliver the highest quality of care across settings" (p. 7).

Accrediting and regulatory bodies such as The Joint Commission (2015) recognize interprofessional collaboration as an essential component of the prevention of medical error. This organization's mission is to continuously improve the safety and quality of care through the measure and evaluation of outcomes data. It has targeted improved communication and collaboration among providers, staff, and patients as a means to better protect patients from harm. Improved patient safety outcomes can be additionally facilitated through collaborative efforts such as development of interdisciplinary clinical guidelines and interprofessional curricula that incorporate proven strategies of team management and collaboration processes. APNs/DNPs are well positioned to participate in and lead interprofessional collaborative teams in efforts to improve health outcomes of the individual patient or target population (American Association of Colleges of Nursing [AACN], 2021).

Effective collaborative partnerships promote quality and cost-effective care through an intentional process that allows members to exchange pertinent knowledge and ideas and subsequently engage in a practice of shared decision making. The purpose of this chapter is to generate a better understanding of interprofessional collaboration, distinguish the elements that APNs/DNPs must possess to successfully collaborate with other professionals to improve the health status of persons or groups, and provide an overview of models of interprofessional collaboration in the real world.

Selected Concepts for Nursing Practice Represented in the Domain

Concepts that are most prominent for this domain include communication, diversity, equity, inclusion, and health policy. The importance of communication is featured as the first competency for this domain and is crucial for effective interprofessional partnerships that result in high quality of care. The performance and effectiveness of a healthcare team is also dependent on the quality of communication among team members. The principles of team dynamics include the need for development of trust which stems from communication that provides a sense of belonging and safety.

Diversity, equity, and inclusion are reflected in the varying backgrounds working together as interprofessional partners. Team members must reflect on their biases toward their own profession in order to function in a partnership. The work of the team must be distributed equitably and all team members must experience a sense of inclusion as a valued member of the team.

The concept of health policy is also active in this domain, often providing the environmental structure for interprofessional partnerships' existence. Health policy is embedded within the mission and values of the interprofessional partnership. Understanding the mission and values of the team are integral to the development of trust in the performance of the interprofessional partnership.

Level II Competencies of the Domain

Communicate in a Manner That Facilitates a Partnership Approach to Patient Care Delivery

Remember not only to say the right thing in the right place, but far more difficult still, to leave unsaid the wrong thing at the tempting moment.

— **Benjamin Franklin**

The Institute for Healthcare Improvement (2017) has identified two foundational domains of effective and safe care: culture and the learning system. The Institute's white paper describes the crucial role of psychological safety needed for promoting a culture of teamwork. They recommend that all team members feel safe enough to "ask the 'stupid' question, elicit feedback without looking incompetent, be respectfully critical without appearing negative, and suggest new ideas or innovations without appearing disruptive" (p. 11).

The issue of "disruptive behavior" in the workplace has been studied in light of the connection between poor communication and adverse events (The Joint Commission, 2021). Rosenstein's (2002) qualitative study of physician–nurse relations found that almost all nurses in the study experienced some sort of "disruptive physician behavior," including verbal abuse. Maddineshat et al. (2016) repeated this work, expanding it to include disruptive behavior by both nurses and physicians. This second report concluded that there are adverse consequences to both the healthcare team and to the patients when disruptive behaviors occur (Maddineshat et al., 2016). It has also been demonstrated that nurses' satisfaction with communication positively affects healthcare delivery, leading to improved patient safety (Noviyanti et al., 2021).

All the work of interprofessional collaborations involves communication. Success or failure of the team is dependent on the effectiveness of the communication processes. Communication is a complex process of transmitting a message between a sender and receiver. The sender must effectively deliver the content, and the receiver must in turn correctly interpret or decipher the message. Many sources of error can occur within this exchange, and skilled communicators must make a concerted effort to deliver clear, consistent messages to prevent misinterpretation and loss of meaning. Communication is more than the exchange of verbal information; in fact, the majority of communication is nonverbal. The APN/DNP must be accomplished not only in the art of verbal and written communication but also in the interpretation and effective use of nonverbal communiqués such as silence, gestures, facial expressions, body language, tone of voice, and space (Sullivan, 2013).

In addition to sending congruent verbal and nonverbal messages, it is vital for APNs/DNPs to employ strategies that enhance communication within the interprofessional team setting. Determining the timing and best medium for what, how, and when to deliver a message is a necessary skill (Sullivan, 2013). Appropriate timing of key messages increases the likelihood that the message will have the desired impact on the recipient. The message may be phrased well but rejected if the intended audience is not receptive. Consider the availability and state of mind of the recipient. Is there adequate time for the discussion? Is the recipient distracted, emotionally or physically? Are other issues more pressing now? Such factors may contribute to misinterpretation or lack of objectivity regarding the communication. Reflect as to whether an alternative time, venue, or medium may provide a more appropriate means by which to deliver the message. For instance, if the message is of a sensitive, confidential matter, face-to-face communication would be preferable to an email, voicemail correspondence, or team discussion (Sullivan, 2013). In group settings, it is imperative to allow participants enough time to provide objective information and express thoughts, viewpoints, and opinions about the situation in order for meaningful collaboration to occur.

Evaluate Effectiveness of Interprofessional Communication Tools and Techniques to Support and Improve the Efficacy of Team-Based Interactions

In an interprofessional team, there are members from diverse professions, each with its own culture and language. An important first task of an interprofessional team is to discuss and understand the scope of each profession represented (Oelke et al.,

2013). It is likely there will be both overlap and diversity of function and skills among the professions. It is also important to develop a sense of shared language by reducing the use of professional jargon. Although it may be unintentional, jargon can prevent knowledge sharing, hinder communication, and promote power imbalances. Standardized tools such as SBAR (situation, background, assessment, and recommendation) developed and used by Kaiser Permanente, should be introduced in the education setting to give interprofessional learner teams the opportunity to practice discussion and problem solving regarding patient situations (Cuchna et al., 2021). SBAR is a simple, easy-to-remember, and useful tool developed to promote patient safety. It can also be used for daily huddles, which are often used for interprofessional collaboration (Agency for Healthcare Research and Quality [AHRQ], 2013). Many successful teams utilize the SBAR process as a common language means to convey critical information to be shared. It provides clear expectations as to what and how information is to be communicated among the team members and by its use promotes patient safety (Cuchna et al., 2021; RWJF, 2015). Effective communication involves the use of a common, shared language that is understood by all members of the team.

Facilitate Improvements in Interprofessional Communications of Individual Information (e.g., EHR)

Organizations and systems may pose additional obstacles to effective interprofessional communications. Outdated, limited, or unavailable technologies—such as videoconferencing, messaging, or paging systems—or lack of electronic health record interoperability between systems can significantly impair the ability of team members to communicate on a timely basis. This can be of vital importance to patient safety when attempting to communicate critical changes in patient status, medications, or lab values. The system further contributes to communication problems when the roles and responsibilities of team members are unclear. Participants may be hesitant or resistant to engage in exchanges or knowledge sharing. Clear designation of roles is of particular importance in virtual organizations and teams (i.e., electronically linked providers). In these collaborative environments, risks can be mitigated if members have a clear understanding of what is expected of each other and have a preestablished path of communication (Grabowski & Roberts, 1999) (see **Box 6-1**).

Box 6-1 Measures to Improve Communication

Maintain eye contact: Convey interest, attentiveness. (United States/Canada)
Speak concisely: Avoid jargon.
Use questions wisely: Clarify or elicit further information.
Avoid qualifiers or tags (e.g., "sort of," "kind of," "I don't know if you would be interested"): These reduce the effectiveness of your message.
Be aware of gestures, facial expressions, and posture: Send positive nonverbal signals (e.g., smiling conveys warmth, leaning forward indicates receptivity, and open-palm gestures suggest accessibility).
Avoid defensiveness.
Avoid responding emotionally: Never raise your voice, yell, or cry.

Role Model Respect for Diversity, Equity, and Inclusion in Team-Based Communications

Transformational leadership, developed first by Burns (1978), is based on the concept of empowering all team members (including the leader) to work together to achieve a shared goal. This fits with Covey's (2004) definition of leadership: "Leadership is communicating to people their worth and potential so clearly that they come to see it in themselves" (p. 98).

The transformational leader need not be in a formal position of administration, but can lead from any position within the organization and operates through an ethical and moral perspective. Transformational leaders lead with a clear vision and use coaching, inspiring, and mentoring to transform themselves, followers, and organizations (Burns, 1978; Kelly, 2012).

As healthcare teams become more global and virtual, the potential for language and cultural communication barriers increases. Misreading body language or misinterpretation of the spoken or written message often results from a lack of understanding regarding language (especially in translation) and cultural differences (Sullivan, 2013). What one group finds acceptable another may consider offensive, such as eye contact, physical touch, or the use of space. Room for misinterpretation exists in translation. Language used by Western cultures typically is direct and explicit, in which the background is not necessarily required to interpret the meaning of the message. This may differ from cultures that use indirect communication, in which the intent of the message often relies on the context in which it is used (Brett et al., 2006). APNs/DNPs and interprofessional colleagues have an obligation to increase their cultural competence and understanding of health issues and healthcare disparities to dispel any misconceptions, particularly if the team is comprised of persons from diverse cultures or if the recipient of care is from another culture.

Jargon is another "language" that can pose a barrier to understanding (Drinka & Clark, 2016; Sullivan, 2013). Unfamiliar terms can lead to confusion and error and should be avoided to prevent unfavorable outcomes. Although professional jargon may serve as a type of verbal shorthand among some group members, it can also be a form of intimidation or exclusion and contribute to an imbalance of knowledge or power within the team (Drinka & Clark, 2016). Lindeke and Block (2001) stress that collaborative teams communicate with a shared, inclusive language (i.e., "we," "our") to prevent this imbalance and promote participation of all members.

Communicate Nursing's Unique Disciplinary Knowledge to Strengthen Interprofessional Partnerships

Buresh and Gordon, in their book *From Silence to Voice: What Nurses Know and Must Communicate to the Public* (2013), suggest use of the "voice of agency" when communicating the role of nursing to others. Within the collaborative team, it is imperative that APN/DNP members clearly communicate nursing's involvement in a patient care scenario or clinical project and, more important, articulate the level of clinical judgment and rationale required for such actions. It is important and necessary to embrace the opportunity to communicate to the team the role of the APN/DNP in enhanced care delivery. This voice of agency is not boastful nor an attempt to be superior, but rather an accurate acknowledgment of the unique contributions, value added, and improved patient outcomes resulting from expert nursing care. Conversely, it may reflect the negative consequences or potential for error averted as a result of the expertise, skills, and knowledge of doctorally prepared nurses.

Buresh and Gordon (2013) went on to discuss the role that self-presentation plays in communicating information regarding the competency and credibility of the APN/DNP to team members, patients, or the public. Attire and manner of address influence the perceptions of others. What does dress communicate if Mary wears teddy bear scrubs rather than street clothes and a lab coat to a committee meeting? How might the ANP/DNP's role be valued if she is introduced as Mary from pediatrics versus Dr. Mary Jones, pediatric nurse practitioner? How are physician colleagues addressed in similar workplace encounters? Introductions using one's full name and credentials convey professionalism, respect, and credibility on par with other healthcare professional colleagues (Buresh & Gordon, 2013).

Nursing and medicine were and are often considered central players in healthcare teams; an examination of the issues related to these two professions is prudent. Nurse and physician role differences are easier to understand in light of the historical roles of gender (Price et al., 2014). In *The Essentials: Core Competencies for Professional Nursing Education*, the AACN (2021) discussed the need for interprofessional healthcare teams to function as high-performance teams. High-performance teams are those that emphasize the skills, abilities, and unique perspective of each team member. If the nurses (or other team members) remain invisible, the overall effectiveness of the team will be impaired.

In the 19th century, nurses, considered a female profession, cared for patients in hospitals, while physicians, considered a male profession, cared for patients in their offices or patients' homes. According to Reverby's *Ordered to Care: The Dilemma of American Nursing 1850–1945* (1987), whereas physicians were "welcome visitors," hospitals were run by lay boards and often staffed by "live in" nurses. That changed when medicine became more science oriented and doctors realized that hospitals were full of sick patients to whom they could apply their newly developed knowledge of science. Medicine soon controlled hospitals and defended this control with the argument that physicians owned "special knowledge" to diagnose and treat. Physicians were able to convince the public that nurses (often because of the menstrual cycle) were not trustworthy enough to manage medications or capable of obtaining the "special knowledge" that physicians had. Nurses soon became handmaidens to physicians; they needed to be "self-less, knowledgeless and virtuous" (Gordon, 2005, p. 63). Nursing education in the 20th century was designed to provide cheap labor for hospitals while educating its new workforce. Nurses came to view themselves as working for doctors, not patients. Nurses were valued for their virtue, not for their knowledge (Buresh & Gordon, 2013). Most nurse leaders either accepted this subjugated role or were unable to change it. As nursing lost power, medicine increased its social status by high-tech innovations in acute care (along with reimbursement for them). Healthcare delivery became fragmented based on physician specialty care for patients with acute care needs. Indeed, medicine dominated health care in the 20th century. The APN/DNP graduate must understand this past and work to eliminate any influence it has on the present.

To work on interprofessional teams, nurses must articulate the role they play in improving patient care. Each team member has experience and specialized knowledge that when shared, can positively improve team decisions (Kreps, 2016). The work that nurses perform is often not recognized by other healthcare professionals and reimbursement systems nor found within the nomenclature of electronic health records. Many tasks that nurses perform are difficult to quantify, such as supporting a family through a crisis. A vital responsibility of the APN/DNP (likely collaborating with other nursing PhD colleagues) is to articulate to the public, insurers, and policy makers the role that nurses play in promoting positive patient and family outcomes.

Another key factor in empowering nurses in interprofessional collaboration is the importance of role identification and clarity. In the United States, there is confusion about the education and titling of nurses. Although many states protect the title of "nurse," the public (including other healthcare professionals) continues to be confused about just who nurses are. Nurses in administration may not identify themselves as nurses, whereas some medical assistants may call themselves "nurses." Although the work that medical assistants do with patients is valuable, it is not nursing; however, it is important to recognize how the medical assistant's knowledge is different but also valuable to the healthcare team. The first step to getting our voices heard is to identify who we are and call ourselves "nurses" at all levels. It is important that as nurses work to gain visibility and voice, they remain open to listening to other voices on the team.

Provide Expert Consultation for Other Members of the Healthcare Team in One's Area of Practice

Understanding the expertise that each unique profession brings to the healthcare team will enhance consultation among team members. DNP-prepared APNs are often seen as experts in their area of study and are now offering consultations to other members of the team. This consultation with other members of the interprofessional team is recognized in the American Association of Nurse Practitioners (AANP) standards of practice (AANP, 2022).

According to Barratt and Thomas (2018) nurse practitioners are "engaging in clinical consultation activities once mostly associated with medical doctors" (p. 2). Many of these consultations occur within the specialty care environment. For successful consultations to occur there must be knowledge of interprofessional specialty competencies, clear communication, trust in each other, and a shared responsibility for a positive outcome (McDarby & Carpenter, 2019).

Demonstrate Capacity to Resolve Interprofessional Conflict

As both leaders and members of interprofessional teams, APNs/DNPs will need to develop and continue to refine skills related to conflict resolution. Conflicts are inevitable and are even vital for interprofessional team effectiveness. *Conflict* is defined in many ways but generally includes disagreement, interference, and negative emotion (Barki & Hartwick, 2001). If conflict is disruptive or dysfunctional to team efforts it can decrease communication and thus team functioning. On the other hand, conflict that is constructive leads to superior results by including the "shared pool of meaning" of all team members. According to Grenny et al. (2022), the "larger the shared pool, the smarter the decisions" (p. 26).

APNs/DNPs need to lead nurses and other professionals in techniques that promote dialogue and thus collaboration between professionals. The purposes of collaborative conflict management are to promote win–win versus win–lose solutions. The skills for conflict resolution and improving dialogue can be learned. According to Grenny et al. (2022) in their book *Crucial Conversations*, conflict resolution includes methods such as starting with the heart, making conversation safe, staying in dialogue when emotions are high, using persuasion, and promoting positive actions. Most of the skills related to collaborative conflict management are intertwined with effective communication skills and the development of emotional intelligence (EI).

Black et al. (2019) suggest that EI is integral to team cohesion, which will improve team effectiveness. Healthcare providers may be highly skilled in practicing emotionally intelligent interactions with their patients and families, but may receive little preparation in promoting emotionally intelligent, healthy communication and functioning between professionals. K. L. Miller et al. (2008) specifically explored the role of EI in nursing practice as it relates to interprofessional team functioning. In this qualitative study, the ability of the nurse to effectively collaborate on interprofessional teams was influenced by his or her degree of EI. Nurses who engaged in *esprit de corps* (significant role embracing, to the exclusion of other professionals) were considerably less able to function successfully on the team, less able to have other members appreciate nursing's contribution to patient care, and generally less engaged in team processes. These researchers support the need to address not only the cognitive aspects of interprofessional teamwork but also the emotional aspects of optimal team functioning. APN/DNP leaders versed in EI work are well suited to recognize individual and personality differences among team members and can build on them, mentor colleagues, and use EI to influence the effectiveness of the team and improve patient outcomes and satisfaction among interprofessional team members.

Chinn (2013) offered suggestions that are foundational for the transformation of conflict into solidarity and diversity. These recommendations begin before there is any conflict in a group or team and include rotating leadership, practicing critical reflection, and adopting customs to value diversity. By rotating leadership, the team members all have a stake in the outcome of the team goals and processes. When a conflict arises, involved parties can step back while other members rise up to help lead the team. Critical reflection can be accomplished by incorporating a closing time at which all team members can share their thoughts and feelings about the team process. By practicing ways to value diversity, such as developing team processes during meetings that show appreciation and value for each individual, conflict can move from violence to peaceful recognition of the diversity of alternative views.

Ineffective communication is a major obstacle in interprofessional collaboration, is directly related to quality of patient care, and contributes to adverse health outcomes (Burgener, 2020; IOM, 1999; RWJF, 2015). Some barriers that lead to communication breakdowns are specific to interactions between the sender and receiver, whereas others relate to the organizational system. Defensiveness on the part of either participant can hamper communications (Sullivan, 2013). These behaviors may result from lack of self-confidence, a fear of rejection, or perceived threat to self-image or status. Defensiveness impedes communication by displacing anger via verbal aggression or conflict avoidance. Awareness of this mechanism and developing an approach to manage it in the context of the collaborative team are necessary attributes of an effective APN/DNP leader.

Perform Effectively in Different Team Roles, Using Principles and Values of Team Dynamics

For a team to be effective, there must be a shared purpose or vision (Kouzes & Pozner, 2023). The purpose of the interprofessional healthcare team is based on improving some aspect of patient or population health outcomes. Competing needs of team members must be tabled in favor of the greater purpose. Turf wars and politicized thinking have no place in an effective interprofessional healthcare team. The leader must inspire this shared vision and elicit buy-in from each member. As Wheatley (2005) suggested, creativity is unleashed in people when they find "meaning" or purpose in "real" work. Meaningful teamwork can create synergistic solutions from members when the team has shared meaning or vision. Grenny et al. (2022) describe how free-flowing dialogue helps "fill the pool" of shared meaning. By allowing dialogue to be safe, more people can add their meaning to the "shared pool," giving the group a higher IQ. Learning to make dialogue safe is a skill that drives trust.

Integrate Evidence-Based Strategies and Processes to Improve Team Effectiveness and Outcomes

The literature of the past 2.5 decades well documents the numerous benefits of collaborative practices, including reduced error, decreased length of stays, improved health, better pain management, improved quality of life, and higher satisfaction (Brita-Rossi et al., 1996; Cowan et al., 2006; D'Amour & Oandasan, 2005; Drinka & Clark, 2016; Green & Johnson, 2015; IOM, 1999; RWJF, 2015; Yeager, 2005; Noviyanti et al., 2021). Nelson et al. (2002) and Sierchio (2003) note the additional benefits to healthcare systems of cost savings and healthy work environments. High-performing collaborative teams promote job satisfaction (D'Amour & Oandasan, 2005; Hall, et al., 2007; Sierchio, 2003; Kreps, 2016), support a positive workplace atmosphere, and provide a sense of accomplishment while valuing the unique work and contributions of team members. Additionally, Weller et al. (2014) note "interventions to improve teamwork in healthcare may be the next major advance in patient outcomes" (p. 149).

Interprofessional collaboration is not limited to efforts in the United States. In two reports to the Minister of Health in Canada, the Health Professions Regulatory Advisory Council (2008, 2009) reviewed the scope of practice of nurse practitioners and the need for interprofessional collaboration as a means to address primary care provider shortages and comprehensive, quality care. As a result, the Minister of Health supported initiatives for innovative practice models to improve access and quality of care for underserved Canadian residents. In the DNP-led project, "A Nurse Practitioner-Led Clinic in Thunder Bay" (Thibeault, 2011), a team of nurse practitioners, RNs, a social worker, a dietitian, a pharmacist, an administrator, and a community representative designed and implemented a comprehensive primary care clinic that opened its doors to Thunder Bay residents in November 2010. The clinic's primary focus is comprehensive care across the life span, with a focus on health promotion, disease prevention, and chronic care delivery. The clinic has exceeded initial goals of increasing access for unattached patients and reducing costly emergency department visits. Nurse-led clinics are expanding both in Canada and in the United States and have shown improvements in patient outcomes (White-Williams & Shirey, 2022). It is important to look to this body of evidence to determine strategies to improve team effectiveness. Nurse-led clinics have demonstrated the importance of continuous monitoring of team function and collaboration, ongoing teamwork assessment, and formal evaluation of the interprofessional team (Schentrup et al., 2019; White-Williams & Shirey, 2022; Schentrup, et al., 2019).

Evaluate the Impact of Team Dynamics and Performance on Desired Outcomes

An effective team must include the development of reciprocal trust between members. According to Kouzes and Pozner (2023), members of a high-trust team must continue to work to maintain interpersonal relationships with one another. In addition to the group mission and goals, the work of the group must also include getting to know one another. The leader or facilitator who is willing to trust others in the group enough to show vulnerability and give up control often begins a culture of trust. The leader must have enough self-confidence to be the first to be transparent; because trust is contagious, others will likely follow. Team members and leaders need to listen intently and value the unique viewpoints of others in the group. If the group fails to develop trust or to listen to and value each other, it is likely that group members will resist and sabotage the group's efforts (Thomas & Winter, 2020). Many authors describe this aspect of team leadership as leading with the heart: looking at how the heart can help shape dialogue and goals (Kouzes & Pozner, 2023; Grenny et al., 2022).

What are the stages of development that transform groups of disparate professionals into high-performance teams? Tuckman and Jensen (1977) and many others believe that teams go through stages, including forming, storming, norming, performing, and adjourning. Amos, Hu, and Herrick (2005) recommend that nurses understand these developmental stages in order to promote the development of a successful team.

Forming is the stage when the team first comes together to serve a specific purpose. Team members come into the group as individuals and get to know each other while determining the mission of the team, along with their roles and responsibilities. The development of trust is key in this stage. Lacerenza et al. (2018) suggest incorporating activities that are designed to improve team building, such as icebreakers, which can be beneficial in the short term, but research indicates that goal setting is important for the long term.

In the *storming* stage, team members have not fully developed trust, and conflict inevitably arises. Within interprofessional teams, members come from diverse disciplines and worldviews. It is highly likely that there will be a wide range of opinions and thoughts related to the issues and work of the team. It is important to face this conflict directly, however, to move on to the next stage. During the storming stage, it is vital that members learn to listen to one another with tolerance and patience (Thomas & Winter, 2020). If the team does not go through this stage successfully, differences between individuals will not be brought into the team process and will often adversely impact outcomes. Conflict resolution will be discussed at length later in this chapter.

Norming is the stage in which team members begin to develop a team identity. It is still important for the team to elicit differences of opinion in order to prevent "groupthink." During this phase, team members develop a comfort level at which they can express their ideas freely and begin to gain respect for others on the team. Constructive criticism is acceptable, and members begin to resolve problems.

In the *performing* stage, team members work together to achieve team goals. Individual and professional turf needs will be set aside for the team to be effective in its mission. At this stage, the team members also learn to be flexible in tasks and roles in order to achieve the team's goals. There should now be a sense of commitment to the tasks and goals of the team.

Finally, the stage of *adjourning* concludes the formation of a team. The team evaluates its performance and progress by reviewing whether outcomes were met. Occasionally team members may lose focus on the actual task. It can, however, be a time of celebration of accomplishments.

The following factors assist teams to progress through the stages of team development:

- Shared purpose, goal, and buy-in of members
- Reciprocal trust in team members
- Recognition and value of the unique role or skills each brings
- Functioning at the highest level of skill, ability, or practice
- Clear understanding of roles and the responsibilities of team members to meet goals
- Work culture and environment that embrace the collaborative process
- Collective cognitive responsibility and shared decision making

During the forming stage of the team (and beyond), it is vital that each team member understand his or her role and responsibilities. Role uncertainty can lead to conflict among team members and decrease team functioning (Campbell, 2014; Thomas & Winter, 2020). The leader should be certain that each team member has a clear understanding of his or her role by having the members restate their role to the team. This type of candid discussion can occur only if the team feels that open communication is safe. A clear understanding of each team member's role helps to prevent role overlap as well as tasks falling through the cracks (Thomas & Winter, 2020).

Reflect on How One's Role and Expertise Influences Team Performance

Lucas et al. (2019) talk about the importance of interprofessional reflection to build team collaboration. Learning how to use reflective practice to enhance clinical decision making and clinical judgment when working interprofessionally is important. Development and reflection on these collaborative skills before entering the "real world" can be beneficial (Lucas et al., 2019, p. 459). As collaborative skills improve among interprofessional team members, it is believed that patient outcomes will also improve.

As fundamental as it is for each team member to have a clear understanding of individual roles and responsibilities, it is also essential for high-performance teams to have a culture of shared decision making or collective cognitive responsibility. Scardamalia (2002) describes collective cognitive responsibility in terms of team members having responsibility not only for the outcome of the group but also for staying cognitively involved in the process as things unfold. She describes the functioning of a surgical team, in which members not only perform their assigned tasks but also stay involved in the entire process. The responsibility for the outcome lies not just with the leader of the surgical team but with the entire team as a whole.

A key component of shared decision making is that it usually occurs at the point of service (Davidson et al., 2022; Grad et al., 2017; Porter-O'Grady et al., 1997). Porter-O'Grady et al. state that "the point of decision making in the clinical delivery system is the place where patients and providers meet" (p. 41), which has implications for including patients as collaborators on the interprofessional team.

Teams within healthcare organizations in the 21st century will need to practice continuous reflective learning (developed by Senge, 1990) to adapt to the rapid changes taking place. Interprofessional teams can utilize the vast organizational behavior research on the significance of continuous reflective learning. Edmonson (2019) describes two types of learning behavior, "learning-what" and "learning-how" (p. 36). Learning-what is very individual, like reading current evidence, compared to learning-how which is team-based learning when suggestions are offered, knowledge is shared, and brainstorming occurs (Edmondson, 2019). Spending some time on reflection regarding team functioning will be vital to learning. Structural practices that foster team learning include providing time during each meeting for reflection, leaving the worksite for retreats, conducting "critical incident" evaluations, discussing errors and failures, using patient satisfaction surveys and interviews, and celebrating successes.

Foster Positive Team Dynamics to Strengthen Desired Outcomes

The drivers of effective interprofessional teams discussed in this chapter will evolve over time. Knowing the drivers is the first step in the development of both personal and team skills, but individual team members, and the team as a whole, will need continuous reflection to reach desired outcomes. Each leader and follower should develop habits that build over time for personal reflection and growth. Many find that reading sacred texts or poetry, listening to music, practicing yoga, praying, meditating, exercising, connecting with spiritual leaders, or being in nature allows for deep reflective thinking and learning. Covey (1991) calls this "sharpening the saw" (p. 38) and recommends that people proactively plan for daily time to renew themselves. The wholeness of each team member is vital for the best functioning of the entire team.

As an effective leader, it is imperative to foster a system of open, timely communication—whether by face-to-face communication, phone, or electronic means—to meet the desired outcomes for the project, patient, or population successfully. Fostering these characteristics is especially important when working in interprofessional teams (Drinka & Clark, 2016). Regularly practicing calming relaxation techniques and rehearsing responses before anticipated stressful encounters allows one to manage reactions in an emotionally intelligent manner. APNs/DNPs can develop these skills with regular practice, self-reflection, coaching, and feedback from colleagues and can use "EQ" (emotional intelligence quotient) (Dhani & Sharma, 2016) as a tool to gauge their performance as leaders (Black et al., 2019).

The concept of interprofessional collaborations to improve health outcomes is not new; it has been and continues to be the cornerstone of public health practice. Effective public health system collaborations are critical to protect populations from disease and injury and to promote health. Public health collaborations have involved not only vested professionals but also systems of communities, governmental agencies, nonprofit organizations, and private-sector groups to address a common goal or complex health outcome (Shahzad et al., 2019). APNs/DNPs can benefit from the experiences of public health colleagues and expand the definition of interprofessional panel collaboration. This is particularly relevant when considering potential stakeholders and in assembling the team. Successful implementation of a system or organizational improvement may require collaborations outside the typical healthcare team. The purpose or outcome of the project may dictate the need to include patient or family representation in accordance with their ability and willingness to participate, as well as professionals from information and technology, health policy, administration, governing boards, and library science.

Use Knowledge of Nursing and Other Professions to Address Healthcare Needs

The terms *interdisciplinary* and *interprofessional* are often interchanged in the literature about collaborative teams, but each has a slightly different connotation. Interprofessional collaboration, occurring "in the field," describes the interactions among individual professionals who may represent a particular discipline or branch of knowledge but who additionally bring their unique educational backgrounds, experiences, values, roles, and identities to the process (Flores-Sandoval et al., 2021, p. 61). Each professional may possess some shared or overlapping knowledge, skills, abilities, and roles with other professionals with whom he or she collaborates. Hence, the term *interprofessional* offers a broader definition than *interdisciplinary*, which is more specific to the theoretical knowledge ascribed to a particular discipline (Flores-Sandoval et al., 2021).

Given the current complexity and expense of health care, it is not possible for one group to do it all. This realization has led to the concept of having all healthcare providers work to the top of their licenses. This involves a shifting of tasks, often with each discipline giving up some tasks that can be done by another care provider more cost effectively. An example of working to the top of one's license is for APNs to take more responsibility for routine chronic and acute care and health maintenance, while physicians perform the diagnosing and treatment of more complex unstable patients, and registered nurses (RNs) assume the role of care coordinator (including pre- and post-visit planning), coach, and educator. In this example, all disciplines may need to give up some tasks to be cost effective. An exemplar of a program that utilizes healthcare providers at the top of their licenses is the DIAMOND (Depression Improvement Across Minnesota, Offering a New Direction) project (ICSI, 2014). At the center of the DIAMOND project is a case manager (typically an RN) who has 150 to 200 patients with depression in an outpatient setting. The case manager works with a consulting psychiatrist to review patients on a weekly basis (typically 2 hours per week). This has proved to be a cost-effective model that provides better depression outcomes than standard care. The challenge is to provide a payment structure that rewards this type of innovative care.

Direct Interprofessional Activities and Initiatives

APNs/DNPs are suited to serve as effective collaborative team leaders and participants not only because of the scientific knowledge, skills, and abilities related to their distinctive advanced nursing practice disciplines but also because of their comprehension of organizational and systems improvements, outcome evaluation processes, healthcare policy, and leadership. This new skillset will be critical for APNs/DNPs leading teams in the complex and ever-changing health arena.

Draye, Acker, and Zimmer (2006), in their article on the practice doctorate in nursing, propose that the educational preparation of APNs/DNPs include opportunity for the student to convene an interprofessional team. This experience allows the student to incorporate strategies to promote effective team functioning while communicating the unique contributions of nursing required for the improved health outcome.

Many APN/DNP programs are now embedding meaningful interprofessional activities in the learners' education experience in the hopes of preparing learners who are ready for collaborative practice. These experiences range from interprofessional simulations in the classroom to collaborative experiences during clinical rotations (Iverson et al., 2018; Carney et al., 2021; Stidham, 2020). In one specific example, learners were intentionally placed in an interprofessional practice environment and were given the opportunity to engage, observe, and reflect as part of the interprofessional team. Learners were clearly able to identify effective and ineffective interprofessional collaborative practice (Carney et al., 2021). Observations and experience such as this will prepare health professionals to effectively engage on collaborative interprofessional teams.

Work With Other Professions to Maintain a Climate of Mutual Learning, Respect, and Shared Values

Many healthcare practitioners indicate that they practice within an interprofessional team. Often this involves each professional addressing a particular portion of patient or population care, working *independently* and in parallel or in sequence with one another, with the physician frequently assuming the role of team leader (RWJF, 2015). Drinka and Clark (2016) reinforce the need to function *interdependently* and engage in collaborative problem solving. All too often, competition exists between roles, with each discipline holding to the belief that it is the most qualified to manage the patient or problem, thus negatively influencing the functioning of the team. In effective interprofessional teams, members recognize and value dissimilar professional perspectives and overlapping roles, put the patient first, communicate effectively, and share decision making and leadership to best meet the needs of the patient or problem at hand (Drinka & Clark, 2016; Interprofessional Education Collaborative [IPEC], 2016; RWJF, 2015). To achieve optimal health outcomes, it is essential for APNs/DNPs and other health professionals to engage in true collaborative interprofessional practices. These types of collaborative practices will be most successful when (1) the complexity of the problem is high; (2) the team shares a common goal or vision for the outcome; (3) members have distinctive roles; (4) members recognize the value of each other's positions; (5) each member offers unique contributions toward the improved patient or population outcome; and (6) systems provide mechanisms for continuous communication (ACP, 2009; Drinka & Clark, 2016; IPEC, 2016; RWJF, n.d., 2015). This model for interprofessional healthcare teams will require APNs/DNPs to have a thorough understanding of effective collaboration—in addition to a firm grounding in effective communication, team processes, and leadership—to bring forth innovative strategies to improve health and health care.

Practice Self-Assessment to Mitigate Conscious and Implicit Biases Toward Other Team Members

Implicit biases are unconscious and may exist even though not recognized as present in oneself (Mkandawire-Valhmu, 2018; Luther & Flattes, 2022). Therefore, it is important to engage in a deep self-assessment of conscious and implicit biases. Such assessment includes acknowledging the biases exist and then working on mitigating the biases. One method for mitigating is by being deliberate in counteracting them by replacing any negative associations with positive associations (Fiarman, 2016; Mkandawire-Valhmu, 2018). Another approach, beyond self-reflection, to discover personal biases is the Project Implicit Social Attitudes Test (Project Implicit, 2011). Identifying and acknowledging biases is the first step toward mitigating them and improving team function.

Additionally, preconceived assumptions and biases prevent the listener from tuning in and focusing on the content (Sullivan, 2013). This hinders the communication process because the receiver has formulated a predetermined judgment or drawn a conclusion, most likely related to conscious or implicit bias, before all the information is shared or facts validated. Effective communicators need to suspend judgments until all viewpoints are shared. Edmondson (2019) has identified how such biases also have the potential for negative impact on interprofessional team performance.

As previously stated in this chapter, the medical profession has historically been dominated by men with the nursing profession historically being dominated by women. Gender differences in style and approach to communication can pose obstacles (Sullivan, 2013). Subtle differences exist in how men and women perceive the same message. In collaborative teams, women may strive for consensus, whereas men may place emphasis on hierarchy and "leading the team." Differences exist in the use of questions and interruptions in communications. An appreciation and understanding of these dissimilarities can prepare the APN/DNP to function more effectively in interprofessional teams of mixed gender.

Foster an Environment That Supports Constructive Sharing of Multiple Perspectives and Enhances Interprofessional Learning

According to Burkhardt and Nathaniel (2019), every individual is their own moral agent and worthy of dignity and respect. Without respect, the work of the group cannot move forward; dialogue is halted. Respect among team members is vital because, as Grenny et al. (2022) note, "Respect is like air. If it goes away, it is all people can think about" (p. 138). Each member's voice must be heard and respected regardless of whether he or she is the highest educated member. To do this, team members must recognize the moral agency of each member and his or her unique skills and abilities, often based on the individual's professional skill set.

Using structure in interprofessional team dialogue may be called for as a result of the entrenched perceived power and authority of individual members and the professions they represent. Methods such as the Indian talking stick and Johari window can be used proactively to be sure that all team members feel they have a voice, are understood, and are free to share their thoughts and feelings. The concept behind the talking stick is that only the person who is holding the stick may speak. When the person finishes speaking, the stick is passed to the next speaker. That next person may not argue or disagree with the former speaker but is to restate what has been said. This process allows for all team members to be heard and feel understood (Covey, 2004).

Integrate Diversity, Equity, and Inclusion Into Team Practices

Integration of diversity, equity, and inclusion (DEI) is vital to the function of interprofessional teams and improvements in healthcare outcomes related to such teamwork. The focus on the need for equity in health care is not new. The IOM included the need to focus on health equity as an aim in their 2001 report, *Crossing the Quality Chasm: A New Health System for the 21st Century*. However, the COVID-19 pandemic heightened understanding of health inequities through the increased mortality experienced by marginalized populations (Bishop et al., 2022; Corbie et al., 2022; Nundy et al., 2022). Nundy et al. (2022) have proposed that the current quadruple aim, which expanded Berwick's triple aim of improving population health, enhancing the care experience, and reducing cost, to include wellness of health professionals, be expanded again to a quintuple aim with the fifth aim being equity. A clear focus on equity in quality improvement teams should help address the root causes of health disparities (Nundy et al., 2022).

Development of awareness of the need for integration of DEI into team practices can be fostered through a team workshop (Bishop et al., 2022). Leadership programs can also be considered to support integration of DEI. Corbie et al. (2022) evaluated their interprofessional team's experience with a Robert Wood Johnson funded equity-focused Clinical Scholars leadership program and noted significant growth in DEI competencies by their team after participation in the program. Unfortunately, this Clinical Scholars program is no longer accepting applicants; however, an eBook focused on equity centered leadership is available at the following website: https://clinicalscholarsnli.org/book/.

Manage Disagreements, Conflicts, and Challenging Conversations Among Team Members

Some of the components of a work culture that embraces collaboration are (1) providing psychological safety (Edmundson, 2019); (2) interprofessional teamwork; and (3) supportive organizational culture (Körner et al., 2015); as well as (4) physical space design that promotes collaboration, such as rooms for interdisciplinary interaction (Lindeke & Sieckert, 2005).

According to Gilbert (2006), organizations that support "upward voice" promote a culture of psychological safety. She goes on to state that "upward voice is communication directed to someone higher in the organizational hierarchy with perceived power or authority to take action on the problem or suggestion" (p. 1). Some tangible evidence of this are leaders who walk around the organization and initiate conversation, suggestion boxes placed around the organization, and an open-door policy. Individuals must have the sense that they can readily ask questions, try out new ideas and innovations, and ask for support from others.

Another way to promote psychological safety within an organization centers on employee confidence that there will not be a penalty for admitting to mistakes. Safety culture research is shifting from focusing on only the role of individuals in errors to the role of systems. Healthcare leaders have had to explore other industry successes that promote safety, such as aviation, where the focus of safety improvement is on the systems in which individuals operate (Feldman et al., 2012). The Joint Commission (TJC) has recommended a nonpunitive incident reporting system, that still includes accountability for error (also known as a Just Culture), to improve safety standards (TJC, 2017; TJC, 2021). A nonpunitive incident reporting system helps ensure that issues are brought to the forefront so that improvements can be made. It is also important to ensure a psychologically safe environment where system changes can be properly addressed (Edmonson, 2019). Since 2001, the Agency for Healthcare Research and Quality (AHRQ) (2022) has developed evaluation tools for primary care offices, nursing homes, and hospitals with questions related to psychological safety and communication. However, in many institutions individuals may still be discouraged from reporting adverse events. It should be recognized that this fear could cause a decrease in safety (AHRQ, 2022). DNPs will be required to provide leadership and recommend resources to champion the culture of both psychological and systems safety within the organizations they serve.

Promote an Environment That Advances Interprofessional Learning

There continues to be a growing body of evidence regarding the benefits of collaboration among professions in the delivery of optimal patient care; however, many healthcare professionals continue to receive their education taught primarily from a uniprofessional lens. Learners in health professional programs are often taught in both the classroom and clinical setting by faculty from the same professional background. They have little opportunity to learn about the work of other professions or participate in any shared learning experience. Spetz and Chapman (2019) describe this pattern of education as "silo" preparation, in which each discipline believes it is best qualified to care for the patient. Without a formal structure and support for learning and practicing a team approach to care delivery in the educational setting, negative attitudes, prejudices, and misunderstanding of roles can occur. This contributes to an inability to collaborate effectively and consult with other providers as practicing professionals and may lead to discipline overlap and competition rather than collaboration for delivery of care.

Currently there is minimal connection between the interprofessional experiences that occur in these "siloed" formal education settings and the health outcomes of patients. To strengthen this connection, it is clear that collaboration in practice improves when learners have the opportunity to work together in the clinical setting. The interprofessional learner continuum model (IOM, 2015) (see **Figure 6-1**), developed through a consensus report from the IOM, illustrates how the learning continuum grows from foundational education to continuing professional development, postgraduation. This model also highlights the enabling and interfering factors and the connection between health system outcomes and learning outcomes.

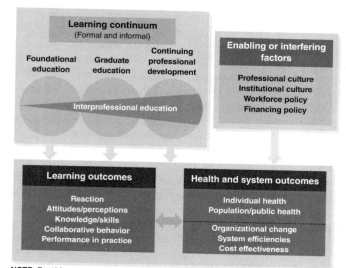

NOTE: For this model, "graduate education" encompasses any advanced formal or supervised health professions training taking place between completion of foundational education and entry into unsupervised practice.

Figure 6-1 The Interprofessional Learning Continuum (IPLC) Model

Reproduced from Institute of Medicine (IOM). (2015). Measuring the impact of interprofessional education (IPE) on collaborative practice and patient outcomes. Ch. 3, p. 29. Washington, DC: National Academies Press.Figure 3-2

The World Health Organization has been a leader in promoting interprofessional collaborative educational efforts. In 2010, a WHO study group was formed to develop a framework for interprofessional education and collaborative practice. This framework highlights the current status of interprofessional collaboration worldwide, identifies key elements of effective teams, and formulates strategies for educating future healthcare professionals in interprofessional work in an effort to build successful collaborative practices in their respective communities. Educational efforts in interprofessional collaboration have flourished in the United States over the past decade. In 2009, educational leaders in medicine, nursing, dentistry, public health, and osteopathic medicine convened and formed the Interprofessional Education Collaborative (IPEC, 2011). The purpose of IPEC is to move beyond the silos of linear profession-specific education to that of learning alongside other healthcare disciplines. IPEC developed a set of core educational competencies refined in 2016 to engage health professional learners across disciplines to learn together with the vision to enter the workforce collaborative practice ready, ultimately improving healthcare delivery. The four core IPEC competency areas are: teams and teamwork, values and ethics, communication, and roles and responsibilities. Since its initial release IPEC has expanded to include the professions of physical therapy, occupational therapy, psychology, podiatry, optometry, social work, and physician assistants. The competencies are widely endorsed by accrediting bodies and have spawned a number of interprofessional practice demonstration projects (IPEC, 2016).

In an effort to increase the ability of health professional teams to deliver optimal patient care, RWJF funded educational programs (Partnerships for Quality

Education [PQE]) designed to improve interprofessional collaboration, chronic disease management, systems-based care, and quality (RWJF, n.d.). These initiatives were developed to provide nurse practitioners, physicians, and other allied healthcare providers with educational experiences, skills, and attitudes to deliver better quality care than could be provided by any single discipline. One funded model was Collaborative Interprofessional Team Education (CITE); the objective of this program was to design collaborative clinical and educational interventions for health professional learners from medicine, nursing, social work, and pharmacy (RWJF, n.d.). The program did make some strides toward improvement in participants' understanding of and attitudes toward other professions.

Whitehead (2007) offered some insight into the challenges of engaging medical students in interprofessional educational programs. Real and perceived power, high degree of status, professional socialization, and decision-making responsibility can limit the ability of physicians to collaborate with other members of the healthcare team unless efforts to change the culture, flatten hierarchy, and share responsibility are promoted. A number of additional obstacles prevented full implementation of the CITE initiative, including differing academic schedules and a lack of faculty practicing in teams to effectively mentor and model for students (RWJF, n.d.).

The primary objective of Achieving Competence Today (ACT), another PQE initiative, was to promote interprofessional collaboration and quality improvement in the curriculum of healthcare professionals within two academic health centers (Ladden et al., 2006; RWJF, n.d.). Four disciplines worked jointly to plan and implement a quality improvement project. As a result, core competencies necessary (IPEC, 2016) for successful interprofessional teams were identified, and researchers suggested measures for incorporating these competencies into the educational preparation of future students as a means to improve quality and safety in health care.

DNP programs can build on concepts of interprofessional education by allowing and encouraging programs to use faculty from a variety of professions to prepare APN/DNP students. Interprofessional faculty can add a depth and richness to the DNP curriculum by bringing and sharing skills, knowledge, and the highest level of expertise in areas of clinical practice—whether it be business and management, pharmacy, public policy, psychology, medicine, or informatics (AACN, 2021). Educational experience related to interprofessional collaboration as a means to improve quality or promote safety should be highly visible within the DNP project.

Summary

In spite of the mandates and recommendations by the IOM, the RWJF, the ANA, and The Joint Commission, effective interprofessional collaboration has yet to be adopted in any widespread form in the United States to improve patient or population outcomes (Goldsberry, 2018). Literature from both Canada and Britain also makes recommendations for interprofessional collaboration to improve care (D'Amour & Oandasan, 2005), along with current thinking as to why healthcare systems have not adopted interprofessional healthcare teams. Some of the barriers to interprofessional collaboration include (1) gender, power, socialization, education, status, and cultural differences between professions (Brandt, 2015; Whitehead, 2007); (2) lack of a payment system and structures that reward interprofessional collaboration; (3) the misunderstanding of the scope and contribution of each profession; (4) turf protection (Grenny, et al., 2022); and the existence of individual discipline-based teams (Weller et al., 2014). The APN/DNP will need a comprehensive understanding of these barriers to provide fresh, creative thinking and leadership for the healthy development and sustainment of collaboration.

Given their advanced preparation, APNs/DNPs are well positioned to participate and lead interprofessional teams. Recognizing obstacles and developing strategies to reduce such barriers are key functions of interprofessional team leadership. All members of the interprofessional team need to have preparation and opportunities to rehearse this new approach to patient care delivery. Incorporating shared interdisciplinary learning experiences into the educational preparation of healthcare professionals provides the foundation for forming partnerships rather than competition for patient care delivery. Continued studies are needed to demonstrate the most effective educational interventions to prepare healthcare providers for successful collaborative work.

References

Agency for Healthcare Research and Quality (AHRQ). (2022). *Surveys on patient safety culture.* https://www.ahrq.gov/sops/about/patient-safety-culture.html

Agency for Healthcare Research and Quality (AHRQ). (2013). *TeamSTEPPS 2.0: Team strategies and tools to enhance patient safety* (No. 14-0001-2). https://www.ahrq.gov/sites/default/files/publications/files/pocketguide.pdf

American Association of Colleges of Nursing (AACN). (2021). *The essentials: Core competencies for professional nursing education.* Author.

American Association of Nurse Practitioners (AANP). (2022). *Standards of practice for nurse practitioners.* Author.

American College of Physicians (ACP). (2009). *Nurse practitioners in primary care* [Policy monograph]. Author.

American Nurses Association (ANA). (2008, February). *Nursing's agenda for health care reform.* Silver Spring, MD: Author.

Amos, M., Hu, J., & Herrick, C. (2005). The impact of team building on communication and job satisfaction of nursing staff. *Journal for Nurses in Staff Development, 21*(1), 10–16.

Bankston, K., & Glazer, G. (2013, November 4). Legislative: Interprofessional collaboration: What's taking so long? *OJIN: The Online Journal of Issues in Nursing, 19*(1).

Barki, H., & Hartwick, J. (2001). Interpersonal conflict and its management in information system development. *MIS Quarterly, 25*(2), 195–228.

Barratt J., & Thomas, N. (2018). Nurse practitioner consultations in primary health care: Patient, carer, and nurse practitioner qualitative interpretations of communication processes. *Primary Health Care Research & Development 20*(e42): 1–9. https://doi.org/10.1017/S14634236 18000798

Black, J., Kim, K., Rhee, S., Wang, K., & Sakchutchawan, S. (2019). Self-efficacy and emotional intelligence: Influencing team cohesion to enhance team performance. *Team Performance Management, 2*(1/2), 100–119. https://doi.org/10.1108/TPM-01-2018-0005

Bishop, K. L., Abbruzzese, L. D., Adeniran, R. K., Dunleavy, K., Maxwell, B., Oluwole-Sangoseni, O., Simon, P., Smith, S. S, & Thurston, L. A. (2022). Becoming an anti-racist interprofessional healthcare organization: Our journey. *Journal of Interprofessional Education & Practice, 27.* https://doi.org/10.1016/j.xjep.2022.100509.

Brandt, B. (2015, March). Interprofessional education and collaborative practice: Welcome to the "new" forty-year-old field. *The Advisor.*

Brett, J., Behfar, K., & Kern, M. (2006, November). Managing multicultural teams. *Harvard Business Review, 84*(11), 84–91.

Brita-Rossi, P., Adduci, D., Kaufman, J., Lipson, S. J., Totte, C., & Wasserman, K. (1996). Improving the process of care: The cost-quality value of interdisciplinary collaboration. *Journal of Nursing Care Quality, 10*(2), 10–16.

Buresh, B., & Gordon, S. (2013). *From silence to voice: What nurses know and must communicate to the public* (2nd ed.). Cornell University Press.

Burgener, A. (2020). Enhancing communication to improve patient safety and to increase patient satisfaction. *The Health Care Manager, 39*(3), 128–132. https://doi.org/10.1097/HCM.0000000 000000298

Burkhardt, M., & Nathaniel, A. K. (2019). *Ethics and issues in contemporary nursing: Nursing ethics for the 21st century.* Elsevier.

Burns, J. (1978). *Leadership.* Harper & Row.

Campbell, G. M. (2014). *Idiot's guides: Project management* (6th ed.). Alpha.

Carney, P., Guzman, C., Taylor., C., Cole, D., Hollander-Rodriquez, J., Rose, T., Wiser, E. (2021). Health professional students' observations about interprofessional collaborative practice during rural clinical rotations. *Journal of Interprofessional Education and Practice, 25.* https://doi .org/10.1016/j.xjep.2021.100471

Chinn, P. (2013). *Peace and power* (8th ed.). Jones and Bartlett.

Collaborate. (2022). In *Merriam-Webster.com.* https://www.merriam-webster.com/dictionary/collaborate

Corbie, G., Brandert, K., Noble, C. C., Henry, E., Dave, G., Berthiume, R., Green, M., & Fernandez, C. S. P. (2022). Advancing health equity through equity-centered leadership development with interprofessional healthcare teams. *Journal of General Internal Medicine, 37*(16), 4120–4129.

Covey, S. (1991). *Principle-centered leadership.* Summit Books.

Covey, S. (2004). *The eighth habit: From effectiveness to greatness.* Free Press.

Cowan, M. J., Shapiro, M., Hays, R. D., Afifi, A., Vazirani, S., Ward, C. R., & Ettner, S. L. (2006). The effect of a multidisciplinary hospitalist/physician and advanced practice nurse collaboration on hospital costs. *Journal of Nursing Administration, 36*(2), 79–85.

Cuchna, J., Manspeaker, S., & Wix, A. (2021). Promoting interprofessional communication through situation, background, assessment, and recommendation (SBAR): An educational technique. *Athletic Training Education Journal, 16*(4), 255–261. https://doi.org/10.4085/1947 -380X-19-079

D'Amour, D., & Oandasan, I. (2005). Interprofessionality as the field of interprofessional practice and interprofessional education: An emerging concept. *Journal of Interprofessional Care, 19*, 8–20.

Davidson, K. W., Mangione, C. M., Bary, M. J., Nicholson, W. K., Cabana, M. D., Caughey, A. B., Davis, E. M., Donahue, K. E., Doubeni, C. A., Kubik, M., Ogedegbe, G., Pber, L., Silverstein, M., Stevermer, J., Tseng, C., & Wong, J. B. (2022). Collaboration and shared decision-making between patients and clinicians in preventive health care decisions and US Preventive Services Task Force recommendations. *JAMA, 327*(12), 1171–1176.

Dhani, P., & Sharma, T. (2016). Emotional intelligence, history, models, and measures. *International Journal of Science Technology and Management, 5*(7), 189–201.

Draye, M. A., Acker, M., & Zimmer, P. A. (2006). The practice doctorate in nursing: Approaches to transform nurse practitioner education and practice. *Nursing Outlook, 54*(3), 123–129.

Drinka, T., & Clark, P. (2016). *Health care teamwork: Interdisciplinary practice and teaching* (2nd ed.). Praeger.

Edmonson, A. (2019). *The fearless organization: Creating psychological safety in the workplace for learning innovation and growth.* Wiley.

Feldman, H. R., Greenberg, M. J., Jaffe-Ruiz, M., McClure, M. L., McBride, A. B., Smith, T. D., & Alexander, G. R. (Eds.). (2012). Patient safety. *Nursing leadership: A concise encyclopedia* (2nd ed., pp. 297–299). Springer.

Fiarman, S. (2016). Unconscious bias: When good intentions aren't enough. *Educational Leadership, 74*(4), 10–15.

Flores-Sandoval, C., Sibbald, S., Ryan, B., Orange, J. (2021). Healthcare teams and patient-related terminology: A review of concepts and uses. *Scandinavian Journal of Caring Sciences, 35*(1), 55–66.

Gilbert, S. J. (2006). Do I dare say something? *Harvard Business School Working Knowledge.* http:// hbswk.hbs.edu/item/do-i-dare-say-something

Goldsberry, J. W. (2018). Advanced practice nurses leading the way: Interprofessional collaboration. *Nurse education today, 65*, 1–3. https://doi.org/10.1016/j.nedt.2018.02.024

Gordon, S. (2005). *Nursing against the odds*. Cornell University Press.

Grabowski, M., & Roberts, K. (1999, November). Risk mitigation in virtual organizations. *Organization Science, 10*(6), 704–721.

Grad, R., Légaré, F., Bell, N. R., Dickinson, J. A., Singh, H., Moore, A. E., Kaperavicius, D., & Kretschmer, K. L. (2017). Shared decision making in preventive health care: What it is; what it is not. *Canadian Family Physician, 63*, 682–684.

Green, B., & Johnson, C. (2015). Interprofessional collaboration in research, education, and clinical practice: Working together for a better future. *Journal of Chiropractic Education, 29*(1), 14–36.

Grenny, J., Patterson, K., McMillan, R., Switzler, A., & Gregory E. (2022). *Crucial conversations: Tools for talking when stakes are high* (3rd ed.). McGraw-Hill.

Hall, P., Weaver, L., Gravelle, D., & Thibault, H. (2007). Developing collaborative person-centered practice: A pilot project on a palliative care unit. *Journal of Interprofessional Care, 21*(1), 69–81.

Health Professions Regulatory Advisory Council. (2008). *A report to the Minister of Health and Long Term Care on the review of the scope of practice for registered nurses in the extended class (nurse practitioners)*. Toronto, Ontario, Canada: Author.

Health Professions Regulatory Advisory Council. (2009). *Critical links: Transforming and supporting patient care: A report to the Minister of Health and Long Term Care on mechanisms to facilitate and support interprofessional collaboration and a new framework for the prescribing and use of drugs by non-physician regulated health professions*. Toronto, Ontario, Canada: Author.

Institute for Clinical Systems Integration (ICSI). (2014). ICSI's DIAMOND (Depression improvement across Minnesota: Offering a new direction). https://www.icsi.org/programs/legacy-work/diamond-for-depression/

Institute for Healthcare Improvement (IHI). (2017). *Safe & Reliable Healthcare*. http://www.ihi.org/resources/Pages/IHIWhitePapers/Framework-Safe-Reliable-Effective-Care.aspx

Institute of Medicine (IOM). (1999). *To err is human: Building a safer health system*. National Academies Press.

Institute of Medicine (IOM). (2001). *Crossing the quality chasm: A new health system for the 21st century*. National Academies Press.

Institute of Medicine (IOM). (2015). *Measuring the Impact of Interprofessional Education (IPE) on Collaborative Practice and Patient Outcomes*. National Academies Press.

Interprofessional Education Collaborative Expert Panel (IPEC). (2011) *Core competencies for interprofessional collaborative practice: Report of an expert panel*. Author.

Interprofessional Education Collaborative (IPEC). (2016). *Core competencies for interprofessional collaborative practice: 2016 update*. Author. https://ipec.memberclicks.net/assets/2016-Update.pdf

Iverson, L., Bredenkamp, N., Carrico, C., Connelly, S., Hawkins, K., Monaghan, M., & Malesker, M. (2018). Development and assessment of an interprofessional education simulation to promote collaborative learning and practice. *Journal of Nursing Education, 57*(7), 426–429.

The Joint Commission. (2015). *Accreditation program: Ambulatory health care national patient safety goals*. https://www.nationaljewish.org/getattachment/professionals/education/pro-ed/Medication-Reconciliation/Overview/Resources-for-Professionals/Jt-Comm-Natl-Pt-Safety-Goals-2015.pdf.aspx

The Joint Commission (TJC). (2017). *Sentinel event alert 57: The essential role of leadership in developing a safety culture*. https://www.jointcommission.org/resources/sentinel-event/sentinel-event-alert-newsletters/sentinel-event-alert-57-the-essential-role-of-leadership-in-developing-a-safety-culture/#.Y_Np23bMI2w

The Joint Commission (TJC). (2021). *Sentinel event alert 40: Behaviors that undermine a culture of safety*. https://www.jointcommission.org/resources/sentinel-event/sentinel-event-alert-newsletters/sentinel-event-alert-issue-40-behaviors-that-undermine-a-culture-of-safety/#.Y_NpY3bMI2w

Kelly, P. (2012). *Nursing leadership and management* (3rd ed.). Cengage Learning.

Körner, M., Wirtz, M. A., Bengel, J., & Göritz, A. S. (2015). Relationship of organizational culture, teamwork and job satisfaction in interprofessional teams. *BMC Health Services Research, 15*, 243. https://doi.org/10.1186/s12913-015-0888-y

Kouzes, J., & Pozner, B. (2023). *The leadership challenge: How to make extraordinary things happen in organizations* (7th ed.). Wiley.

Kreps, G. (2016). Communication and effective interprofessional health care teams. *International Archives of Nursing and Health Care 2*(3). https://doi.org/10.23937/2469-5823/1510051

Lacerenza, C. N., Marlow, S. L., Tannenbaum, S. I., & Salas, E. (2018). Team development interventions: Evidence-based approaches for improving teamwork. *American Psychologist, 73*(4), 517–531. https://doi.org/10.1037/amp0000295

Ladden, M., Bednash, G., Stevens, D., & Moore, G. (2006). Educating interprofessional learners for quality, safety and systems improvement. *Journal of Inter-professional Care, 20*(5), 497–509.

Lindeke, L. L., & Block, D. E. (2001). Interdisciplinary collaboration in the 21st century. *Minnesota Medicine, 84*(6), 42–45.

Lindeke, L. L., & Sieckert, A. M. (2005). Nurse-physician workplace collaboration. *Online Journal of Issues in Nursing, 10*(1). http://ojin.nursingworld.org/MainMenuCategories/ANAMarketplace /ANAPeriodicals/OJIN/TableofContents/Volume102005/No1Jan05/tpc26_416011.html

Lucas, C., Power, T., Hayes, C., & Ferguson, C. (2019). Development of the RIPE-N model (reflective interprofessional education model) to enhance interprofessional collaboration. *Research in Social and Administrative Pharmacy, 15*(4), 459–464.

Luther, B. & Flattes, V. (2022). Bias and psychological safety in healthcare teams. *Orthopedic Nursing, 41*(2), 118–122.

Maddineshat, M., Rosenseein, A., Akaberi, A., & Tabatabaeichehr, M. (2016). Disruptive behaviors in an emergency department: The perspective of physicians and nurses. *Journal of Caring Science 5*(3), 241–249. https://doi.org/10.15171/jcs.2016.026

McDarby, M., & Carpenter, B. (2019). Barriers and facilitators to effective inpatient palliative care consultations: A qualitative analysis of interviews with palliative care and nonpalliative care providers. *American Journal of Hospice & Palliative Medicine, 36*(3) 191–199. https://doi.org/10 .1177/1049909118793635

Miller, K. L., Reeves, S., Zwarenstein, M., Beales, J. D., Kenaszchuk, C., & Gotlib Conn, L. (2008). Nursing emotion work and interprofessional collaboration in general medicine wards: A qualitative study. *Journal of Advanced Nursing, 64*(4), 332–343.

Mkandawire-Valhmu, L. (2018). *Cultural safety, healthcare and vulnerable populations: A critical theoretical perspective.* Routledge.

Nelson, E. C., Batalden, P. B., Huber, T. P., Mohr, J. J., Godfrey, M. M., Headrick, L. A., . . . Wasson, J. H. (2002). Microsystems in health care: Part 1. Learning from high-performing front-line clinical units. *The Joint Commission Journal on Quality Improvement, 28*(9), 472–493.

Noviyanti, L., Ahsan, A., & Sudartya, T. (2021). Exploring the relationship between nurses' communication satisfaction and patient safety culture. *Journal of Public Health Research, 10*(2). https://doi.org/10.4081/jphr.2021.2225

Nundy, S., Cooper, L. A., & Mate, K. S. (2022). The quintuple aim for health care improvement: A new imperative to advance health equity. *JAMA, 327*(6), 521–522.

Oelke, N. D., Thurston, W. E, & Arthur, N. (2013) Intersections between interprofessional practice, cultural competency and primary healthcare. *Journal of Interprofessional Care, 27*(5), 367–372.

Porter-O'Grady, T., Hawkins, M. A., & Parker, M. L. (1997). *Whole systems shared governance: Architecture for Integration.* Aspen.

Price, S., Doucet, S., & McGillis Hall, L. (2014). The historical social positioning of nursing and medicine: Implications for career choice, early socialization and interprofessional collaboration. *Journal of Interprofessional Care, 28*(2), 103–109. https://doi.org/10.3109/13561820.2013 .867839

Project Implicit (2011). *Project Implicit Social Attitudes Test.* https://implicit.harvard.edu/implicit/

Reverby, S. (1987). *Ordered to care: The dilemma of American nursing 1850–1945.* Cambridge University Press.

Ring, P. (2005, January). Collaboration. In N. Nicholson, P. G. Audia, & M. N. Pillutla, (Eds.), *Blackwell encyclopedic dictionary of organizational behavior* (2nd ed., pp. 43–44). Blackwell.

Robert Wood Johnson Foundation (RWJF). (n.d.). *Partnerships for quality education.* http://www.pqe .org/about.html

Robert Wood Johnson Foundation (RWJF). (2015). *Lessons from the field: Promising interprofessional collaboration practices* (White paper). https://www.rwjf.org/en/insights/our-research/2015/03 /lessons-from-the-field.html

Rosenstein, A. (2002). The impact of nurse-physician relationships on nurse satisfaction and retention. *American Journal of Nursing, 102*(6), 26–34.

Scardamalia, M. (2002). Collective cognitive responsibility for the advancement of knowledge. In B. Smith (Ed.), *Liberal education in a knowledge society* (pp. 67–98). Open Court.

Schentrup, D., Whalen, K., Black, E., Blue, A., Chacko, L. (2018). Building interprofessional team effectiveness in a nurse-led health center. *Journal of Interprofessional Education and Practice, 12,* 86-90.

Schentrup, D., Black, E., Blue, A., Whalen, K. (2019). Interprofessional team: Lessons learned from a nurse-led clinic. *The Journal for Nurse Practitioners, 15,* 351–355.

Senge, P. (1990). *The art and discipline of the learning organization.* Doubleday.

Shahzad, M., Upshur, R., Donnelly, P., Bharmal, A., Wei, X., Feng, P., & Brown, A. D. (2019). A population-based approach to integrated healthcare delivery: A scoping review of clinical care and public health collaboration. *BMC Public Health, 19,* 708. https://doi.org/10.1186/s12889 -019-7002-z

Sierchio, G. P. (2003). A multidisciplinary approach for improving outcomes. *Journal of Infusion Nursing, 26*(1), 34–43.

Spetz, J., & Chapman, S. A. (2019). The health workforce. In J. Knickman & B. Elbel (Eds.), *Jonas & Kovner's health care delivery in the United States* (12th ed., pp. 231–256). Springer.

Stidham, A. (2020). Developing interprofessional clinical rotation in low income areas: Learned strategies for healthcare educators. *New Directions for Teaching and Learning, 162,* 45–56. https:// doi.org/10.1002/tl.20390

Sullivan, E. J. (2013). *Becoming influential: A guide for nurses* (2nd ed.). Pearson.

Thibeault, L. (2011). *A nurse practitioner-led clinic in Thunder Bay* (Unpublished doctoral dissertation). College of St. Scholastica, Duluth, MN.

Thomas, P. L., & Winter, J. E. (2020). Synergistic interprofessional teams: Essential drivers of person-centered care. In J. L. Harris, L. Roussel, C. Dearman, & P. L. Thomas, (Eds.), *Project planning and management: A guide for nurses and interprofessional teams* (3rd ed., pp. 103–118). Jones & Bartlett Learning.

Tuckman, B. W., & Jensen, M. A. C. (1977). Stages of small-group development revisited. *Group & Organization Management, 2*(4), 419–427. https://doi.org/10.1177/105960117700200404

Weller, J., Boyd, M., & Cumin, D. (2014). Teams, tribes and patient safety: Overcoming barriers to effective teamwork in healthcare. *Postgraduate Medical Journal, 90*(1061), 149–154.

Wheatley, M. (2005). *Finding our way: Leadership for an uncertain time.* Berrett-Koehler.

Whitehead, C. (2007). The doctor dilemma in interprofessional education and care: How and why will physicians collaborate? *Medical Education, 41*(10), 1010–1016.

White-Williams, C., & Shirey, M. (2022). Taking an interprofessional collaborative practice to the next level: Strategies to promote high team performance. *Journal of Interprofessional Education and Practice, 26*(86–90), 1–8.

World Health Organization (WHO). (2010). Framework for action on interprofessional education and collaborative practice. https://apps.who.int/iris/bitstream/handle/10665/70185/WHO_HRH _HPN_10.3_eng.pdf;jsessionid=1E172DD9947906CC0DF6BBDB9DA46549?sequence=1

Yeager, S. (2005). Interdisciplinary collaboration: The heart and soul of healthcare. *Critical Care Nursing Clinics of North America, 17*(2), 143–148.

CHAPTER 7

Systems-Based Practice

Sandra Petersen, DNP, APRN, FNP-BC, GNP-BC, PMHNP-BE, FAANP
Amy Roberts, PhD, APRN, FNP, FAANP
Diane M. Schadewald, DNP, MSN, RN, WHNP-BC, FNP-BC, CNE

"All systems produce results which incentivize their continuation. Systems are living beings—by nature, they prioritize self-preservation. That's why it's important to apply data and wisdom to the design of systems."

—**Hendrith Vanlon Smith Jr.**, CEO of Mayflower-Plymouth

Introduction

No matter whom voters supported to represent them in the White House, Congress, or state legislatures, 2020 candidates at all levels promised that the issues plaguing health care would be addressed in one way or another, either by mending the current flaws or dismantling the entire system. However, in the time since the elections and the ensuing COVID-19 pandemic, legislators have been unable to agree on healthcare policy. The chasm has grown wider, so this promise has yet to be realized, especially in the fields of primary care and mental health (Cunningham et al., 2022). This makes for an unpredictable healthcare landscape in which many of the existing challenges the public faces in health care have been exacerbated.

The healthcare system in the United States is multi-faceted and multilayered. This multifaceted, multilayered healthcare system is prone to unintended consequences when faced with change. That is, even apparently "inconsequential" changes in healthcare systems at any level will almost always produce unintended consequences. It is predictable that unintended consequences will likely emerge, but what those consequences will be and whether they will be beneficial or destructive are often unpredictable at best and could, at worst, result in unintended harm. Margaret Wheatley (1992) espoused an interesting perspective on unintended consequences, seeing them as unintended opportunities to find new ways of looking at things and redesigning poor processes. In her book *Turning to One Another: Simple Conversations to Restore Hope to the Future*, written in 2002, Wheatley notes that failures within systems are the signal that more connections need to be made within the organization; she contends that the solution lies within untapped conversations and undiscovered connections.

Advanced practice nurses (APNs) have become increasingly elevated to a station of independent practice, autonomy, flexibility, and leadership to meet system failures. Those in advanced nursing practice specialties who are prepared at the doctor of nursing practice (DNP) level also are often called on to address system failures. As legislators struggle to make sense of a dwindling budget and an ever-expanding deficit, coupled with an outcry for increased access to care for all, the National Academy of Medicine (NAM, formerly the Institute of Medicine [IOM]), The Joint Commission (TJC), and other authorities, along with the American Association of Colleges of Nursing (AACN), have called for recasting health professions education and development to meet the needs of the overburdened healthcare delivery system in the United States while maintaining quality, safety, and ethical practice. Advanced-level nursing education is answering that call by moving to prepare transformational leaders well versed in evidence-based practice and systems design to shape the evolution of health care.

Selected Concepts for Nursing Practice Represented in the Domain

The AACN *Essentials* (2021) concepts that can be considered as most prominent for this domain are communication, evidence-based practice, diversity, equity, inclusion, health policy, and social determinants of health. Communication is the "glue" that holds any system together and promotes collaboration of all individuals of varied disciplines functioning within the system to promote effective and efficient operation. The importance of communication is underscored as a competency for this domain and is critical to the achievement of optimal outcomes and high quality of care within any system. The performance and effectiveness of a healthcare team is also dependent on the quality of communication among team members (Drinka & Clark, 2016). Communication is an integral part of systems design and function.

Evidence-based practice (EBP) is prominent as the most successful advocates for any systems change are strong proponents of EBP. That is, as advanced practice leaders work at addressing system issues, they must use EBP to be able to correctly define the underlying clinical issues, appraise the appropriate body of evidence, and practically apply it within the targeted system in order to achieve the anticipated outcomes. Today's healthcare environment demands translational scientists who are well versed in the EBP process and its swift application to healthcare issues such as access to care and cost-effectiveness (Tucker & Gallagher-Ford, 2019). APNs/DNPs must be able to make data-driven decisions backed by vetted research so they may predictably and systematically effect change.

Systems thinking inherently supports the concept of diversity, equity, and inclusion. Gorman (2023) posits that when thinking systematically one will ask better questions to get to the heart of an issue before jumping to conclusions. Goodman (2023) describes systems thinking as moving from observing events/data to identifying patterns over time that bring to the surface structures that impact the events.

Systems must be crafted or re-tooled to address health care for those in *all* walks of life—not just those of means. The burden of health care requires a systems thinking approach—one that reaches across all professions and all cultures when developing health policy.

Social determinants of health (SDOH) is a fairly new concept in health care. As defined by the World Health Organization (WHO, n.d.), SDOH, which transcend well beyond healthcare proper, are "the conditions in which people are born, grow, live, work and age, and the wider set of forces and systems shaping the conditions of daily life" (para 1). SDOH are shaped by the distribution of money, power, and resources at global, national, and local levels. The SDOH also can determine access to and quality of medical care. Magnan (2017) maintains that "clinicians, given their intuitive recognition that health outcomes are affected by patients' conditions outside the clinical walls (i.e., SDOH) may raise several concerns about involvement in the SDOH" (para 2). First, there is concern of a lack of expertise in the area of SDOH. Additionally, some are worried about an already overburdened healthcare system and how to manage efforts to ameliorate adverse impacts of SDOH. Lastly, they wonder if there is an adequate evidence base that addressing SDOH is effective. However, some providers consider that there is enough evidence to include efforts to address SDOH and that healthcare systems need to be concerned about population health (Magnan, 2017). The AACN (2021) includes SDOH as one of the eight concepts to be integrated in nursing curriculums at all levels and the most recent NAM report on the future of nursing also identifies that the SDOH are mandatory to address to improve the health of the nation (NAM, 2021).

Level II Competencies of the Domain

Apply Knowledge of Systems to Work Effectively Across the Continuum of Care

The AACN (2021) essentials statement on systems-based practice noted, "Understanding of systems-based practice is foundational to the delivery of quality care and incorporates key concepts of organizational structure, including relationships among macro-, meso-, and microsystems across healthcare settings" (p. 44). Microsystems of health care are the people, equipment, and data at the level of direct patient care. Microsystems have both clinical and business aims that support linkages to processes of care, shared information, and the production of services and care that may be measured and leveraged as performance outcomes. A mesosystem consists of two or more microsystems. These microsystems and mesosystems are subsystems within macrosystems such as hospitals, nursing homes, and clinics.

Health and well-being are promoted when primary care teams partner with patients and provide care coordination to mitigate risks and promote optimal health across the continuum of care. Identification of patients for care coordination is typically based on claim-driven risk assessments. Evidence shows that a systems approach incorporating SDOH decreases risk for adverse health outcomes but is generally lacking in today's health care. Missed opportunities for care coordination contribute to increased healthcare costs, poorer health outcomes, and reduced patient well-being.

Addressing the gap of risk-informed care coordination across the continuum of care includes addressing SDOH through a systems thinking approach. Singer and Porta (2022) clearly illustrated the verity of this when they conducted a non-randomized care coordination quality improvement project at a community health center. Criteria for inclusion was the presence of risk attribution score and completion of an SDOH questionnaire. Care coordination was offered to 540 patients. Of these 540 patients, 216 accepted at least one month of care coordination; the other 324 patients maintained usual care. Descriptive statistics distinguished patient demographics, frequency of care coordination contact, and specific SDOH insecurities for both groups. Patients who received care coordination noted improvement in level of anxiety (well-being) ($t = 4.051$; $p < 0.000$)], food access ($t = 4.662$; $p < 0.000$) and housing ($t = 2.203$; $p = 0.008$)] that was significantly different from those in the non-intervention group.

As early as 2002 in *The Ingenuity Gap: Facing the Economic, Environmental, and Other Challenges of an Increasingly Complex and Unpredictable Future,* author Homer-Dixon presented evidence that the demand for ingenuity arising from the ever-increasing complexity of our world is far outstripping our capacity. In the past we have been able to find solutions—and, in Homer-Dixon's words, "throw huge amounts of energy at our problems"—to keep our ever-expanding complex systems glued together. As a result, we will almost certainly find it necessary to accept some large breakdowns in human and natural systems and to develop radical new ways of running things. Homer-Dixon explains that human capacity to deal with the complexity of what lies ahead may not be sufficient because of cognitive characteristics of humans and the self-reinforcing nature of our economic systems.

When Homer-Dixon refers to "cognitive characteristics," he underscores the fact that societies adapt easily to small-scale, incremental change. It is this slow evolution that makes it possible for humanity to face each day and not feel as though our foundations have been shaken. It is part of self-preservation. And yet, according to Homer-Dixon, this human capacity is a real handicap when it comes to dealing with "slow-creep" problems. Humans don't perceive the change, and so slow-creep problems may slow-creep for a while, but then all of a sudden there's a non-linear shift and a crisis.

How well this describes our current crisis in health care and the need for APNs/DNPs to be competent and well versed in systems thinking across the continuum of care and steeped in competency with regard to essential core skills such as data analytics can be argued. At the turn of the century, when the term *big data* was first acknowledged, it was often defined by the "three V's" of volume, velocity, and variety, and consisted of massive amounts of data in widely varying file formats. The APN/DNP leader must be able to discern what metrics are useful to the organization with regard to internal data and to utilize it quickly to make effective decisions.

Nursing innovators within the healthcare industry have continued to push for more education around the introduction of healthcare analytics and the critical part it plays not only in quality improvement but also in the implementation of best practices throughout the organization in both the clinical and leadership realms. In part, clinical documentation improvement initiatives, such as integration of electronic medical records (EMRs) that share data across systems, which encourage meaningful outcomes have played a vital role in the acceptance of new technology across the continuum of care.

Participate in Organizational Strategic Planning

The advanced practice nurse must be able to discern issues quickly and effectively and contribute to effective and efficient strategic planning, evidence-based implementation, and system redesign. This phenomenon is perhaps best described by Senge (2006) in *The Fifth Discipline* when he conveys the development of the *mental model* as, "turning the mirror inward; learning to unearth our internal pictures of the world, to bring them to the surface and hold them rigorously to scrutiny. It also includes the ability to carry on 'learningful' conversations that balance inquiry and advocacy, where people expose their own thinking effectively and make that thinking open to the influence of others" (pp. 8-9).

The evolution of the APN/DNP leader, and, indeed, leaders within all disciplines, is the by-product of concerted efforts to align personal behavior with values and to learn how to listen and appreciate others' talents, abilities, and insights. Without this diligent effort launched toward the development of the capacity to lead, the lack of personal charisma, personal mastery, information sharing, and mental mastery renders one ineffective in the pursuit of shared vision and the transformational leadership so vital to the survival of health care in the future.

Once personal mastery is achieved, however, one must transcend the traditional activity of management as most of us know it to wielding power within a system and participating in organizational strategic planning. This endeavor encompasses not only the balancing of structures within an organization or system but also embodies shared vision and empowerment, inducing people and resources to migrate from the current state to the desired state while seeking their own personal mastery. While this sounds very noble, the reality is that as the *current state* approaches the *desired state*, promotion of the activity and motivation typically decline; this goes on until someone takes notice and raises the red flag of organizational panic and reactive decision making (which rarely produces good results). So, the task of the leader becomes sustaining the effort long enough to close the gap between what *was* and the present, while avoiding panic, reactivity, and ultimately, disaster.

Participate in System-Wide Initiatives That Improve Care Delivery and/or Outcomes

The development of the ANP/DNP to be a strategic systems thinker and visionary for health care lies largely within the profession's commitment to lifelong learning and the realization that people and organizations do not exist as islands unto themselves, but rather as part of a larger network, web, or matrix of systems that all function more or less independently yet *inter*dependently to improve care delivery and outcomes through shared system-wide initiatives. One must realize the necessity of developing a dedication to disrupting the system as we know it, while at the same time retaining flexibility, balance, connectivity and a sense of social intelligence and responsibility across the larger realm of health care. The ANP/DNP can do so by participating in system-wide initiatives to improve care.

Additionally, evidence-based practice supports the utilization of the body of evidence to address system-wide issues and ensure the provision of high-quality care. Such highly effective systems inevitably promote access to care through inclusion, equity, and diversity—systems in which all are valued for their unique needs and contributions to the larger system.

Analyze System-Wide Processes to Optimize Outcomes

Senge (2006) noted that there are multiple levels of explanation in any complex situation, including the analysis of system-wide processes, as leaders seek to optimize outcomes. These include *reactive*, *responsive*, and *generative* explanations for system failures. As leaders begin to look for patterns of events, explanations related to poor outcomes typically "lay blame" or result in a reactive stance to problems. To further explore this concept, let's take the example of the patient who has a fall. A reactive stance might be to immediately restrain the patient in response to that event. We assume in this instance that, because the patient can move and has fallen, we must keep him from moving. As one can quickly see, the reactive stance leaves no room for discussions about why the fall occurred or what could be done to improve the patient's fall risk, if possible. There are no discussions regarding quality of life for the patient, and, certainly, there are no explorations of root cause or how falls (or even such a narrow approach) might affect other patients. This type of explanation tied to a single event is the most likely type of explanation to reinforce the flaws within a reactive system, maintaining the status quo. Little room is left for problem solving or quality improvement.

Approaching this same scenario from a *responsive* stance, we might look at patterns of behavior, asking if the patient has incurred falls in the past. And, if he had multiple falls, at what times did the falls occur? We might also look at fall risk and prevention for this patient and, ultimately, for other patients within the system, tracking and trending in response. The responsive approach focuses on explaining patterns of behavior and envisioning long-term results and trends that can benefit the larger system. The responsive approach allows for quality improvement in response to data gathered through tracking and trending within a system, thus breaking the hold of reactivity and the "short-term fix."

Generative explanation, the most powerful of the three approaches, focuses on finding the root cause(s) for patterns of behavior. In the case of the falling patient, for example, we might look at the types of situations in which the falls occur. We could ask, "Under what circumstances did the falls occur?" We could consider falls occurring during transfers; perhaps staff are not using appropriate transfer techniques or appropriate equipment. Perhaps there are critical steps missing from transfer procedures that result in the failure of the process. It is at this level of explanation that patterns of behavior can actually be *changed*—not just reacted to or responded to, but actually *changed*!

Design Policies to Impact Health Equity and Structural Racism Within Systems, Communities, and Populations

Designing policy to address the concerns of health equity and structural racism must become the focus of APNs/DNPs with a worldview (Porter et al., 2020). We must look across the globe, appraising the evidence fully and effectively, to find policy solutions that lead to the implementation and maintenance of systems that address the dire need for healthcare solutions that present with an eye to the future for meeting healthcare concerns of generations to come.

Structural racism within systems needs to be addressed through system-wide policies that support health equity. One of the first steps in creating such policies could be to establish system goals that include diversity, equity, and inclusion as well as identification of goals to address racial disparities noted in the communities and populations the system serves (Cunningham et al., 2022). Application of health equity frameworks, such as the *American Academy of Nursing Social Determinants of Health for Nursing Action* (Kuehnert et al., 2022) or the *Health Equity Measurement Framework* (Dover & Belon, 2019) for example, in addressing structural racism is another policy approach that can be considered (Cunningham et al., 2022).

It may be tempting to believe the notion that current healthcare policy is beyond repair. Yet, a look back reveals countless metamorphoses of an externally different, but eternally fundamentally flawed healthcare entity (Winasti et al., 2023). Thus, transformational ANPs/DNPs can drive the avoidance of this abysmal cycle through full dissection and understanding of the underlying structure and root cause analysis of the dysfunction. Is it indeed acceptable to deny people health care based on their ability to pay? Or is health care a basic need that should be provided to every American as a matter of course? If the latter is the solution, we must ensure that the ANP/DNP is well armed to overcome the remarkably complex inertia of the American healthcare system and spearhead policy to drive the effort to create a society in which health care is available to all.

Incorporate Consideration of Cost-Effectiveness of Care

The consideration of cost-effectiveness of care inherently engenders the insecurity of health care. As the outcry for a single-payer source for care grows louder, few solutions have proven effective. Health spending is projected to continue to grow and be 19.7% of the gross domestic product (GDP) by 2028 (Keehan et al., 2020). As these concerning developments unfold, the APN/DNP leader must be prepared to look at the provision of care to the masses, while optimizing outcomes and supporting value-based care. The focus for the future must be on cost-effective provision of care without sacrificing quality (Schneider et al., 2021).

Analyze Relevant Internal and External Factors That Drive Healthcare Costs and Reimbursement

In 2017, the Senate made an attempt to replace the Affordable Care Act (ACA). The attempt was unsuccessful. Also that year, the Commonwealth Fund released an evaluation of the ailing U.S. healthcare system and once again, the think tank found the U.S. medical system performed the worst among 11 similar countries, all while spending more. The United States performed poorly on measures of affordability, access, health outcomes, and equality between the rich and poor. The United Kingdom ranked first in comparison with other countries included in the comparison such as Australia, Switzerland, Sweden, the Netherlands, New Zealand, Norway, Germany, Canada, and France. Analysis continually underscored the fact that America spends more on health care than any other country in the world, yet the nation still suffers from rampant lack of insurance, poor outcomes, inconsistency in quality, and excessive administrative waste (Schneider et al, 2017).

An external factor that impacts reimbursement is the presence or absence of insurance or other designated payer. Any erosion of employer-based coverage in the last few years has been partially offset by increased enrollment in Medicaid, ACA's marketplace insurance plans, and lower-cost insurance products that are designed to provide a safety net for the lowest-income Americans. According to the Kaiser Family Foundation (KFF) (2023) only 10 states still have not adopted Medicaid expansion in which those up to 138% of the federal poverty level are eligible for Medicaid. In these non-expansion states Medicaid has been the subject of relentless funding cuts. Nationally, Medicaid is also at risk from Congressional representatives who are ideologically opposed to welfare programs. Healthcare systems and providers look to the federal government to reimburse about two-thirds of the costs stemming from those who are uninsured (uncompensated care) with the other one-third of reimbursement for uncompensated care being sought from state and local governments if the individual can't pay for the care on their own (Coughlin et al., 2021). That is, healthcare systems do seek reimbursement in some form for services provided. However, according to the American Hospital Association (AHA), systems have reported that any reimbursement they receive for uncompensated care is only equivalent to about 10 cents per dollar of cost (AHA, 2017).

Schneider et al. (2021), in a later Commonwealth report, noted that the United States continues to spend more on health care than other countries and continues to have some of the poorest outcomes for the most vulnerable individuals. Care delivery can be described as "too little, too late" when one reviews the data in the 2021 Commonwealth report. Many process measures focus on the care available to people who actually have access to care; but for many vulnerable people, who are often the most sick, the most vulnerable, and not reflected in these measures, outcomes are very poor. For example, a measure of care quality for hospitalized patients focuses on those who had access to hospital care in the first place and does not reflect the number who died before reaching a hospital. Schneider et al. (2021) note that it is possible to deliver high-quality care to the population that has access to care and that can afford such care, while delivering poor-quality care to the smaller share of the population that lacks those means. The result may be an average level of performance overall, but a health system that nevertheless inadequately serves the most vulnerable of patients.

Design Practices That Enhance Value, Access, Quality, and Cost-Effectiveness

The increasing scrutiny on both the quality and the cost of health care continues to demand value-driven health care that promotes access, quality, and cost-effectiveness. As the U.S. healthcare system grapples to reshape itself, APN/DNP leaders will continually be challenged to balance high-quality care with return on investment and optimal cost-effectiveness. Newer payment models, such as accountable care organizations (ACOs), accountable health communities (AHCs), and value-based payment (VBP), provide healthcare organizations the flexibility to pursue these goals. The term *cost-effective* does not mean *never* spending any money or resources to diagnose, treat, and manage diseases, but it does require evidence-based, data-driven decisions on how, when, and where to invest resources. The "shotgun" approach—ordering an entire battery of tests to rule out a multitude of diagnoses, for example, does not generate cost-effective or even high-quality care. Targeting the right tests at the right time to safely diagnose conditions without needless waste requires critical thinking, asking the right questions to get the right information, and providing easily accessible decision-making support and multidisciplinary teamwork.

Advocate for Healthcare Economic Policies and Regulations to Enhance Value, Quality, and Cost-Effectiveness

Delivering cost-effective care in a complex system-based endeavor means coordinating lots of moving parts. Success means recognizing the relationship between the moving parts and consistently identifying opportunities for improvement. The APN/DNP must be able to demonstrate how communication, multidisciplinary teamwork, and measurement can be incorporated into successful systems to deliver cost-effective care. Nurse leaders across the country in a wide variety of organizations, both nonprofit and for-profit are aware of the need to provide leadership in the development of healthcare economic policies to enhance value, quality, equity, and cost-effectiveness.

One such organization is the National Health Council (NHC) which is made up of more than 150 member organizations from all sectors. It is a nonprofit association of health organizations. Its membership includes leading patient advocacy groups such as the American Cancer Society, the American Heart Association, the American Diabetes Association, and the Alzheimer's Association. The NHC is committed to promoting a society in which all people have equitable access to high-quality health care designed around the health outcomes most important to patients (NHC, n.d.).

NHC's Reducing Health Care Costs (HCC) Initiative, launched in 2016 and reviewed every 5 years, takes a hard look at a variety of policy proposals designed to curb healthcare costs and established policy recommendations. The HCC Initiative prioritized patient-centered policies that contribute to equitable healthcare access. Under the most recent analysis, the NHC screened a diverse set of policy proposals against a patient-centered framework using four driving principles. The four driving principles are that the policy must:

- Promote high-value care;
- Stimulate research and competition for healthcare products and services;
- Curb costs responsibly; and
- Ensure health equity.

Once policies are screened, the NHC's focus is to develop a set of policy recommendations that: (1) align with the above principles, (2) demonstrate the potential to result in cost savings for patients and/or the healthcare system, and (3) have a reasonable likelihood of gaining sufficient political support. Across its various programs and policy priorities, the NHC is committed to increasing access to sustainable, affordable, high-value care. As such, for each policy the NHC recommends, the savings achieved through policy reforms must be directly reinvested to benefit patients and the systems that support them. While many of the NHC's recommendations would include upfront costs to the government or healthcare system, it is felt that these investments are crucial to ultimately reduce costs patients pay to manage their chronic conditions. The NHC strongly opposes policies that achieve savings if they negatively impact patient safety, quality, or access to existing or future care. Additionally, it is important that any efforts designed to reduce healthcare costs must be predicated on promotion of value as defined by the patient. The NHC actively supports efforts to better incorporate patients into the ongoing debate on defining value in health care (NHC, September 2021).

Formulate, Document, and Disseminate the Return on Investment for Improvement Initiatives Collaboratively With an Interdisciplinary Team

Health systems primarily concentrate performance improvement initiatives around critical areas, including clinical outcomes, patient experiences, and organizational costs. While this high-value improvement approach has the potential for significant impact, its long-term success relies on strategic execution and return on investment (ROI) to continually fund the efforts. Unfortunately, performance improvement efforts often fall short of their desired results when organizations approach improvement as a series of one-off projects; effective and sustainable performance improvement requires development and performance of structured initiatives within an ongoing performance infrastructure and program.

In health care, determination of ROI needs to consider the value of any improvement initiative in regard to benefits to both patients and the organization. The APN/DNP needs to understand that benefits need to be considered overall and not necessarily only as they relate to an individual improvement initiative. Thusini and colleagues (2022) have proposed a conceptual framework based on a systematic review that can be used to consider both unintended and intended benefits in determining ROI. The proposed conceptual framework includes organizational performance, organizational development, external outcome, and unintended outcomes (both positive and negative).

The development of a system infrastructure for ongoing performance improvement initiatives is necessary for the APN/DNP leader to formulate, document, and disseminate the return on investment for improvement activities across disciplines. An analytics system to measure improvement, whether clinical, financial, or operational facilitates quick, accessible data sharing. An adoption system must be crafted to create permanent cross-functional workgroup teams that focus on identifying, deploying, and monitoring the effectiveness of quality improvements. Interdisciplinary teams must then be formulated to analyze the data and discover patterns that lead to insights and progress through different levels of healthcare analytics. Lastly, a best-practice system, driven by appraisal of the evidence and appropriate internal data, must be utilized to deploy a data-driven, evidence-based approach to implementing best practices.

Recommend System-Wide Strategies That Improve Cost-Effectiveness Considering Structure, Leadership, and Workforce Needs

Most healthcare finance experts recommend the expedited adoption of advanced value-based payment models. Value-based payment in Medicare has grown, but most value-based payments remain anchored in a fee-for-service structure. Exploring value-based insurance design may further assist promotion of cost-effectiveness (Dzau et al., 2017). Another approach could be expanding on existing pilot programs in Medicare Advantage. The CMS Administrator could use the authority of the Center for Medicare and Medicaid Innovation (CMMI) to reduce cost sharing for cost-effective, high-value services in traditional Medicare and Medicare Advantage. APNs/DNPs can advocate for these strategies to be pursued by membership and leadership in professional nursing organizations.

In addition, Medicare Advantage could be strengthened. More than a third of Medicare beneficiaries are now enrolled in Medicare Advantage plans. The program benefits from strong bipartisan support and has catalyzed the adoption of advanced value-based payment models. Strengthening the program could position it to serve as a foundation for coverage expansion, increasing flexibility for Medicare Advantage plans to design new benefit packages while incentivizing healthy choices, and redistributing funding to reduce disparities and improve equity. As voluntary enrollment in Medicare Advantage begins to outpace that in traditional Medicare in some regions, the administrator will need to reconsider financial models that determine benchmark payments as well. Sustainable risk adjustment for Medicare Advantage plans must also be considered.

Stabilizing independent primary care providers may be a key piece to meeting workforce needs. COVID-19 has placed significant financial strain on independent primary care providers. This strain is especially troubling, as these clinicians provide critical access to health care for much of the U.S. population and have been uniquely successful at delivering value-based care. Taking action to stabilize finances for independent primary care providers by providing prepayment to offset lost fee-for-service revenue as a path to population-based payment may be helpful.

Evaluate Health Policies Based on an Ethical Framework Considering Cost-Effectiveness, Health Equity, and Care Outcomes

It has been estimated that approximately one quarter of annual healthcare spending in the United States is unnecessary and wasteful. This amounts to almost nine and one-half billion dollars that could be saved annually and which, if saved, could reduce increasing U.S. healthcare expenditures (Shrank et al., 2019). A number of strategies have been proposed to decrease unnecessary spending, such as driving policy to focus on preventive care, eliminating unnecessary tests and procedures, and controlling costs of prescription drugs. Healthcare system instability and vital resource depletion in crises, such as the recent COVID-19 pandemic, make it necessary to evaluate and create policies that promote the allocation of limited healthcare resources to maximize overall population health benefits while minimizing risk and harm. Resource allocation decisions about which interventions to invest in are fraught with complexity and uncertainty. Therefore, analytic models that drive decision making must be used to synthesize evidence from multiple sources and help inform decisions that must be made while navigating the ethical challenges of such complexity.

Healthcare economic decision models aim to quantify clinical and economic benefits and harms associated with interventions to help policy makers and organizational leaders forecast prospective costs and manage likely trade-offs (Keehan et al., 2020). In 1977, for example, Weinstein and Stason proposed that resource allocation should be based on indices of the costs relative to anticipated benefits. Although vast improvements have occurred in medicine and in our ability to analyze data and conduct health economic analyses since that time, little attention has been given to the ethical and social dimensions of using economic decision models and analyses in health care. As a result, APN/DNP leaders must consider how economic modeling can motivate good decision making about improving health systems performance, clinical practice, and patients' healthcare experiences.

Decision makers in health care often face challenging questions. Shrank and colleagues (2021) discussed an approach that involves conducting a cost-effectiveness analysis (CEA) that explicitly quantifies the relative costs and benefits of alternative interventions. This approach seeks to highlight the potential trade-offs and inform discussions of whether the additional resources demanded by an intervention (over an alternative) are worth the additional gain in health outcomes produced by it.

A CEA expresses this "trade-off" using a metric called the incremental cost-effectiveness ratio (ICER). The ICER can be regarded as a "price tag" for an additional unit of health gained through any given intervention. A smaller ratio, like a low price, is considered optimal because it implies that an intervention can produce an incrementally superior health gain at a lower cost. ICERs are often compared to a range of predetermined threshold values that reflect the willingness to pay for an additional unit of health gain from the perspective taken. For example, the willingness-to-pay threshold usually ranges from $100,000 to $150,000 per additional unit of health gain measured by quality-adjusted life-years (QALYs) in the United States. It implies that if the ICER for the intervention lies below the chosen threshold, it is deemed cost-effective.

Since the 1990s, the number of CEAs has grown substantially, covering a wide range of diseases and interventions across the globe. In the United States and abroad, many public and private organizations have formally adopted a health technology assessment (HTA) process that uses ICERs to inform reimbursement decisions, benefit designs, and price negotiations. While many nations around the world have developed formal HTA processes, the United States has categorically refused to do so. The one exception in the United States is for the use of cost-effectiveness evidence by the Centers for Disease Control and Prevention's Advisory Committee on Immunization Practices to inform national recommendations on immunization policy. As healthcare leaders have voiced a growing concern about inefficient healthcare spending, the incorporation of value as the measure of health gain into healthcare system decisions and practice guidelines has become more prevalent (Shrank et al., 2021).

Nevertheless, the use of cost-effectiveness evidence to inform healthcare decisions faces challenges and opposition from policy makers, the drug industry, and patient advocates. Shrank and colleagues (2021) noted that the fragmented health care system with its various key players diminishes the incentive to consider the broader implication of allocation of resources. Some resistance to CEA pertains to Americans' aversion to rationing and unwillingness to accept limits in the delivery of health care. Methodological challenges, often based on poor appraisal of the evidence or failure to adhere to evidence-based principles, have resulted in CEA's limited applicability in assessing effectiveness and have contributed to the mistrust of results. Although how well and how widely CEA will be accepted and implemented in the United States remains to be seen, CEA methods have been substantially improved to meet some of these challenges.

Variations among standards of care, evidence-based care, and value-based care may complicate ethical and economic decision modeling guidance when designing and implementing models and interpreting results generated by those models. Model structures, data sources, and assumptions, for example, influence the validity of what clinicians and organizational leaders can learn from them and are, therefore, ethically, socially, and culturally relevant. APN/DNP leaders must drive transparency in modeling, thereby motivating equity, cost-effectiveness, good resource stewardship, and value (NAM, 2021).

Optimize System Effectiveness Through Application of Innovation and Evidence-Based Practice

In order to optimize system effectiveness and consider application of innovation and evidence-based practice to improve system effectiveness it would be helpful for the ANP/DNP to be knowledgeable about theories that describe systems thinking as applied to organizations. In *The Fifth Discipline*, Peter Senge (2006) describes five basic disciplines that support shared vision and empowerment, but places systems thinking as the primary discipline. He calls it "the fifth discipline" because it is the conceptual cornerstone that underlies all of the other learning disciplines. As he points out, all are concerned with a shift of mind from seeing parts to seeing wholes, from seeing people as helpless reactors to seeing them as active participants in shaping their reality, from reacting to the present to creating the future.

When it comes to operationalizing and applying systems thinking concepts within the learning organizations or across many organizations, C. West Churchman (1913–2004), a pragmatic philosopher with a deep concern for the welfare of humanity, laid the groundwork for the most practical approach to creatively shaping the future. In the 1950s he worked with R. L. Ackoff and E. L. Arnoff to develop and describe the philosophical and methodological aspects of operations research, designed as an interdisciplinary approach to "real-world problem solving" (Ulrich, 2016).

Early in 1971, Churchman adapted the design of what he called *inquiring systems*—systems capable of facilitating learning and organizational change. The purpose of these inquiring systems is to create knowledge, thereby "creating the capability of choosing the right means for one's desired ends" (Churchman, 1971, p. 200). Churchman's Model for the Design of Inquiring Systems provides the basis for sustaining evolving organizations. Churchman's theoretical work was driven by his unrelenting interest in determining whether it is "possible to secure improvement in the human condition by means of the human intellect" (Ulrich, 2009, p. 4). One of his significant contributions to the development of systems theory was his recognition that "problem solving often appears to produce improvement, but the so-called 'solution' often makes matters worse in the larger system" (Churchman, 1982, p. 19f). He argued that "simple, direct, head-on attempts to 'solve' system problems don't work and, indeed, often turn out to be downright dangerous" (Churchman, 1979, p. 4). No problem exists in isolation; rather, problems are inextricably linked to each other and to the environment, thus requiring an approach to the "whole."

Churchman's inquiry systems model is centered around the *client* as the "complex of persons whose interests ought to be served" (Churchman, 1971, p. 48). Clients can be described by their value structure. Each client has a set of possible futures (i.e., goals or objectives) and a preference for one future over others. Clients have trade-off principles that reveal how much of one objective they would relinquish in order to achieve or increase another objective, establishing a means of "balancing" a given system.

For Churchman, the *environment* is limitless. It consists of all things outside the system that may, in some direct, indirect, or even barely comprehensible way, affect—or be affected by—what happens within the system. Also within the model, a *decision maker* controls system resources. He or she "*co-produces* the future along with the environment, which he[/she] does not control" (Churchman, 1971, p. 47). The decision maker's preferred future may not be identical to that of other stakeholders (clients) and his/her trade-off principle may not be the same.

The system *planner* is the person who should at all times be working toward improvement in the human condition. Churchman (1971, 1979) envisions a planner who seeks to identify the clients' underlying principles and trade-offs, to create measures of performance based on those principles, and to trace out all potential consequences of action. The planner's intentions are presumed to be "always good with respect to the client" (Churchman, 1971, p. 47) and the planner assumes the role of trying to assure that the decision makers' value structure also supports those of the client.

The *measure of performance* is, in simple form, the degree of attainment of a stated goal, purpose, or objective, sometimes measured by the probability or amount of attainment and sometimes by evaluating benefits and costs (Churchman, 1979). Agents and factors both within and without the system may be said to *co-produce* the measures of performance. By their influence, co-producers may either help to achieve or to block the achievement of the clients' objectives. Following the work of Edgar A. Singer, Churchman states that, "Something is a producer of an event if at least one description of the event would be different were the producer not there" (Churchman, 1979, p. 87). Churchman goes on to note that "in the case of organizational decision making, the co-producers are many but often operate in subtle and non-formalized manners." Indeed, "part of an organization's 'unconscious' is the existence of co-producers who block the implementation of 'good' ideas, but are never mentioned" (Churchman, 1979, p. 87).

Apply Innovative and Evidence-Based Strategies Focusing on System Preparedness and Capabilities

The aforementioned roles fail to give a true impression of Churchman's dedication to creating learning systems within organizations. Foremost in these systems is the recognition that decision makers must be as open minded and creative as possible, so that their problem identifications and proposed innovative solutions reflect not merely the concerns of interest to the decision makers, but also the implications of the problem and its solutions for the whole system—indeed, for the environment itself (Ulrich, 2016).

To create a learning system, leaders, acting as planners, must move away from focusing on the obvious (i.e., data, hard facts). For planners who focus on the obvious—*goal planners*—"reality stops at the boundaries of the problem" (Churchman, 1979, p. 108). In contrast, *objective planners* attempt to reframe the obvious within the context of a larger problem. For the objective planner, "reality stops at the boundaries set by feasibility and to some extent by responsibility" (Churchman, 1979, p. 106). Although this larger perspective moves the system in the direction of learning, Churchman ponders another level: *ideal planning*. Where goals are deemed short-term and objectives long-term, ideals are considered to stretch indefinitely into the future, approaching the essential question of how to improve the human condition. The ideal planner moves past the feasible and the realistic and attempts to define purposes that could hold if these restraints were removed. In the ideal system, planners and decision makers work not with the obvious and the tangible but with limitless imagination (Churchman, 1979). Because the bounds of creativity can never fully be known, Churchman's model (1979) for inquiring systems is one constructed not of answers but of questions. Inquiry, and its corollary, decision making, are conducted in a learning system through a process of unfolding questions. Application of the inquiry model begins with the following questions and can be readily utilized in problem solving (Churchman, 1979, pp. 79–80) (**Table 7-1**).

Within any human service organization dedicated to benevolent purposes, the APN/DNP can readily see how Churchman's model could be utilized to provide organizational assessment and a blueprint for a holistic systems approach to problem solving. The complexities of healthcare issues lend themselves to the use of Churchman's design of inquiring systems and provide the transformational leader with a solid, methodical approach that promotes engagement by all parts and all disciplines within the organization.

Table 7-1 Churchman's Problem-Solving Model

The Client

- What is his/her purpose(s)?
- What should be his/her purpose(s)?
- How is the variety of his/her purposes unified under a measure of performance?
- How should the variety of his/her purposes be unified under a measure of performance?

The Decision Maker

- What is the decision maker able to use as resources?
- What should the decision maker be able to use as resources?
- What can the decision maker not control, which nonetheless matters—the environment?
- What should the decision maker not control, which nonetheless matters—the environment?

The Planner

- How is the planner able to implement his/her plans?
- How should the planner be able to implement his/her plans?
- [Ideally]What is the guarantor that his/her planning will succeed (i.e., will secure improvement in the human condition)?
- [Ideally]What should be the guarantor that his/her planning will succeed (i.e., will secure improvement in the human condition)?

Reproduced from Churchman, C. W. (1971). *The design of inquiring systems: Basic concepts of systems and organization.* New York, NY: Basic Books.

If we consider the example of an organization providing primary family care, the construction of a simple spreadsheet could readily identify key stakeholders whose purposes and counterpurposes the organization must consider in addressing problems. The spreadsheet might list each stakeholder as a *client* with particular needs and objectives—purposes—relating to optimal health care. For example, geriatric clients served by the practice are identified as having several purposes, including a desire for fulfilling quality of life, for the attention of a cost-effective, skilled medical provider, and for the cost-effective provision of medication. In Churchman's model, client purposes are both those things the client desires (e.g., fulfilling quality of life) and those things the client *should* have (e.g., safe, cost-effective care and medications).

Continuing with the example, a stakeholder may be represented by more than one client category. Young adult clients of the primary care practice, for example, may have purposes both as "parents"—concerned about their children's health— and as "patrons" who may themselves access the healthcare system. In addition, every stakeholder has the potential to act as a *co-producer* of the solution to the problem posed. They may do so by assisting the decision maker, or by laying obstacles in the decision maker's path. It is important to note that the decision makers are also clients, in that they too have purposes to be served. As one completes the inquiry noted in the example above, it becomes easier to observe patterns within the desires and needs of clients at all levels of the system. It is these patterns that become the basis for the understanding of the overall system; leaders, as a result, can then target innovation (change) efforts more effectively. This is where the approach of systems thinking is fundamentally different from that of traditional methods of analysis. Instead of isolating smaller parts of a system (e.g., individual clients), systems thinking looks at the whole, considering larger numbers (patterns) of interactions in order to gain understanding. If we continue our consideration of the primary care clinic noted, we might, for instance, through traditional analysis, make a change in practice that would benefit one group of clients at the detriment of another. Let's say that we decide to see all pediatric sick cases in the morning to accommodate working mothers and move geriatric chronic cases to the afternoon. We find, however, in examining *feedback* from the geriatric clients that they are only able to get public transportation to appointments in the morning, the latest senior bus picking up at 11:30 a.m. If the senior clients catch the earlier buses to make an afternoon appointment, they have a long wait time AND they are exposed to the sick children! Over time, if we continued with this plan (sans the feedback), we would see that the benefits of this innovation would begin to quickly evaporate and our organization and patients would suffer. Avoiding this global failure is a key advantage of systems thinking. By closely examining all the interactions created by a decision, potential problems can be detected and avoided.

Design System Improvement Strategies Based on Performance Data and Metrics

System improvement strategies that promote interoperability (information sharing) are critical to supporting care coordination, delivery of high-quality, cost-effective care, and optimal care outcomes (Koznik & Espinoza, 2003). Additionally, evidence-based practice (EBP) is a well-documented methodology that supports improved patient safety, quality of care, and practice initiatives that reduce costs.

The benefits of EBP underpinned the Institute of Medicine's (IOM, now NAM) Roundtable on Evidence-Based Medicine 2008 goal: "by the year 2020, 90% of clinical decisions will be supported by accurate, timely, and up-to-date clinical information that reflects the best available evidence" (para 1). In addition to this goal, the critical nature of EBP is demonstrated by the general expectation of the public that healthcare teams utilize current and best available evidence and that they share information. Despite the IOM goal, the current literature states that it still takes an average of 17 years from new knowledge generation to its translation into routine healthcare practices (Tucker & Gallagher-Ford, 2019).

Many healthcare organizations claim that evidence is utilized within their healthcare delivery practices. However, given the reported length of time it takes for evidence to reach practice, and given the current state of reported outcomes, it is clear that evidence does not yet produce timely organizational practice changes or contribute significantly to system design (Kouzes & Posner, 2023). Implementation of EBP within organizational structures and processes that support nursing EPB remain the most-cited reasons that adoption of current evidence into practice remains low. Structures are defined as factors or building blocks that affect the context in which care is provided. This includes library resources, physical facilities, technologies, equipment, and individuals available and dedicated to nursing EBP and optimum outcomes for patients. Although structures, such as dedicated academic time, are built into many faculty appointments for physicians, dedicated structured time incorporated into nursing workflows is rare, yet essential, for optimum outcomes (NAM, 2021).

Outcomes are the impacts of healthcare teams' actions and center on changes to patient health status. Nurse-led, EBP outcomes are exemplified by nursing care interventions that result in reduced pressure injury, reduced central line–associated blood stream infections, reduced falls with injury, and increased patient satisfaction with discharge instructions (Warren et al., 2016). Analysis of data and key metrics reviewed by leadership on an ongoing basis, effectually "inspecting what is expected," drive continual redesign of the system in response to the data and key performance metrics.

Manage Change to Sustain System Effectiveness

The APN/DNP may manage change by understanding driving forces and restraining forces surrounding any change as described by Kurt Lewin's early work developing a model of change. According to the theory, until the driving forces exceed the restraining forces, change will not occur (Lewin, 1951). Therefore, system effectiveness can be sustained by enhancing the driving forces and developing plans to overcome and/or manage the restraining forces to change that may be present within the system in which the change is occurring.

Everett Rogers's Diffusion of Innovation theory can also be helpful for the APN/DNP to use to maintain system effectiveness during any change initiative. Rogers describes individual's response to change as innovators, early adopters, early majority, late majority, and laggards (Rogers, 2003). Innovators are the individuals who provide leadership in the system in planning change. By leveraging early adopters in promoting the change while also listening to and examining any cautions expressed about the change by individuals in the late majority and laggard categories, the APN/DNP can sustain the effectiveness of the system.

Table 7-2 Dynamic Network Theory—Eight Social Network Roles

Role	Characteristics of Role
Goal striving	Independent in goal pursuit
System supporting	Support others in goal pursuit
Goal preventing	Independently obstruct or resist goal
Supportive resisting	Support others in obstructing or resisting goal
System negating	Upset about those pursuing goal
Constructive system reacting	Constructive reaction to conflicts with others involved with goal pursuit
Observing	Not interacting nor helping or hurting process of goal pursuit
Interacting	Interacting but not impacting goal pursuit process or focusing on those pursuing the goal

Data from Westaby, J. D. (2012). *Dynamic Network Theory: How social networks influence goal pursuit*. Washington, DC: American Psychological Association; Westaby, J. D., Woods, N., & Pfaff, D. L. (2016). Extending dynamic network theory to group and social interaction analysis: Uncovering key behavioral elements, cycles, and emergent states. *Organizational Psychology Review*, 6(1), 34–62. https://doi.org/10.1177/2041386614551319; Westaby, J. D. & Parr, A. K. (2020). Network goal analysis of social and organizational systems: Testing dynamic network theory in complex social networks. *Journal of Applied Behavioral Science*, 56(1), 107–129.

Dynamic network theory can also be used in change management to identify social networks within an organization to understand behaviors, person interactions, and goal achievements of individuals within the system. This depth of understanding of the system's social networks can be helpful for the APN/DNP to consider during any change process. The social network theory details eight social network roles that individuals and groups within the system may play in pursuit of a goal (Westaby, 2012; Westaby et al., 2016; Westaby & Parr, 2020). **Table 7-2** lists the roles and behaviors associated with the roles. Identifying the network role of individuals and groups in response to any goal of the system can be very valuable in promoting smooth transitions when change is needed.

Design System Improvement Strategies That Address Internal and External System Processes and Structures That Perpetuate Structural Racism and Other Forms of Discrimination in Healthcare Systems

The evolution of the APN/DNP as that of strategic systems thinker and visionary for health care lies largely within the profession's commitment to lifelong learning and the realization that people and organizations do not exist as islands unto themselves, but rather as part of a larger network, web, or matrix of systems that all function more or less independently yet *inter*dependently to improve care delivery and outcomes through shared system-wide initiatives (Winasti et al., 2023). One must realize the necessity of developing a dedication to disrupting the system as we know it, while at the same time retaining flexibility, balance, connectivity and a sense of social intelligence and responsibility across the larger realm of health care (Taylor et al., 2007). Designing policy to address the concerns of health equity and structural racism must become the focus of APNs/DNPs with a worldview. We must look broadly, appraising the evidence fully and effectively, to find policy solutions that lead to the implementation and maintenance of systems that address the dire need for healthcare solutions that present with an eye to the future for meeting healthcare concerns of generations to come.

Summary

Advanced practice leadership must acknowledge the healthcare system as an open system affected by, and to some degree dependent upon, larger systems of which it is a part. Employing a systems approach to seeking solutions in health care will ultimately alter the role of the various disciplines within health care. This reconsideration of roles will become the purview of leaders at all levels. These advanced systems thinkers will ultimately lead the way as we seek to begin the inquiries expressed by these questions: What are the human vulnerabilities with respect to our capacity to keep up with new knowledge, to remember, or to analyze large amounts of data? How might the principles of distributed cognition (interaction and feedback) and information-sharing technology protect us from these vulnerabilities? How might system redesign as a result of a shared vision protect us from making fatal design errors? What are the human vulnerabilities with respect to our thinking, emotions, and actions?

These challenges ahead require that the ANP/DNP be well prepared in the application of systems thinking to the healthcare environment. Through careful analysis of the structure of both microsystems and macrosystems, how their performance is best measured, and how they interrelate, one can make a determination of their vulnerabilities and strengths within the context of structural explanation. Detection of behavioral patterns in the underlying structure may assist in optimizing system components to maximize results of the system. Additionally, detection of behavioral patterns can be used to address structural racism and other discriminatory practices. Systems thinking may further provide the tools for identifying and monitoring unintended consequences and illuminate the possible interventions to prevent harm from such consequences. The unique preparation of APN/DNP nurse leaders makes them well suited as translational catalysts for the implementation of systems that can and must transform health care for a future of quality and equitable care provision.

References

American Association of Colleges of Nursing (2021). *The Essentials: Core competencies for professional nursing education.* https://www.aacnnursing.org/Essentials
American Hospital Association (2017). *Fact sheet: Hospital billing explained.* https://www.aha.org/system/files/2018-01/factsheet-hospital-billing-explained-9-2017.pdf

Churchman, C. W. (1971). *The design of inquiring systems: Basic concepts of systems and organization.* Basic Books.

Churchman, C. W. (1979). *The systems approach and its enemies.* Basic Books.

Churchman, C. W. (1982). *Thought and wisdom.* Intersystems Publications.

Coughlin, T. A., Samuel-Jakubos, H., & Garfield, R. (2021). Sources of payment for uncompensated care for the uninsured. *KFF Issue Brief.* https://www.kff.org/uninsured/issue-brief /sources-of-payment-for-uncompensated-care-for-the-uninsured/

Cunningham, R., Polomana, R. C., Wood, R. M., & Aysola, J. (2022). Health systems and health equity: Advancing the agenda. *Nursing Outlook, 70,* S66–S76. https://www.nursingoutlook.org /article/S0029-6554(22)00097-5/fulltext

Dover, D. C., & Belon, A. P. (2019). The health equity measurement framework: A comprehensive model to measure social inequities in health. *International Journal for Equity in Health, 18*(36). https://doi.org/10.1186/s12939-019-0935-0

Drinka, T., & Clark, P. (2016). *Health care teamwork: Interdisciplinary practice and teaching* (2nd ed.). Praeger.

Dzau, V. J., McClellan, M., McGinnis, J. M., & Finkelman, E. M. (Eds.). (2017). *Vital directions for health & health care: An initiative of the National Academy of Medicine.* National Academy of Medicine.

Goodman, M. (2023). *Systems thinking: What, why, when, where, and how?* https://thesystemsthinker .com/systems-thinking-what-why-when-where-and-how/

Gorman, S. (2023). *Developing the craft of collaboration: Stretching, weaving, designing and mapping better collaboration.* https://static1.squarespace.com/static/5d3f1017387fd200018e0e29/t/63f3 453b0dfbbb6b8184d6c4/1676887357631/Developing+the+Craft+of+Better+Collaboration +-+Part+2+200223.pdf.

Homer-Dixon, T. (2002). *The ingenuity gap: Facing the economic, environmental, and other challenges of an increasingly complex and unpredictable future.* Vintage Books.

Kaiser Family Foundation (KFF). (2023). *Status of state Medicaid expansion decisions: An interactive map.* https://www.kff.org/medicaid/issue-brief/status-of-state-medicaid-expansion-decisions -interactive-map/

Keehan, S. P., Cuckler, G. A., Poisal, J. A., Sisko, A. M., Smith, S. D., Madison, A. J., Rennie, K. E., Fiore, J. A., & Hardesty, J. C. (2020). National health expenditure projections, 2019–28: Expected rebound in prices drives rising spending growth. *Health Affairs (Millwood) 39*(4): 704–714. https://doi.org/10.1377/hlthaff.2020.00094. Epub 2020 Mar 24. PMID: 32207998.

Kouzes, J., & Pozner, B. (2023). *The leadership challenge: How to make extraordinary things happen in organizations* (7th ed.). Wiley.

Koznik, L & Espinoza, J. (2003). Microsystems in health care: Part 7. The microsystem as a platform for merging strategic planning and operations. *Joint Commission Journal on Quality and Safety. 29*(9), 452–459.

Kuehnert, P., Fawcett, J., DePriest, K., Chinn, P., Cousin, L., Ervin, N., Flanagan, J., Fry-Bowers, E., Killion, C., Maliski, S., Maughan, E. D., Meade, C., Murray, T., Schenk, B., & Waite, R. (2022). Defining the social determinants of health for nursing action to achieve health equity: A consensus paper from the American Academy of Nursing. *Nursing Outlook. 70*(1):10–27. https:// doi.org/10.1016/j.outlook.2021.08.003. Epub 2021 Oct 8. PMID: 34629190.

Lewin, K. (1951). *Field theory in social science.* Harper Row.

Magnan, S. (2017). Social Determinants of Health 101 for Health Care: Five Plus Five. *NAM Perspectives.* Discussion Paper, National Academy of Medicine, Washington, D.C. https://doi.org/10 .31478/201710c

National Academies of Sciences, Engineering, and Medicine (NAM). (2021). *The future of nursing 2020-2030: Charting a path to achieve health equity.* The National Academies Press. https://doi .org/10.17226/25982

National Health Council (NHC) (nd). *Putting patients first.* https://nationalhealthcouncil.org/

National Health Council (NHC). (2021, September). *Policy recommendations for reducing health care costs.* https://nationalhealthcouncil.org/wp-content/uploads/2021/09/NHC-Health-Care-Costs -2021-Recommendations-1.pdf

Porter, K., Jackson, G., Clark, R., Waller, M., & Stanfill, A. G. (2020). Applying social determinants of health to nursing education using a concept-based approach. *Journal of Nursing Education 59*(5), 293–296.

Rogers, E. M. (2003). *Diffusion of innovations* (5th ed.). Free Press.

Schneider, E. C., Sarnak, D. O., Squires, D., Shah, A., & Doty, M. M. (2017). *Mirror, mirror 2017: International comparison reflects flaws and opportunities for better U.S. health care.* The Commonwealth Fund.

Schneider, E. C., Shah, A., Doty, M. M., Tikkanen, R., Fields, K., & Williams II, R. D. (2021). *MIRROR, MIRROR 2021: Reflecting poorly: Health care in the U.S. compared to other high-income countries.* Commonwealth Fund. https://www.commonwealthfund.org/sites/default/files/2021 -08/Schneider_Mirror_Mirror_2021.pdf

Senge, P. (2006). *The fifth discipline: The art and practice of the learning organization.* Doubleday.

Shrank, W., DeParle, N., Gottlieb, S., Jain, S., Orszag, P., Powers, B., & Wilensky, G. R. (2021). Health costs and financing: Challenges and strategies for a new administration. *Health Affairs (Project Hope), 40*(2), 235–242. https://doi.org/10.1377/hlthaff.2020.01560

Shrank, W. H., Rogstad, T. L., & Parekh, N. (2019). Waste in the US health care system. *Journal of the American Medical Association, 322*(15), 1501–1509.

Singer, C., & Porta, C. (2022). Improving patient well-being in the United States through care coordination interventions informed by social determinants of health. *Health & Social Care in the Community, 30*(6), 2270–2281.

Smith, H. V. (2019). The wealth reference guide: An American classic. Author.

Taylor, T. A., Martin, B., Hutchinson, S., & Jinks, M. (2007). Examination of leadership practices of principals identified as servant leaders. *International Journal of Leadership and Education, 10*(4) 401–419.

Thusini, S., Milenova, M., Nahabedian, N., Grey, B., Soukup, T., & Henderson, C. (2022). Identifying and understanding benefits associated with return-on-investment from large-scale healthcare quality improvement programmes: An integrative systematic literature review. *BMC Health Services Research, 22,* 1083. https://doi.org/10.1186/s12913-022-08171-3

Tucker S., & Gallagher-Ford, L. (2019). EBP 2.0: From strategy to implementation. *American Journal of Nursing, 119*(4), 50–52.

Ulrich, W. (2009, March 26). *An appreciation of C. West Churchman* (Rev. ed.). (Original work published 1988 as C. West Churchman— 75 years. *Systems Practice, 1*(4), 341–350). https://wulrich .com/cwc_appreciation.html

Ulrich, W. (2016). *Operations research and critical systems thinking: An integrated perspective Part 2.* https://wulrich.com/bimonthly_september2016.html

Warren, J. L., McLaughlin, M. Bardsley, J., Eich, J., Esche, C. A., Kropkowski, L., & Risch, S. (2016). The strengths and challenges of implementing EBP in healthcare systems. *Worldviews on Evidence-Based Nursing, 13*(1), 15-24.

Weinstein, M.C., & Stason, W.B. (1977). Foundations of cost-effectiveness analysis for health and medical practices. *New England Journal of Medicine. 296*(13), 716–721. https://doi.org/10.1056 /NEJM197703312961304. PMID: 402576.

Westaby, J. D. (2012). *Dynamic Network Theory: How social networks influence goal pursuit.* American Psychological Association.

Westaby, J. D., Woods, N., & Pfaff, D. L. (2016). Extending dynamic network theory to group and social interaction analysis: Uncovering key behavioral elements, cycles, and emergent states. *Organizational Psychology Review, 6*(1), 34–62. https://doi.org/10.1177/2041386614551319

Westaby, J. D., & Parr, A. K. (2020). Network goal analysis of social and organizational systems: Testing dynamic network theory in complex social networks. *Journal of Applied Behavioral Science, 56*(1), 107–129.

Wheatley, M. (1992). *Leadership and the new science: Discovering order in a chaotic world.* Berrett-Koehler.

Wheatley, M. (2002). *Turning to one another: Simple conversations to restore hope to the future.* Berrett-Koehler.

WHO (World Health Organization). (n.d.). *Social determinants of health.* https://www.who.int /health-topics/social-determinants-of-health#tab=tab_1

Winasti, W., Berden, H., & van Merode, F. (2023). Hospital Organizational Structure and Information Processing: An Entropy Perspective. *Entropy* (Basel, Switzerland), *25*(3), 420. https://doi .org/10.3390/e25030420

CHAPTER 8

Informatics and Healthcare Technologies

Michelle Ullery, DNP, APRN, CNP

Introduction

The American Association of Colleges of Nursing (AACN, 2021) *Essentials: Core Competencies for Professional Nursing Education* identifies ten domains that are essential for nursing education. The advanced-level nursing education subcompetencies build the foundation for education of all advanced nursing practice specialties and advanced practice nursing (APN) roles with the doctor of nursing practice (DNP) degree in mind (AACN, 2021). This chapter explores Domain 8: Informatics and Healthcare Technologies. AACN Domain 8 is described as:

> Information and communication technologies and informatics processes are used to provide care, gather data, form information to drive decision making, and support professionals as they expand knowledge and wisdom for practice. Informatics processes and technologies are used to manage and improve the delivery of safe, high-quality, and efficient healthcare services in accordance with best practice and professional and regulatory standards. (p. 46)

The chapter will define informatics and nursing informatics (NI), review a model for NI framework, consider nursing terminologies and standards, describe the nursing informatics specialty, and define healthcare technology. The relationship of informatics and health information with key concepts communication, clinical judgment, ethics, and health policy will be explored. The AACN Advanced-Level Nursing Education Domain 8 Competencies will be identified and the Domain 8 sub competencies will be interpreted.

What Is Informatics and Healthcare Technologies?

Informatics

The American Medical Informatics Association (AMIA) describes informatics as a science "of how to use data, information and knowledge to improve human health and the delivery of health care services" (AMIA, 2023, para. 2). Health informatics is a broad term that includes the application of research and informatics practice in health care (AMIA, 2023). Health informatics combines health science, computer science, and information science. AMIA identifies five domains under the umbrella of biomedical and health informatics: translational bioinformatics, clinical research informatics, clinical informatics, consumer health informatics, and public health informatics (AMIA, 2023).

Clinical informatics "is also referred to as applied clinical informatics and operational informatics" (AMIA, 2023, para. 6). Although informaticists are often thought of as the electronic health records (EHR) clinical documentation experts, clinical informaticists are skilled to work with other software applications used in health care (e.g., imaging, administrative, and financial systems), clinical technologies (e.g., patient monitoring, nurse call, IV pumps), clinical decision support, and analytics. Informaticists are experts in workflow evaluation, systems design, build, testing, implementation, adoption, and optimization of health information technology (HIT).

Nursing Informatics

NI is a specialty that combines nursing science with multiple information and analytical sciences to use, process, understand, and evaluate data to inform decision making (ANA, 2022). It is important to make the distinction that NI is not solely concerned with information science or technology. A core component of NI is the synthesis of data and information to generate knowledge and wisdom (ANA, 2022). **Figure 8-1** illustrates the intersection of nursing and NI. Understanding how NI is used to support and promote nursing practice provides the foundation to build and give nursing a voice within the digital and technological advances in the healthcare environment. A DNP-prepared nurse is expected to have knowledge and understanding of the crosswalk between nursing and informatics and how to support and lead efforts to improve health systems through the use of data.

Model for NI Framework. Nursing informatics is guided by a meta-model called the Data, Information, Wisdom, and Knowledge Model. This model was originally created by Nelson and Staggers (2016) (**Figure 8-2**).

Nurses gather a plethora of data from patients and then turn this data into information. For example, a simple patient temperature data point, 101°F, in isolation is not enough information without context. The nurse determines if this data of 101°F temperature is down from 103°F or elevated from 98.6°F. This single data point is now information when evaluated in the context of additional data. Next, a nurse may use knowledge to integrate and understand what this data and information means in relationship to everything that is happening with the patient to determine

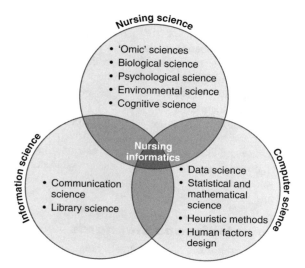

Figure 8-1 Core of Nursing Informatics Expanded to Intersect Multiple Sciences

Adapted to include additional sciences that influence nursing informatics in today's healthcare environment.

Data from American Nurses Association (ANA). (2022). *Nursing informatics: Scope and standards of practice* (3rd ed.). Silver Spring, MD: Author

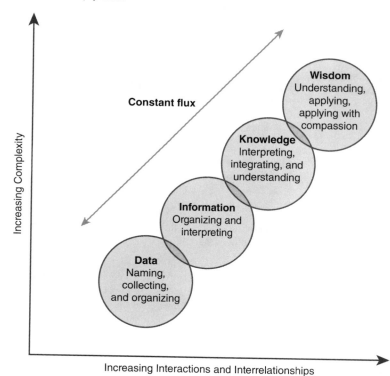

Figure 8-2 Data, Information, Wisdom, and Knowledge Model

Data from Nelson, R., & Staggers, N. (2016). *Health informatics: An interprofessional approach.* Elsevier Health Sciences

next steps, select appropriate interventions, and interpret health outcomes. Finally, the nurse will apply wisdom to assess the patient for increasing complexity and understand interrelationships between data, information, and knowledge related to care of the patient. This example is specific to the nurse–patient relationship but also can be applied to many scenarios within healthcare settings, public health services, and whole populations (**Table 8-1**).

Table 8-1 provides examples of nursing and nursing informatics in relation to the Nursing Informatics Meta-Model Data, Information, Knowledge, and Wisdom. In the current health environment, data-driven decisions backed by evidence-based practice and clinical knowledge are critical for health improvement. As a DNP-prepared nurse, it is essential to use clinical nursing skills in combination with informatics knowledge and skills to improve health and health care for individuals, families, and populations.

Nursing Terminologies and Standards

For more than 10 years there has been extremely rapid implementation of EHRs, in part due to national initiatives and incentives. The Health Information Technology for Economic and Clinical Health (HITECH) Act of 2009 rewarded hospitals and eligible providers for attesting to meaningful use (MU) of certified EHRs, with incentives paid by the Centers for Medicare and Medicaid Services (CMS) (McCormack et al., 2015). In turn, 6 years after HITECH, 96% of non-federal acute care

Table 8-1 Nursing and Nursing Informatics

Nursing Informatics Meta-Model	Nursing	Nursing Informatics
Data	Patients (individuals), families, communities, caregivers, environment	Data quality, user interface, create information data models
Information	Information management and support	Information user and/ or recipient, data exchange/interoperable
Knowledge	Using system applications and technology for patient care and documentation	Design, structure, interpret, and represent data and information
Wisdom	Combine expert clinical judgment and system usability to improve experience and influence health outcomes	Develop, design, implement, and evaluate clinical applications of increasing complexity and understand/evaluate the interrelationships of health systems

Data from American Nurses Association (ANA). (2022). *Nursing informatics: Scope and standards of practice* (3rd ed.). Silver Spring, MD: Author.

hospitals had implemented certified EHRs. EHRs are certified by the U.S. Department of Health and Human Services once the EHR meets requirements for capabilities, functionality, and security. All hospital types (small rural, small urban, critical access, medium, large) achieved 94% or greater adoption (Henry, Searcy, & Patel, 2016).

The rise of EHRs has created massive amounts of data that can be used for health improvement and research. Unfortunately, a majority of data from the electronic health record systems are not readily available or easily interpretable for clinical decision making and/or research. The current electronic health system has been referred to as data-rich-information-poor (DRIP) (McCormack et al., 2015). Data standards must be adopted across HIT and EHRs to have accessible, interpretable data, and facilitate interoperability or exchange of information. Specific to the nursing profession, standardized nursing data should be incorporated within the EHR. Furthermore, nursing data, which represents the largest portion of EHR documentation, is seldom included in clinical data repositories and is not often used for translational research (Westra et al., 2015). Nurses' voices need to be visible and represented within the EHR to provide a whole picture of patient health. The nursing profession can contribute an enormous amount of valuable data related to the care of the patient and the nursing process (Welton & Harper, 2016; Westra et al., 2015). However, if nursing data are not stored in a standardized electronic format, or easily translated to a vocabulary used by interdisciplinary care team members, the value and contributions of nursing to patient outcomes may not be measurable or retrievable (Welton & Harper, 2016). The Office of the National Coordinator (ONC) of Health Information Technology put forth recommendations to incorporate standardized nursing terminology into the EHR (Welton & Harper, 2016; Westra et al., 2015).

Currently, the ANA recognizes two minimum data sets, two reference terminologies, and eight interface terminologies for facilitating documentation of nursing care and interoperability of nursing data between multiple concepts and nomenclatures within IT systems (ANA, 2018) (**Table 8-2**). The ANA released a 2013 position statement identifying SNOMED-CT (nursing problems, interventions, and observations) and LOINC® (nursing assessments and outcomes) as the terminologies of choice to support data interoperability across systems (ANA, 2018).

Understanding the basis of informatics and standardized terminologies allows the APN/DNP graduate to see the broader picture and implications of their work at a systems level within an organization and across populations and communities. Informatics skills provide a foundation to understand the relationship between data and information. Combined with clinical expertise, informatics furthers the ability to apply knowledge and wisdom to improve quality care and patient outcomes.

Nursing Informatics Specialty

NI is a special field of study recognized by the ANA and American Nurses Credentialing Center (ANCC). The ANCC informatics nursing board certification is a competency-based examination that provides a valid and reliable assessment of the entry-level clinical knowledge and skills of registered nurses in the informatics specialty after initial RN licensure (ANCC, 2018). The DNP-prepared graduate specializing in nursing informatics is the foundational level for students to take this exam. In 2017, the Health Information Management Systems Society (HIMSS)

Table 8-2 ANA Recognized Standard Nursing Terminologies

ANA Recognized Nursing Terminology	Content	Year Recognized
Minimum Data Sets (2)		
Nursing Management Minimum Data Set (NMMDS)	Nursing administration data elements	1999
Nursing Minimum Data Set (NMDS)	Clinical data elements	1999
Reference Terminologies (2)		
SNOMED-CT	Diagnosis, interventions, and outcomes	1999
Logical Observation Identifiers Names and Codes (LOINC®)	Outcomes and assessments	2002
Interface Terminologies (8)		
ABC Codes	Interventions	2000
Clinical Care Classification System (CCCS)	Diagnosis, interventions, and outcomes	1992
NANDA (Nursing Diagnoses, Definitions, and Classification)	Diagnosis	1992
Nursing Interventions Classification System (NICS)	Interventions	1992
Nursing Outcomes Classification (NOC)	Outcomes	1997
International Classification for Nursing Practice (ICNP®)	Diagnosis, interventions, and outcomes	2000
Omaha System	Diagnosis, interventions, and outcomes	1992
Perioperative Nursing Data Set (PNDS)	Diagnosis, interventions, and outcomes	1999

Data from American Nurses Association (ANA). (2022). *Nursing informatics: Scope and standards of practice* (3rd ed.). Silver Spring, MD: Author.

conducted a workforce survey to capture professional status and practice trends within the nursing informatics workforce (HIMSS, 2017). The survey suggests nurse informaticists play a crucial role in the development, implementation, and optimization of clinical applications within the healthcare infrastructure (HIMSS, 2017).

See **Table 8-3** for a list of nursing informatics resources.

Table 8-3 Nursing Informatics Resources

Resource	Link
Alliance for Nursing Informatics (ANI)	www.allianceni.org/
American Medical Informatics Association (AMIA)	www.amia.org/
American Medical Informatics Association (AMIA) Nursing Informatics Working Group	https://amia.org/community /working-groups/nursing-informatics
American Nursing Informatics Association (ANIA)	www.ania.org/
Health Information Management and Systems Society (HIMSS)	www.himss.org/
Nursing Knowledge Big Data Science Initiative	https://nursing.umn.edu/centers/center -nursing-informatics/nursing-knowledge -big-data-science-initiative

Data from American Nurses Association (ANA). (2022). *Nursing informatics: Scope and standards of practice* (3rd ed.). Silver Spring, MD: Author.

Healthcare Technology

The definition of healthcare technology has evolved over the last 40 years. The initial definition of healthcare technology was narrower when defined in the United States in 1982. Healthcare technology was defined as, "all drugs, devices, and medical and surgical procedures used in medical care, and the organizational and supportive systems within which such care is provided" (Bozic, Pierce, & Herndon, 2004, p. 1305). Since then, health information and technology has expanded and grown beyond the technology used in medical care and within healthcare systems. The U.S. Department of Health and Human Services has updated the term from healthcare technology to health information technology (Guide to Community Preventive Services, 2022). Health information technology is defined as, "digital tools and services (e.g. mobile phone apps, mail messaging) that can be used to enhance patients' self-care, facilitate patient-provider communication, inform health behaviors and decisions, prevent health complications, and promote health equity" (Guide to Community Preventive Services, 2022, para. 2). Concepts around enhancing health, facilitating communication, and promoting health equity align with current national health priorities.

The World Health Organization (WHO) defines health technology as, "the application of organized knowledge and skills in the form of devices, medicines, vaccines, procedures and systems developed to solve a health problem and improve quality of life" (WHO, 2011). The WHO recognizes that new interventions and technologies impact health and also have implications for health systems (WHO, n.d.). This leads to the value of assessing the impact of healthcare technology on health and systems. The WHO has developed a process called the Health Technology Assessment (HTA) and defined it as "a systematic and multidisciplinary evaluation of the properties of

health technologies and interventions covering both their direct and indirect consequences" (WHO, n.d., para. 1). Broadly speaking, this identifies the need to assess
both the intended and unintended consequences of health technology. DNP-prepared
APNs are expected to do this, as evidenced by the advanced-level competencies.

Selected Concepts for Nursing Practice Represented in the Domain

The concepts of communication, clinical judgment, ethics, and health policy are
highlighted as they relate to advanced level practice in this domain. The concept
of communication is at the core of informatics and healthcare technologies. Communication is defined by AACN (2021) as, "an exchange of information, thoughts,
and feelings through a variety of mechanisms" (p. 12). Methods of communication
are recognized by interaction through verbal, written, behavioral, body language,
touch, and emotion. The various forms of communication are at the core of the
nurse–patient relationship. The growing field of informatics and health technology
has shifted our communication from in-person interaction that encompasses all
forms of communication to just a few types of communication, primarily written
and verbal communication. Written communication is the primary type of communication used in electronic health records (EHR) between members of the health
care team through documentation. EHR portals increase written communication
between patients and the healthcare team. Verbal communication is often time
maintained through telehealth and patient care technologies. When video technology replaces face-to-face interaction with patients, interaction through touch is lost
and communication through behavior, body language, and emotion is less. Health
technology can be a useful tool to facilitate communication but APNs must recognize limitations and when face-to-face interaction is indicated. APNs must be
mindful to use technology as a bridge to maintain the therapeutic APN–patient
relationship rather than to replace it.

Informatics and healthcare technologies provide APNs with valuable tools to
support clinical judgment. As the clinical complexity of patients has increased,
healthcare technology has grown by using artificial intelligence to help APNs and
other providers understand and interpret information. Examples include using clinical decision support (CDS) systems and emerging technologies such as genomics
and artificial intelligence (AI) to improve care of patients.

The concept of ethics underpins informatics and healthcare technology. When
individual and aggregate patient health information is reduced to data sets this
highlights social injustices and inequities in historically and intentionally excluded
populations. These populations include people from racial, ethnic, sexual/gender/
linguistic/religious minority groups and people living with mobility/cognitive/vision/
hearing/independent living/self-care disabilities. The study of informatics and utilization of health technology can help APNs/DNPs to consciously support the bioethical principles of autonomy, beneficence, nonmaleficence, and justice for all patients.

Health policy relies on the use of informatics to form information to drive
decision making. Health policy is often driven by data, and informatics supports
the collection of data to support health policy in patient care. Health policy encompasses all system levels including local health systems, state, regional, national, and
global. When health technology supports better outcomes, data is used to drive
health policy change.

Level II Competencies of the Domain

Describe the Various Information and Communication Technology Tools Used in the Care of Patients, Communities, and Populations

Identify Best Evidence and Practices for the Application of Information and Communication Technologies to Support Care

New technologies are emerging constantly to support patient care. APNs/DNPs need to be skilled in identifying best evidence and practices before implementing new technologies into practice. New technologies may be introduced by patients, vendors, colleagues, or self-inquiry when trying to solve a clinical problem. It is important to evaluate any new technology thoroughly before implementing it into practice.

The Systems Development Life Cycle (SDLC) is a framework that can guide the application of information technology into practice (McBride & Tietze, 2022). The phases of the SDLC are (1) System planning, (2) System analysis, (3) System design, (4) System implementation and testing, and (5) System evaluation, maintenance, and support (McBride & Tietze, 2022). The components of the five phases vary depending on whether the technology tool will be implemented with patients, communities, or with a population. The planning phase encompasses project management, identifying the goal and ensuring alignment with the organization, product analysis, assessing return on investment, and identifying the team (McBride & Tietze, 2022). The planning phase aligns with the need to first identify how the technology will support care.

Evaluate the Unintended Consequences of Information and Communication Technologies on Care Processes, Communications, and Information Flow Across Care Settings

The *Analysis Phase* of the SDLC framework (phase 2) includes doing a needs assessment, feasibility assessment, process analysis, process development, and selection of the technology (McBride & Tietze, 2022). The process analysis phase of the SDLC is the first opportunity to analyze unintended consequences of information and communication technologies. By addressing it in the planning phase work can be done to prevent unintended consequences. This is a priority for patients, communities, and populations who have been historically marginalized. Unintended consequences should be considered again later in the final phase, phase five, *System Evaluation, Maintenance, and Support* (McBride & Tietze, 2022). In this phase, enhancements can be made to further ensure equity of access to information and communication technologies.

Some of the most vulnerable patients are often subject to unintended consequences of technology. For example, access to health technology on a smartphone application assumes one has access to a smartphone and a level of physical and cognitive ability to utilize it. Often, individuals, communities, and populations that have been historically marginalized are excluded from healthcare services available through technologies, further creating health inequities (Miller et al., 2016; Nahm et al., 2017). APNs/DNPs need to first anticipate and evaluate the unintended consequences of information and communication technologies. Subsequently, APNs/DNPs are called to follow through with mitigating the effects of unintended consequences of health technologies on historically marginalized communities.

Propose a Plan to Influence the Selection and Implementation of New Information and Communication Technologies

System Planning, step one of the SDLC, is the step in which a new information and communication technology is selected (McBride & Tietze, 2022). This is done after doing a vendor, product, and market analysis. *System Design*, step three in the SDLC, guides the APN/DNP in designing and proposing a plan to implement the new technology (McBride & Tietze, 2022). This step includes critical success factors, algorithms, process redesign, ensuring integrity and securing, and quality assurance (McBride & Tietze, 2022).

Planning is of utmost importance when new information or communication technology is being selected or implemented. Depending on the technology selected, there may be specific frameworks to guide the development of a plan, perhaps an implementation framework will be used as a guide, or the SDLC may be sufficient. For example, multiple frameworks exist to implement telehealth services. One such framework the American Telemedicine Association (ATA) has proposed is *A Framework for Eliminating Health Disparities Using Telehealth* (ATA, 2021). This framework would work well when establishing a telehealth practice. A more broad theory to help guide implementation of a new technology is E. M. Rogers's Diffusion of Innovation (DOI) theory (Rogers, 2003). Rogers's DOI theory recognizes that the adoption of a new idea, behavior, or innovation is a process where people adapt to change at different speeds when new information or communication technology is being selected or implemented. Different categories of adopters are described as innovators, early adopters, early majority, late majority, and laggards (Rogers, 2003). The DOI theory is a relevant theory to apply when implementing a new technology that affects many stakeholders because it seeks to understand the population and influencing factors.

Explore the Fiscal Impact of Information and Communication Technologies on Health Care

The fiscal impact of information and communication technologies is defined with a thorough cost–benefit analysis. This is done in the systems planning phase of the SDLC when considering what resources it will take and analyzing the benefit (McBride & Tietze, 2022). The fiscal impact is revisited in phase five, the *System Evaluation Phase*. Specific costs to consider will vary depending on the technology implemented, the care setting, and the scope of the project. Fiscal impact should include all steps of the SDLC from initial planning all through system evaluation, maintenance, and support. Important categories of cost to consider include the technology start-up and maintenance, overhead expenses, personnel, and the fiscal impact the technology will have directly on patients (McBride & Tietze, 2022).

Identify the Impact of Information and Communication Technologies on Workflow Processes and Healthcare Outcomes

The design of new technology on workflow processes is covered in the *Systems Analysis Phase*, phase 2, of SDLC. In this phase workflows and decision trees are developed. Phase three, systems evaluation, maintenance, and support is where workflows are revisited and operational enhancements are made (McBride & Tietze, 2022). To further evaluate the impact, the Donabedian model provides a useful framework to measure quality of health care. The Donabedian model guides evaluation through three dimensions: structure, process, and outcome (Donabedian, 2005). Structure relates to the content in which care is delivered, the process is how the care is delivered, and the outcome is the quality of care delivered. When a new information or communication technology is implemented, it is important to evaluate the impact from a holistic perspective. The Donbedian model is one framework that can be used as a guide.

Use Information and Communication Technology to Gather Data, Create Information, and Generate Knowledge

Generate Information and Knowledge From Health Information Technology Databases

The term *Big Data* evolved from the massive size and amounts of data and additional characteristics known as the five V's: volume, variety, velocity, veracity, and value (Laney, 2001). As explained, volume refers to the size and amount of data. Variety reflects the diversity of data types, including but not limited to alphanumeric data, image data, and continuous flow data, such as streaming video or blood flow monitoring. Velocity is the unprecedented speed at which data are generated and received. Veracity refers to the level of uncertainty associated with data elements and their source (Brennan & Bakken, 2015; Laney, 2001). A 2014 National Action Plan for Sharable and Comparable Nursing Data for Transforming Health and Healthcare builds on and seeks to coordinate existing but separate long-standing efforts of many individuals and organizations to standardize nursing data (Westra et al., 2015).

As health care shifts to the community, personal health data from devices such as Fitbits, Apple watches, and other mobile health applications (apps) add to Big Data. The ability to enable data capture of clinical nursing data combined with a variety of personal data sources has the power to transform healthcare delivery and health outcomes. To achieve this, it will be instrumental to incorporate nursing data into clinical data repositories for Big Data analysis through the use and implementation of standardized nursing terminologies, common data models, and information structures within EHRs (Westra et al., 2015). The nursing profession is needed within the new era of Big Data. In order to take advantage of Big Data, reliable nurse-sensitive data is needed to highlight and demonstrate the value of nursing; this is essential to drive the future of the profession (Brennan & Bakken, 2015).

Evaluate the Use of Communication Technology to Improve Consumer Health Information Literacy

The U.S. Department of Health and Human Services (DHHS) (2010) has developed a National Action Plan to Improve Health Literacy. This plan identifies two core principles: (1) All people have the right to health information that helps them make informed decisions and (2) health services should be delivered in ways that are easy to understand and that improve health, longevity, and quality of life (U.S. DHHS, 2010). Technology has the ability to work toward these two principles to promote health literacy or conversely the potential of being a barrier to health literacy.

For diverse patients who do not speak the predominant language, access to interpreters through video and telephone capacity improves access to health information. Other forms of communication technology continue to expand depending on the healthcare setting and specialty. Communication technology solutions that have been found to improve digital health literacy in the cardiology field includes artificial intelligence machine learning, voice-activated technology such as Siri or Alexa, wearables for detecting atrial fibrillation, remote monitoring of blood pressure, and smartphone apps (Dunn & Hazzard, 2019). These types of communication technology expand beyond the cardiologist specialty throughout health care. Depending on what communication technology is used, it is necessary for APNs to evaluate its effect on patient health information literacy.

Use Standardized Data to Evaluate Decision Making and Outcomes Across All System Levels

Data standardization is the process of creating standards and converting data from various sources in a consistent format. An example of this is Minnesota (MN) Community Measurement where standardized data is collected from healthcare organizations, analyzed and shared publicly on healthcare quality and cost (MN Community Measurement, 2023). A standardized set of data is collected on clinics and hospitals in the state. Reports are published indicating each clinical quality measure, the measurement year, if the rating was above or below average, and at what rate the quality measure is met (MN Community Measurement, 2023). APNs/DNPs can use this information from a systems level to evaluate decision making and outcomes (MN Community Measurement, MN Health Scores, 2023). Internally, health systems report standardized data to individual providers, including APNs, about their patient panels. APNs can use this data on a practice level to improve quality of direct patient care.

Clarify How the Collection of Standardized Data Advances the Practice, Understanding, and Value of Nursing and Supports Care

The APN/DNP needs to evaluate standardized data critically since standardized data does not take into account unique attributes of individuals, communities, and populations of patients. Standardized data is a collection of objective data measures APNs should consider in patient care, but not be limited to in patient care. For example, it may be unrealistic to expect an APN's patient panel to achieve the blood sugar goal of a glycated hemoglobin (HbA1c) of less than 8. Perhaps health information literacy on diabetes is not available in the primary language of many in the APN's panel, or the patient panel may have many social determinants of health barriers that make meeting a goal HbA1c goal of less than 8 unrealistic. Examining when an individual, community, or population faces barriers to meeting standardized goals can uncover important health inequities. When APNs identifies gaps such as this, APNs are well equipped to lead efforts to overcome these health inequities. Deviations in standardized data are useful to evaluate decision making and outcomes as long as the deviation is evaluated with an understanding of content of the population the data is collected on.

Evidence-based practice merges research evidence, clinical experience, and patient preference to guide APN practice. Middle range theories help to guide APNs in care delivery. Such middle range theories include behavior change theory, harm-reduction theory, and more. These theories help APNs to understand the importance of meeting patients where they are in their health journey, rather than focusing on meeting predetermined outcome measures. The APN has an important role to support patients in their health journey, wherever they are at. Aggregate and standardized data should not undermine the care we provide to the individual patient. Clarification about how to use aggregate and standardized data is a key concept for APNs to consider so the health care we provide to patients, communities, and populations from historically marginalized communities is uplifted.

Interpret Primary and Secondary Data and Other Information to Support Care

Traditionally data is categorized as primary or secondary. Primary data is data that is collected directly from the source whereas secondary data is collected by someone other than the primary user. Gray literature is defined as:

> information that falls outside the mainstream or published journal and monograph literature, not controlled by commercial publishers. Includes: hard to find studies, reports, or dissertations; conference abstracts of papers, governmental or private sector research, clinical trials—ongoing or unpublished, and experts or researchers in the field. (National Institute of Health, n.d., para. 14)

Given the expanse of information available on the World Wide Web, the APN/DNP needs to be skilled in interpreting not only primary and secondary data but also gray literature and other information to support patient care.

Use Information and Communication Technologies and Informatics Processes to Deliver

Evaluate the Use of Information and Communication Technology to Address Needs, Gaps, and Inefficiencies in Care

APNs in practice are well positioned to identify when there is a need in patient care, gaps in care, and inefficiencies in care. Information and communication technology should be evaluated as part of the solution to the clinical problem. Information and communication technologies (ICT) include eHealth, mHealth, telehealth, telemedicine, and more. In March 2020, at the start of the COVID-19 pandemic, state and federal regulation barriers were quickly lifted and the use of telehealth was expanded (CMS, 2020). The APN needs to critically evaluate when ICT is an appropriate solution to augment or address patient care needs and when ICT is inappropriate and other solutions are necessary.

Formulate a Plan to Influence Decision-Making Processes for Selecting, Implementing, and Evaluating Support Tools

Support tools in information and communication technologies are tools that provide the APN and patient the opportunity to track, register, and view gathered/reported information (Randine et al., 2022). Support tools used by patients include smartphone applications, commercial wearable devices, and the Internet of Things (IoT). IoT is a term used to describe the "internet working of different types of physical devices that are entrenched with transducers including sensors, detectors, actuators, electronic components, and equipment and website links, in order to maintain the association and stress-free interchange of data in a real-time environment" (Sharma et al, 2020, p. 153). These support tools provide additional objective data to guide APN care and decision making. The APN needs to develop a plan to select, implement, and evaluate information and communication support tools that align with the practice need.

Appraise the Role of Information and Communication Technologies in Engaging the Patient and Supporting the Nurse-Patient Relationship

Consumer demand and the rise of the patient engagement movement is shifting how patients, families, and communities interact with the healthcare system. Over the last few years, much focus has been placed on patient engagement and has been referred to as the "blockbuster" drug of the century (Kish, 2012). In response to these initiatives and consumer interest, a subspecialty field of health informatics called consumer health informatics (CHI) focuses on the health consumer or patient and the interaction with HIT. CHI uses a patient and consumer perspective of electronic information and communication to improve health outcomes and the healthcare decision-making process (AMIA, 2023). Specific examples of consumer health technologies include telehealth, mobile health technology such as applications (apps), patient monitors and sensor devices, and fitness tracking devices.

National efforts in patient engagement include the recent announcement of data sharing and access across health systems. A recent announcement, My Health Data Initiative to Put Patients at the Center of the U.S. Healthcare System, expands patient's access and allows the patient to have more control of their data. This is a government-wide initiative in collaboration with organizations such as the CMS, the ONC, National Institutes of Health (NIH), and the Department of Veterans Affairs (VA). The goals of this initiative are to remove barriers that prevent patients from accessing their own health records, to improve interoperability between systems, and to empower patients by providing more control of their health data. As national initiatives continue to increase, the field of CHI is increasing in popularity and is seen as an integral component to the overall health systems and informatics strategy for individual, family, and population health strategies. Specific examples of CHI are personal health records, telehealth, mobile health technologies, and the Internet of Things and quantified self-movement.

The patient engagement movement has increased the focus on patient access to their own individual health records. There are national initiatives to support this work and bring much needed access to individuals, families, and caregivers. One specific example of personal health records is the My HealtheVet by the Veterans Administration (VA) (My HealtheVet, n.d.). This program was one of the first to introduce personal health records and it allowed veterans to request and refill medications online, make appointments online, and view their health records online (My HealtheVet, n.d.). Another program derived from the VA is the Blue Button initiative. The Blue Button initiative symbolizes patients being able to view, download, and transmit (VDT) health records (U.S. Department of Veterans Affairs, 2017). Blue Button has grown to include many health organizations and is seen as a symbol for patients to understand the health organization has VDT capabilities. Another initiative, OpenNotes, focuses on patient access to read and view provider notes (OpenNotes, 2018). OpenNotes is a strategy for healthcare professionals and organizations to improve transparency within the system. These initiatives—My HealtheVet, Blue Button, and OpenNotes—focus on the goal and mission to increase access to a patient's own health records or notes to empower patients, families, and caregivers. Research has shown patients feel more in control of their health decisions and can improve the quality and safety of care (Bell et al., 2017; Delbanco et al., 2010).

Evaluate the Potential Uses and Impact of Emerging Technologies in Health Care

The definition of *emerging technology* (ET) varies widely between industries and in healthcare. Whende (2020) defines ET as, "the scientific inventions now used in industries across the modern landscape to help people complete tasks, communicate, make decisions, and find answers" (p. 3). The types of emerging technology that APNs/DNPs will use vary depending on area of practice. ETs in health care range from being accessible, such as telemedicine and health wearables, to more advanced technologies like virtual reality, artificial intelligence, robotics, and 3D printing (Whende, 2020).

Many emerging technologies are influencing APN practice. Two examples are the application of genetics to practice and artificial intelligence. The human genome project was completed in 2003 and new genetic technologies are being developed to apply knowledge related to genetics into practice (National Human Genome Research Institute, n.d.). These technologies are aimed at improving health through reading, manipulating, and even editing the human genome (National Human Genome Research Institute, n.d.). This knowledge is leading to the growing field of precision health (CDC, 2022a). Precision health factors in genetic, environmental, and lifestyle factors of an individual to formulate a unique prevention and treatment plan (CDC, 2022a). Similarly, artificial intelligence has the ability to improve health through analysis, integration, and interpretation of large data sets for specific health conditions. Many ETs are focused on taking large data sets and utilizing them to improve patient care.

The use and impact of emerging technologies is broad depending on the technology. ET can be used to improve the Institute for Healthcare Improvement's (IHI) Triple Aim and the Quadruple Aim. The Triple Aim framework developed by IHI sought to improve population health, reduce cost of care, and enhance the patient experience (IHI, 2023). The Quadruple Aim framework adds in a fourth aim to improve provider satisfaction (Bodenheimer & Sinsky, 2014). As APNs integrate different types of ET into practice, evaluating the use and impact is an important step.

Pose Strategies to Reduce Inequities in Digital Access to Data and Information

Digital access to data and information has rapidly expanded and as a result there are inequities in distribution of healthcare resources. Not all people have equal access to and use of data and information that needs to be accessed digitally. Yao et al. (2022) completed *Inequities in Health Care Services Caused by the Adoption of Digital Health Technologies: Scoping Review* in which they identified key factors that affected digital health inequities. These factors include older adults, Black communities, lower socioeconomic status, poorer health conditions, low eHealth literacy, and rural geographic location due to limited internet broadband coverage (Yao et al., 2022).

It is important for APNs/DNPs to help guide strategies to reduce digital inequities. Ideas to reduce these digital inequities include:

- building patient-centric digital health technology
- leading policy makers to promote equitable access to digital health technology
- supporting healthcare institutions simplifying web-based service processes
- educating and training in health literacy
- encouraging patients affected by inequities to access digital information when available
- and designing digital tools with equitable access in mind. (Bhattacharjee et al., 2022)

Use Information and Communication Technology to Support Documentation of Care and Communication Among Providers, Patients, and All System Levels

Assess Best Practices for the Use of Advanced Information and Communication Technologies to Support Patient and Team Communications

Effective communication is necessary to provide high-quality health care. Advanced information and communication technologies allow for more direct, asynchronous communication pathways between the APN and the patient, the APN and the healthcare team, and the patient and other members of the healthcare team. Communication technologies used between the patient and the APN usually are limited to communication through the EHR and telephone calls. Communication technologies used between the patient and the healthcare team include secure messaging within the EHR, instant messages, email, text messages, and telephone calls.

Although many types of communication technologies exist, it is important for the APN to assess for best practice depending on the nature and urgency of the communication. Despite the multiple types of technology communication, in-person communication should still be valued. In a small survey of primary providers, Norful et al. (2022) found that "in-person communication is more likely to reduce burnout and job dissatisfaction compared to other forms of communication infrastructure in primary care settings" (para. 20). In addition to burnout and job dissatisfaction, APNs and healthcare team members need to be mindful of feeling overburdened by the many types of communication technologies they are expected to keep up with on a day-to-day basis. Streamlining information and communication technologies is an important consideration in assessing best practice.

Employ Electronic Health, Mobile Health, and Telehealth Systems to Enable Quality, Ethical, and Efficient Patient Care

The rise of internet connectivity, wireless technology, and sensor devices has increased the way individuals, families, and communities can connect with health services. Health professionals can use this type of technology to connect, communicate, and collaborate with patients, families, and populations like never before. According to the American Telemedicine Association (ATA), the four foundational benefits to telemedicine include improved access, cost effectiveness, improved quality of care, and patient demand (ATA, 2023). The Center for Connected Health Policy (n.d.) states that *telemedicine* is often used when referring to using technology for a clinical diagnosis and monitoring, and *telehealth*, a more common term, is used to describe a broader range of services in addition to clinical diagnostics such as care management, patient education, and routine follow-up visits (Center for Connected Health Policy, n.d.). The presence of telehealth services continues to increase as organizations are incorporating telehealth services to reach patients who may not have easy access to transportation and also to bring specialty services to rural areas. APNs are in a prime position to take advantage of these services and lead efforts to increase access to care. Resources are readily available for APNs to support the delivery of care via telehealth (**Table 8-4**).

According to Fox (2013), one in three cell phone owners have used their phone to look for health information, and 59% of U.S. adults have searched online for information about a health topic within the past year (Fox, 2013). As of 2015, 64% of the overall U.S. population and 82% of persons aged 18–49 years owned an app-enabled mobile phone (Smith, 2015). Over 40,000 health-related apps were available for download from the Apple iTunes store alone. As of 2013, health, fitness, or medical care (i.e., health apps) are among the most downloaded (IMS Institute for Healthcare Informatics, 2013; Krebs & Duncan, 2015). Specific app features consumers prefer include accomplishing basic tasks such as making and being reminded of appointments, viewing information about their medications, increased interconnectivity with health providers, and accessing their own health data (Krebs & Duncan, 2015). Currently, many health systems lag behind in allowing consumers to upload data in real time into the electronic health records. This is mostly due to data privacy and security concerns. There is tremendous potential in the use of mHealth apps, and the evolving health system is working to integrate this technology in order to offer these services that health consumers are demanding (Krebs & Duncan, 2015).

Table 8-4 List of Resources Available to Support the Delivery of Care via Telehealth for APNs

Resource	Website
American Telemedicine Association	https://www.americantelemed.org/
AMA Telehealth Implementation Playbook	https://www.ama-assn.org/practice-management/digital/telehealth-implementation-playbook-overview
Center for Connected Health Policy	https://www.cchpca.org/
National Consortium of Telehealth Resource Centers (TRC)	https://telehealthresourcecenter.org/
Telehealth Etiquette Video Series by Old Dominion University College of Health Sciences, School of Nursing	https://learntelehealth.org/telehealth-etiquette-series/
Telehealth Interprofessional Practice Module	https://pdp.nursing.nyu.edu/Education/

Michelle Ullery

Evaluate the Impact of Health Information Exchange, Interoperability, and Integration to Support Patient-Centered Care

Health information exchange is the capability to electronically share clinical information between healthcare information systems and maintain the integrity of the data (HIMSS, 2023). Interoperability is defined as:

> the ability of different information systems, devices and applications (systems) to access, exchange, integrate and cooperatively use data in a coordinated manner, within and across organizational, regional and national boundaries, to provide timely and seamless portability of information and optimize the health of individuals and populations globally. (HIMSS, 2023, para. 1)

The interoperability of electronic health records to exchange health information provides more seamless transitions for the delivery of health care to patients in different settings.

Benefits to interoperability and integration of health information exchange include care coordination, improving business and administrative processes, increased patient safety and satisfaction, and value-based care (HIMSS, 2023). In addition to the EHR, the Prescription Drug Monitoring Program (PDMP) is another means of health information exchange. This allows prescribers and pharmacists to assist in managing patient's care by detecting diversion, abuse, and misuse of prescriptions for controlled substances (CDC, 2022b). It is important for the APN to evaluate the impact of different types of health information exchange on patient-centered care.

Use Information and Communication Technologies in Accordance With Ethical, Legal, Professional, and Regulatory Standards, and Workplace Policies in the Delivery of Care

Apply Risk Mitigation and Security Strategies to Reduce Misuses of Information and Communication Technology

Health information is protected by the Health Insurance Portability and Accountability Act of 1996 (HIPAA). The federal law created national standards to protect sensitive patient health information from being disclosed without the patient's consent or knowledge (ASPE, n.d.). The amount of data and number of tools used to collect sensitive patient health information and communication technology are expanding. Like all healthcare professionals, APNs/DNPs need to know and implement protected health information (PHI) policies and procedures. Furthermore, APNs/DNPs need to apply risk mitigation and security strategies to reduce the misuse of information. Risk mitigation and security strategies start with a risk assessment. The Office of National Coordinator of Health Information Technology (ONC) (n.d.) offers guidance with their Online Security Risk Assessment Tool (SRA Tool) for medium to small providers. The basic steps include: (1) reviewing the existing security of PHI; (2) identifying threats and vulnerabilities; (3) assessing risks for likelihood and impact; (4) mitigating security risks; and (5) monitoring results (ONC, n.d.). The SRA tool may be accessed through the following website: https://www.healthit.gov/topic/privacy-security-and-hipaa/security-risk-assessment-tool. In large health systems, APNs/DNPs often work with information technology professionals to mitigate risk and apply security strategies. In smaller health practices, APNs need to be prepared to lead this work to protect patients.

Assess Potential Ethical and Legal Issues Associated With the Use of Information and Communication Technology

There has been a shift in where health information is collected since information and communication technology has expanded. In the past, most patient data was collected within the healthcare system. Now more data is being collected and communicated remotely using information and communication technology. Digital tools and services need to be assessed for ethical and legal concerns before being implemented into practice as well as monitored while used in practice. Assessing for ethical and legal concerns is an important step when formulating a plan to implement new information and communication technology support tools (as reviewed in the subcompetency about formulating a plan to influence decision making). The nine provisions in the Nursing Code of Ethics can be applied by the APN/DNP in the use of information and communication technology (American Nurses Association [ANA], 2015).

APNs need to be aware of how data collected on our patients reflects on our identity as a healthcare professional. It is important to ask the following questions: What data is being collected that reflects the value I bring to a patient's care/the care team? Does the data being collected reflect the value that I bring to patient care/the care team? Are there other measures that better reflect the value I bring to patient care?

Telehealth allows APNs to access patients remotely and across state boundaries and raises legal issues associated with such access. Currently, APN practice is limited to the state they are licensed in. This limits APN telehealth practice to only the states for which an APN has a license. The advanced practice registered nurse (APRN) Consensus Model is a model that will standardize each aspect of the regulatory process for APRNs (NCSBN, n.d.). If adopted by all states, the APRN Consensus Model holds promise to increase mobility for APNs to practice and for patients to access APN care.

Recommend Strategies to Protect Health Information When Using Communication and Information Technology

When using communication and information technology, protecting health information is a top priority. Strategies for APNs to protect health information include using HIPAA compliant telehealth platforms and communicating with patients using secure EHR portals. Telehealth allows APNs to provide care outside of the healthcare organization's physical location. APNs need to assure that privacy is maintained from both the provider's location and the patient's location. Health and Human Services (2022) provides useful information for patients to promote telehealth privacy and can be accessed at https://telehealth.hhs.gov/patients/telehealth-privacy-for-patients/.

Promote Patient Engagement With Their Personal Health Data

Personal health records and patient portals in electronic health records promote patient engagement. Successful implementation of patient portals has been associated with positive patient outcomes in the management of some chronic conditions (McBride & Tietze, 2022). In April of 2021, the federal rule on Interoperability, Information Blocking, and ONC Health IT Certification, also known as the *Cures Rule* were instituted (OpenNotes, n.d.). The Cures Rule requires healthcare providers to provide patients access to their health information including notes, labs, and diagnostics in their electronic health record without delay and without charge (OpenNotes, n.d.). Now patients can easily access and engage with their personal health data. Promoting patient's access to their personal health data is an important role of the APN.

Advocate for Policies and Regulations That Support the Appropriate Use of Technologies Impacting Health Care

APNs/DNPs need to be aware of the appropriate use of technologies in health care and evaluate if policies and regulation are supportive of health care. This need for awareness includes policies at various levels including the local health systems, state, and nationally. When new policies and regulations need to be developed or revised, APNs/DNPs must have a voice at the table. Advocacy for APNs/DNPs can take the form of educating oneself and others on relevant policies and regulations, supporting advocacy organizations, collecting data on the impact of technology on health care, and supporting implementation in the practice setting.

APNs/DNPs can increase their knowledge related to laws, regulations, and policy at the state level by accessing respective state government websites. At the national level, relevant information can be accessed through HealthIT.gov. The Healthcare Information and Management Systems Society (HIMSS) is an additional resource to maintain knowledge of policies and regulations related to information technology and to guide and advocate for change. HIMSS's mission is to "reform the global health ecosystem through the power of information and technology" (HIMSS, n.d., para. 2). Information on HIMSS is accessed at himss.org.

Maintaining membership in professional APN organizations at the state and national level is a means of supporting organizations that advocate for legislative concerns related to health care. APNs/DNPs involved in program development, quality improvement, or other projects involving the use of technologies to improve care can use the data collected to further advocate for change in policy and regulation.

Analyze the Impact of Federal and State Policies and Regulation on Health Data and Technology in Care Settings

Federal policies and regulation are the drivers of change related to health data collected and technology utilized in health care. The purpose of the Health Information Technology for Economic and Clinical Health (HITECH) Act of 2009 was to "promote the adoption and meaningful use of health information technology" (U.S. Department of Health and Human Services, 2017, para. 1). The regulation has largely resulted in healthcare systems transitioning to the use of EHRs. The use of the EHR is a movement toward the triple aim to improve the patient experience, affordability of care, and improve the health of populations (IHI, 2023). This chapter has already noted how federal policy in 2020 transformed care delivery through telehealth and in 2021 the Cures Act changed patient engagement with their personal health information. These are some examples of federal regulations that have had a significant impact on healthcare delivery. It is important for APNs/DNPs to analyze historical and proposed federal policies on health data and technology to understand its impact on patient care and advocate for change.

Similarly, each state has acts, laws, rules, and statutes unique to the delivery of care of patients in the state in which the care is being provided. This includes, but is not limited to, policies and regulations directing Medicaid programs, private health insurers, boards of nursing, and other health care professions, and the activities of the department of health and human services. Depending on where the APN is practicing, state policies and regulations related to health data and technology can be found on the state's department of human services, department of health, and/or legislature websites. The APN/DNP can analyze such data for the impact of the policy/regulation at the state level.

One example of analyzing the impact of policy/regulation at the state level is to access a state PDMP. PDMPs have information on misuse of controlled substance prescription medications. Minnesota Statutes Section 152.126 "governs data collecting, retention, and access to the Minnesota Prescription Monitoring Program database" (MN Board of Pharmacy, 2023, para. 1). On the Minnesota Board of Pharmacy website, the Minnesota Prescription Monitoring Program reports how many controlled substance prescriptions have been reported and how many prescription monitoring program searches have been performed by healthcare providers (MN Board of Pharmacy, 2023). The APN can analyze data such as monitoring trends in utilization and prescribing practices published on the website and state-wide data reported on prescription drug abuse and deaths. With this data, the APN can begin to analyze the impact one state policy (Minnesota Statutes Section 152.126) has on the use of technology (a PDMP health information exchange) in APN practice.

Summary

The advanced-level nursing education competencies in Domain 8: Informatics and Health Care Technology build on the entry-level professional nursing education competencies. In summary, the advanced-level competencies expect APNs/DNPs to evaluate evidence and formulate strategies using technology tools; gather, create, and generate knowledge from data; evaluate and formulate plans to use information and communication technologies and informatics to deliver care; use information and communication technology to communicate care; and analyze and advocate for the use of information and communication technology to deliver care. The concepts of communication, clinical judgment, ethics, and health are threaded throughout the informatics and healthcare technology domain. Health care continues to move toward integrating information and communication technology to support patient care and APNs/DNPs need to ensure the patient's best interest is the driver of change. Advocating for and implementing emerging health technologies and reducing health inequities to health technologies are priority future work for APNs/DNPs in this domain. It is essential that the use of data and technology enhance the experience of care APNs provide, rather than detract from it.

References

American Association of Colleges of Nursing (AACN). (2021). *The essentials: Core competencies for professional nursing education.* Author.

American Nurses Association. (2015). *View the code of ethics for nurses.* https://www.nursingworld.org/practice-policy/nursing-excellence/ethics/code-of-ethics-for-nurses/

American Nurses Credentialing Center (ANCC). (2018). *Informatics nursing certification (RN-BC).* www.nursingworld.org/our-certifications/informatics-nurse/

American Medical Informatics Association (AMIA). (2023). *Why informatics: Informatics research and practice.* https://amia.org/about-amia/why-informatics/informatics-research-and-practice

American Nurses Association (ANA). (2018). *Inclusion of recognized terminologies within EHRs and other health information technology solutions.* https://www.nursingworld.org/practice-policy/nursing-excellence/official-position-statements/id/Inclusion-of-Recognized-Terminologies-Supporting-Nursing-Practice-within-Electronic-Health-Records/

American Nurses Association (ANA). (2022). *Nursing informatics: Scope and standards of practice* (3rd ed.). Author.

American Telemedicine Association (ATA). (2023). *A Framework for Eliminating Health Disparities Using Telehealth.* https://www.americantelemed.org/resources/a-framework-for-eliminating-health-disparities-using-telehealth/

American Telemedicine Association (ATA). (2023). *Telemedicine benefits.* https://www.american telemed.org/resource/why-telemedicine/

Assistant Secretary for Planning and Evaluation (ASPE). (n.d.). *Health insurance portability and accountability act of 1996.* https://aspe.hhs.gov/reports/health-insurance-portability-accountability -act-1996

Bell, S. K., Mejilla, R., Anselmo, M., Darer, J. D., Elmore, J. G., Leveille, S., . . . Walker, J. (2017). When doctors share visit notes with patients: A study of patient and doctor perceptions of documentation errors, safety opportunities and the patient–doctor relationship. *BMJ Quality & Safety, 26*(4), 262–270.

Bodenheimer, T., & Sinsky, C. (2014). From Triple to Quadruple Aim: Care of the patient requires care of the provider. *Annals of Family Medicine, 12*(6), 573–576. https://doi.org/10.1370 /afm.1713

Bozic, K. J., Pierce, R. G., & Herndon, J. H. (2004). Health care technology assessment: Basic principles and clinical applications. *The Journal of Bone and Joint Surgery, 86*(6), 1305–1314.

Brennan, P. F., & Bakken, S. (2015). Nursing needs big data and big data needs nursing. *Journal of Nursing Scholarship, 47*(5), 477–484.

Center for Connected Health Policy. (n.d.). *What is telehealth?* https://www.cchpca.org/what-is -telehealth/

Centers for Disease Control and Prevention. (2022a). *Precision health: Improving health for each of us and all of us.* https://www.cdc.gov/genomics/about/precision_med.htm

Centers for Disease Control and Prevention. (2022b). *Prescription drug monitoring programs (PDMPs).* https://www.cdc.gov/opioids/healthcare-professionals/pdmps.html#:~:text=A%20 prescription%20drug%20monitoring%20program,transitions%20to%20a%20new%20 clinician

Centers for Medicare and Medicaid. (2020). *President Trump expands telehealth benefits for Medicare beneficiaries during COVID-19 outbreak.* https://www.cms.gov/newsroom/press-releases /president-trump-expands-telehealth-benefits-medicare-beneficiaries-during-covid-19-out break

Delbanco, T., Walker, J., Darer, J. D., Elmore, J. G., Feldman, H. J., Leveille, S. G., . . . Weber, V. D. (2010). Open notes: Doctors and patients signing on. *Annals of Internal Medicine, 153*(2), 121–125.

Donabedian A. (2005). Evaluating the quality of medical care: 1966. *The Milbank Quarterly, 83*(4), 691–729. https://doi.org/10.1111/j.1468-0009.2005.00397.x

Dunn, P., & Hazzard, E. (2019). Technology approaches to digital health literacy. *International Journal of Cardiology, 293,* 294–296. https://doi.org/10.1016/j.ijcard.2019.06.039

Fox, S. (2013). *Health and technology in the U.S. Pew Research Center.* https://www.pewresearch.org /internet/2013/12/04/health-and-technology-in-the-u-s/

Guide to Community Preventive Services. (2022). *Health communication and health information technology.* https://www.thecommunityguide.org/topics/health-communication-and-health -information-technology.html

Healthit.gov. (n.d.). *Security Risk Assessment Tool.* https://www.healthit.gov/topic/privacy-security -and-hipaa/security-risk-assessment-tool

Health and Human Services (2022). *Telehealth privacy for patients.* https://telehealth.hhs.gov /patients/telehealth-privacy-for-patients/

Henderson, K., Winkler, Y., & Wyatt, R. (2021). A framework for eliminating health disparities using telehealth. *American Telehealth Association.* https://www.americantelemed.org/resources /a-framework-for-eliminating-health-disparities-using-telehealth/

Henry, J., Searcy, T., & Patel, V. (2016). Adoption of electronic health record systems among U.S. non-federal acute care hospitals: 2008–2015. ONC Data Brief 35. Office of the National Coordinator (ONC)/American Hospital Association (AHA), AHA Annual Survey Information Technology Supplement, 2015. https://www.healthit.gov/sites/default/files/briefs/2015_hospital _adoption_db_v17.pdf

Health Information Management Systems Society (HIMSS). (2017). *HIMSS 2017 nursing informatics workforce survey.* https://www.himss.org/sites/hde/files/d7/2017-nursing-informatics-workforce -full-report.pdf

Health Information Management Systems Society (HIMSS). (2023). *Interoperability in healthcare.* https://www.himss.org/resources/interoperability-healthcare

Health Information Management Systems Society (HIMSS). (n.d.). *Who we are*. https://www.himss.org/who-we-are

IMS Institute for Healthcare Informatics. (2013). *Patient apps for improved healthcare: From novelty to mainstream*. http://ignacioriesgo.es/wp-content/uploads/2014/03/iihi_patient_apps_report_editora_39_2_1.pdf

Institute for Healthcare Improvement. (2023). *Triple aim for population*. https://www.ihi.org/Topics/TripleAim/Pages/default.aspx

Kish, L. (2012). The blockbuster drug of the century: An engaged patient. *Health Standards*. https://hl7standards.com/08-2-5/

Krebs, P., & Duncan, D. T. (2015). Health app use among US mobile phone owners: A national survey. *JMIR mHealth and uHealth, 3*(4), e101.

Laney, D. (2001). 3D data management: Controlling data volume, velocity, and variety. *Application Delivery Strategies*. https://studylib.net/doc/8647594/3d-data-management--controlling-data-volume--velocity--an...

McBride, S., & Tietze, M. (2022). *Nursing informatics for the advanced practice nurse* (3rd ed.). Springer.

McCormick, K., Sensmeier, J., Dykes, P., Grace, E., Matney, S., Schwartz, K., & Weston, M. (2015). Exemplars for advancing standardized terminology in nursing to achieve sharable, comparable quality data based upon evidence. *On-Line Journal of Nursing Informatics, 19*(2).

Miller, D. P., Jr., Latulipe, C., Melius, K. A., Quandt, S. A., & Arcury, T. A. (2016). Primary care providers' views of patient portals: Interview study of perceived benefits and consequences. *Journal of Medical Internet Research, 18*(1), e8. https://doi.org/10.2196/jmir.4953

MN Community Measurement. (2023). *About us*. https://mncm.org/about/

MN Community Measurement. (2023). *MN Health Scores*. https://mncm.org/mnhealthscores/

Minnesota Board of Pharmacy. (2023). *Minnesota prescription monitoring program*. https://pmp.pharmacy.state.mn.us/

Minnesota Board of Pharmacy. (2023). *PMP statue requirements*. https://mn.gov/boards/pharmacy-pmp/requirements/

My HealtheVet. (n.d.). *About My HealtheVet*. www.myhealth.va.gov/mhv-portal-web/home

Nahm, E. , Diblasi, C. , Gonzales, E. , Silver, K. , Zhu, S. , Sagherian, K., & Kongs, K. (2017). Patient-centered personal health record and portal implementation toolkit for ambulatory clinics. *CIN: Computers, Informatics, Nursing, 35*(4), 176–185. https://doi.org/10.1097/CIN.0000000000000318

National Human Genome Research Institute. (n.d.). *The human genome project*. https://www.genome.gov/human-genome-project

National Institute of Health. (n.d.). *Literature search: Databases and gray literature*. https://www.nihlibrary.nih.gov/services/systematic-review-service/literature-search-databases-and-gray-literature

Nelson, R., & Staggers, N. (2016). *Health informatics: An interprofessional approach*. Elsevier Health Sciences.

NCSBN. (n.d.). *APRN Consensus model*. https://www.ncsbn.org/nursing-regulation/practice/aprn/aprn-consensus.page

Norful, A. A., He, Y., Rosenfeld, A., Abraham, C. M., & Chang, B. (2022). Revisiting provider communication to support team cohesiveness: Implications for practice, provider burnout, and technology application in primary care settings. *International journal of clinical practice, 2022*, 9236681. https://doi.org/10.1155/2022/9236681

Office of National Coordinator of Health Information Technology (ONC). (nd). *Security risk assessment tool*. https://www.healthit.gov/topic/privacy-security-and-hipaa/security-risk-assessment-tool

OpenNotes. (2018). *Homepage*. www.opennotes.org/

OpenNotes. (n.d.). *Opennotes for health professionals*. https://www.opennotes.org/opennotes-for-health-professionals/

Randine, P., Sharma, A., Hartvigsen, G., Johansen, H. D., & Årsand, E. (2022). Information and communication technology-based interventions for chronic diseases consultation: Scoping review. *International Journal of Medical Informatics, 163,* 104784. ISSN 1386-5056, https://doi.org/10.1016/j.ijmedinf.2022.104784

Rogers, E. M. (2003). *Diffusion of Innovations* (5th Ed), New York, NY, Free Press.

Sharma, D. K., Bhargava, S., & Singhal, K. (2020). *An industrial IoT approach for pharmaceutical industry growth*. Academic Press. ISBN 9780128213261.

Smith, A. (2015). U.S. smartphone use in 2015. *Pew Research Center*. Pew Internet & American Life Project. https://www.pewresearch.org/internet/2015/04/01/us-smartphone-use-in-2015/

U.S. Department of Health and Human Services, Office of Disease Prevention and Health Promotion. (2010). *National Action Plan to Improve Health Literacy*. Author.

U.S. Department of Health and Human Services. (2017). *HITECH act enforcement interim final rule*. https://www.hhs.gov/hipaa/for-professionals/special-topics/hitech-act-enforcement-interim-final-rule/index.html

U.S Department of Veterans Affairs. (2017). *Blue button*. www.va.gov/bluebutton/

Welton, J. M., & Harper, E. M. (2016). Measuring nursing care value. *Nursing Economic$, 34*(1), 7.

Westra, B. L., Clancy, T. R., Sensmeier, J., Warren, J. J., Weaver, C., & Delaney, C. W. (2015). Nursing knowledge: Big data science—Implications for nurse leaders. *Nursing Administration Quarterly, 39*(4), 304–310.

Whende, C. (2020). *Merging technologies for nurses*. Springer Publishing.

World Health Organization. (n.d.). *Health technology assessment*. https://www.who.int/health-topics/health-technology-assessment#tab=tab_1

World Health Organization. (2011). *Health technology assessment of medical devices*. https://apps.who.int/iris/handle/10665/44564

Yao, R., Zhang, W., Evans, R., Cao, G., Rui, T., & Shen, L. (2022). Inequities in health care services caused by the adoption of digital health technologies: Scoping review. *Journal of Medical Internet Research, 24*(3), e34144. https://doi.org/10.2196/34144

CHAPTER 9

Professionalism

Lauren Petersen, DNP, MPH, APRN, CPNP-PC
Stephanie Gingerich, DNP, RN, CPN

Background

Nursing has a circuitous, storied history in its journey to becoming a profession and a scientific discipline. While nursing itself is not young and extends throughout history, the evolution to becoming a profession is more a recent endeavor compared to other professions, such as medicine and law (American Association of Colleges of Nursing [AACN], 2021; Fitzgerald, 2020; Grace, 2023a; Godfrey, 2022; Willetts & Clarke, 2014). Within this journey, nursing has developed a specialized body of knowledge, theories, and core values, including but not limited to, ethics, integrity, altruism, humanity, autonomy, and social justice (AACN, 2021). As nursing evolves, so does society's understanding of the nursing role and subsequent expectations regarding care, health education, and the maintenance of dignity and autonomy that occurs in nursing care. Although a consensus definition of a profession is lacking, the discipline of nursing maintains characteristics of a profession by having accountability for actions in service to the public good and a unique body of knowledge and skills that are regulated by organized oversight to ensure members are adequately prepared (Beauchamp & Childress, 2019; Grace 2023a). As the discipline, society, and the workforce changes, a deeper understanding and articulation of the practices of the professional nurse is critical for nursing's full partnership toward healthcare transformation.

Since a unique body of knowledge and skills are foundational for defining a profession, academic institutions are charged with preparing students and providing assurance that graduates have attained the requisite knowledge and skills of the profession. Competency-based models, as reflected in *The Essentials: Core Competencies for Professional Nursing Education*, focus on outcomes attained as opposed to demonstration of knowledge acquisition or time-based training (AACN, 2021; Frank et al., 2010; Giddens et al., 2022). The intent of this educational model is assuring that the professional graduate has attained a base of competence that can be applied to various situations so that employers and the public know what to expect (Frank et al., 2010; Giddens et al., 2022). However, competency-based education models have been critiqued as being reductionist, promoting milestone achievement over excellence, and logistically challenging (Frank et al., 2010; Jarvis-Selinger et al., 2012). Therefore, Jarvis-Selinger et al. (2012) argue that competency-based approaches alone within medical education are insufficient in how the healthcare workforce is trained. Instead, they propose that "including *identity* alongside *competency* allows us to reframe our inquiries toward questions that include a focus on *being* rather than exclusively on *doing*" (Jarvis-Selinger et al., 2012, p. 1185). Thus, *professionalism* is included as one of the ten domains in the new AACN *The Essentials: Core Competencies for Professional Nursing Education* (AACN, 2021). Along with the charge for educational programs to actively engage in the "formation and cultivation of a sustainable professional identity" (p. 49), this domain aims to create synergy between assuring future nurses attain the competencies of what nurses do as well as creating intention around learning what it is to "be" a nurse at all levels of practice and education.

What Is Professionalism?

Through professionalism, nurses convey the unique knowledge, skills, and the patient-centered care valued within the nursing profession. Dictionary.com defines *professionalism* as "the standing, practice, or methods of a professional, as distinguished from an amateur." Although broad and inclusive, this definition, along with others, highlight behaviors or actions as the defining characteristics for a professional; the "doing" aspects of a professional group (Cruess et al., 2014; Godfrey & Young, 2021). But, those who work in health care know that it is not merely the attainment and delivery of technical skills or complex physiologic concepts that determines a healthcare professional. Instead, it is a deeply internalized set of values and attitudes regarded as integral to a profession that ultimately guides actions, decisions, and behaviors consistent with the professional community (Benner et al., 2010; Cruess et al., 2014; Godfrey & Young, 2021). In healthcare professional education, a challenge has been understanding how to educate and evaluate students to not only know and do the work of the profession, but how to "be" a professional. Nursing professionalism is not new, but as healthcare changes, there is a need for clarity in the articulation of the practice and profession of nursing to convey to colleagues, society, and future nurses what it means to be a nurse (Godfrey, 2022).

The concept of *professional identity* is becoming a more widely adopted term to reflect the dynamic processes whereby an individual transitions from a layperson into a mature, experienced professional (Benner et al., 2010; Godfrey & Young, 2021; Hilton & Slotnick, 2005). Professional identity in health professions generally consists of actions and behaviors (what professionals do), knowledge and skills (what professionals know), values, beliefs and ethics (internalized core values), context and socialization (group identification and social influences), and group and personal identity (societal and interprofessional recognition) (Fitzgerald, 2020). Further, the process of professional identity formation is influenced by one's personal identities and beliefs, formal educational experiences, socialization within the community of the profession, and governing bodies (Benner et al., 2010; Cruess et al., 2019; Hilton & Slotnick, 2005; Jarvis-Selinger et al., 2012; Willetts & Clark, 2014). This formation process is consistent with the notion that professional identity is not simply acquiring the ability to complete the tasks and roles of the profession, but includes professional socialization and the integration of the values and characteristics of the profession into one's personal identity (AACN, 2021; Crigger & Godfrey, 2014; Godfrey & Young, 2021). Godfrey and Young (2021) highlight that the concept of professionalism today may be better described as professional identity along with the process of professional identity formation. It is clear that the concept of professionalism is more faceted and complex than simply specialized knowledge or skills in an individual; being a professional nurse is not simply donning a badge that says "nurse."

Professional Identity in Nursing

Colleagues in other healthcare professions started innovative work in changing how students develop their professional identity in the early 2000s and are transforming education for future professionals (Benner et al., 2010; Crigger & Godfrey, 2014; Cruess et al., 2014; Cruess et al., 2019; Jarvis-Selinger et al., 2012). Godfrey (2022), a leader in professional identity formation, asserts that a similar trajectory in the nursing discipline will move the nursing profession forward by developing a new knowledge and a shared language across healthcare disciplines, in pursuit of the overarching goal of improving health outcomes. As health care continues to change under pressures of dynamic population healthcare needs, economics, and politics, the need for healthcare professionals to not only deliver quality care, but to guide the trajectory of health care grounded in the values and ethics of accountability, inclusivity, humanity, advocacy and social justice are paramount. Development of a sound professional identity offers flexibility and innovation through a sense of purpose in a changing healthcare world and may bolster professionals through challenging times, such as burnout and attrition (Owens & Godfrey, 2022). Therefore, the incorporation of learning strategies intentionally focused on professional identity formation in both academic programs and clinical learning environments will support future nursing success in full partnership for healthcare innovation.

In astute awareness of the importance of fostering professional identity in nursing, a seminal "Think-tank on Professional Identity in Nursing" was convened in 2018 to evaluate the state of the science and address the need to articulate what it means to "be" a nurse (Goodolf & Godfrey, 2021). This work has developed momentum and the International Society for Professional Identity in Nursing (ISPIN) was formed (Goodolf & Godfrey, 2021). Key outcomes from this society offer a foundation for understanding and guiding professional identity formation in nursing, both in education and practice (Godfrey, 2022; Goodolf & Godfrey, 2021). First, Godfrey and Young's (2021) concept and definition of Professional Identity in Nursing was confirmed as "a sense of oneself, and in relationship with others, that is influenced by the characteristics, norms, and values of the nursing discipline, resulting in an individual thinking, acting, and feeling like a nurse" (p. 363). Second, four domains for professional identity in nursing were defined including Value & Ethics, Knowledge, Leadership and Professional Comportment (see **Figure 9-1**) (Godfrey, 2022; Goodolf & Godfrey, 2021; Landis et al., 2022). This clarification of the domains of professional identity grounds understanding in what a competent, professional nurse exemplifies and reflects in professional practice. These also offer foci for curriculum development at all levels of nursing preparation that foster understanding about what it means to be a nurse.

Professional identity formation will certainly be dynamic over the course of an individual's career as opposed to "checklist" achievements at the end of an

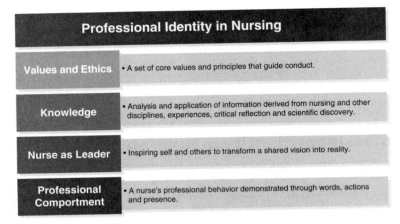

Figure 9-1 Professional Identity in Nursing Domains

Reproduced from Godfrey, N. (2022). New language for the journey: Embracing a professional identity of nursing. Journal of Radiology Nursing, 41(1), 15–17. https://doi.org/10.1016/j.jradnu.2021.12.001

educational program. Nurses at all levels and in any practice setting will continue to have formative experiences that will hone their practice in all domains of their professional identity. As discussed previously, this dynamic nature is consistent with *professionalism*, having both a professional identity and ongoing professional identity formation (Godfrey & Young, 2021). This chapter aims to discuss the domain of professionalism in the new *Essentials* and support the formation of professional identity for the doctor of nursing practice (DNP)–prepared nurse. The overarching goal is to provide insight for students and educators on the expected competencies and subcompetencies for DNP-prepared nurses to achieve in this domain to reflect the nursing profession. In a few cases in this chapter, subcompetencies from more than one competency of this domain are combined. They were determined to be closely interrelated and elaboration on these individually would likely lead to some redundancy. Further, this chapter is not a comprehensive review of Professional Identity in Nursing. We encourage all readers to explore this concept further as nursing is in an exciting time of growth and evolution.

Selected Concepts for Nursing Practice Represented in the Domain

Professionalism and professional identity are reflected in the whole of nursing practice. Professional identity evolves with influences from personal identities and socialization within the community of nursing and among the communities of health care. As the "domains" of the *Essentials* outline the areas of competency expected for professional nurses, the "concepts" capture broad areas of knowledge for nursing practice (AACN, 2021). In this chapter, the following concepts of nursing practice are highlighted: ethics, compassionate care, communication, healthcare policy, and diversity, equity, and inclusion (DEI). These concepts are robust and have overlap within the competencies of the professionalism domain. Throughout this chapter, the work of the DNP-prepared nurse will be reflected as "practice," meaning clinical and nonclinical experiences, encompassing nursing practice across health care.

Currently, nurses are practicing in complex environments that demand skills in navigating ethically challenging situations at an individual, family, interprofessional, and system levels. Based on the *Code of Ethics for Nurses with Interpretive Statements*, practice as a professional nurse in any capacity maintains an ethical responsibility to provide for the best outcomes in human health and well-being, from daily mundane tasks to complex care dilemmas (American Nurses Association [ANA], 2015a; Grace, 2023a; Milliken & Grace, 2017; Robichaux et al., 2022). Likewise, as will be reflected in the discussion of BASE of nursing, *Active caring* is a foundation for compassionate care in nursing practice. As DNP students prepare for a variety of practice settings, the concept of compassionate care may be reflected in how an advanced practice nurse (APN) cares for individuals in an outpatient practice, is translated to nursing students by those in academia, or it may find a broader foothold for those who work in leadership and systems practice. Supporting future DNP graduates in developing competence and confidence in navigating ethical concerns with compassion and striving to create moral communities of practice will create professional nurses who reflect the values and commitments of nursing.

Sharing of nursing's perspective and expertise is imperative for enhancing the public's understanding of the necessary contributions of nursing in health care. Nurses who are prepared to clearly communicate the profession of nursing to society and actively challenge long-standing stereotypes will help move the nursing profession into full interprofessional partnership. Using this same voice, DNP-prepared nurses can be change agents for patient care and nursing practice through active engagement in health policy. All DNP-prepared nurses will witness the impacts of policy in any practice environment as it permeates throughout all aspects of nursing. DNP-prepared nurses are ready for a future of influence and advocacy in the advancement of the profession and in healthcare innovation.

The concept of DEI in the new *Essentials* should be an integral part of professional identity and at the forefront in the formative process of advanced nursing competency. By integrating the core values of diversity, equity, and inclusion in all competency domains of advanced practice, the nursing profession may more fully realize its commitment to "the inherent dignity, worth, and unique attributes of every person," both to those served by nurses and those within the nursing profession (ANA, 2015a, p. v). Through intentional practice and actions, all nurses can contribute to ending the negative impact of discrimination and marginalization of people based on, but not limited to, race, culture, gender, sexual identity, age, and/or disabilities that lead to health disparities, unsafe work and learning environments, and traumatic experiences within communities. As a concept with research and literature to guide learning, knowledge sharing, best practice, and interventional skills, this chapter will not be comprehensive or address all perspectives of this concept. Instead, the intent is to highlight examples to guide students and educators toward resources for deeper exploration of this concept within their own professional identity development and lifelong learning.

In the end, professional nurses are accountable for their practice. Nurses are accountable to ourselves in developing a sound professional identity that generates innovation, excellence, and provides fortitude in challenging times. Nurses are accountable to their patients to provide evidence-based, compassionate care. Nurses are accountable to health care and society in their commitment to health promotion and the reduction of health disparities. Through competencies in ethics, compassionate care, accountability, health policy, communication, and DEI, DNP-prepared nurses will evolve their professional identities in nursing and lead in conveying the values and commitment of the profession to other communities and future nurses.

Level II Competencies of the Domain

Demonstrate an Ethical Comportment in Practice Reflective of Nursing's Mission

The commitment of the nurse to patients and society, as outlined in the *Code of Ethics for Nurses,* is to provide a "good" that aims to protect and promote health and well-being, prevent illness and injury, and alleviate suffering (ANA, 2015a; Grace, 2001; Grace, 2023a). A driving factor for promoting ethically competent nurses is finding that nurses lack confidence in ethical decision making and moral agency in practice (Grace, 2018; Robichaux et al., 2022; Rushton et al., 2016; Storaker et al., 2022). Thus, curricula that supports the development of ethical comportment as a part of professional identity is necessary for students at all levels of practice. Moreover, DNP programs are positioned to prepare influential, transformational nurse leaders who guide ethical practice and "good" nursing care in all spheres of nursing influence (Grace, 2018). In line with this call for fortifying moral agency and ethical comportment, the new *Essentials* have sagely included ethical competencies within the professionalism domain.

"Nursing ethical awareness is the willingness and ability to recognize the ethical nature of nursing practice" (Milliken & Grace, 2017, p. 523). All nurses should have foundational knowledge in biomedical ethics, ethical theories, and, most certainly, the ANA *Code of Ethics for Nurses* (2015a) to ground their ethical awareness. DNP students may have studied the moral principles of biomedical ethics outlined by Beauchamp and Childress (2019) and the *Code of Ethics for Nurses* in undergraduate coursework. As these remain fundamental guides for advanced level practice, it is prudent for DNP students and educators to maintain a working knowledge of these as their ethical practice continues to mature throughout the DNP program and into future practice settings.

In a brief review, Beauchamp and Childress (2019), as leaders in the area of Western biomedical ethics, have described four principles widely used in the healthcare sector for navigating ethical issues. These four principles—Respect for Autonomy, Nonmaleficence, Beneficence, and Justice—are intended to provide guidance for healthcare providers and systems to provide ethical care to all humans. A fuller articulation of these principles can be reviewed in the *Principles of Biomedical Ethics* by Beauchamp and Childress (2019). Of note, Beauchamp and Childress (2019) articulate the difference between moral and ethical, but these terms will be used interchangeably in this chapter. Similarly, over the last 65 years, the American Nurses Association (ANA) has developed and promulgated the *Code of Ethics for Nurses* (2015a). The code is a guiding document for daily practice, a concise statement of the ethical responsibilities of individual nurses, the "nonnegotiable" ethical standard of the profession, and an expression of the nursing profession's understanding of its ethical commitment to society (ANA, 2015a; White et al., 2011). The first three provisions affirm what has been described as "the most fundamental values and commitments of the nurse" (ANA, 2015a, p. xiii). These three foundational ethical principles articulate the charge for nursing practice and the right to a seat at the table for discussions about issues of health care that occur on a local, state, national, and international level (White et al., 2011). Provisions 4, 5 and 6 describe the "boundaries of duty and loyalty" (ANA, 2015a, p. xiii). The final three provisions describe the "duties beyond individual patient encounters" (ANA, 2015a, p. xiii, White et al., 2011). In consideration of the concept of ethics and professionalism, the ninth provision upholds that nursing is a distinctive profession, different from other types of healthcare providers. All nurses should be familiar with the *Code of Ethics for Nurses* given these provisions are foundational to the profession of nursing in their articulation of nursing's values and responsibilities.

As professional identity is ever evolving through lifelong learning, so is ethical competency and comportment. In the process of professional identity formation as a DNP-prepared nurse, students engage in knowledge- and skill-building strategies to develop ethical competency and agency from their new perspective and role to navigate the challenges of professional practice. A valuable model for nursing ethics to support moral agency development is Rest's Four-Component Model (FCM) (see **Figure 9-2**) (Grace, 2018; Lee et al., 2020; Rest, 1982; Rest, 1983; Robichaux et al., 2022; Robinson et al., 2014). Rest's model describes four psychological processes for moral behavior which include: recognizing a situation as having a moral concern (moral sensitivity); determining an ideal course of moral action (moral reasoning); evaluating potential outcomes and selecting the moral course of action (moral motivation); and finally, the critical component, taking action and maintaining persistence for the future goal (moral action) (Figure 9-2) (Rest, 1982; Rest,

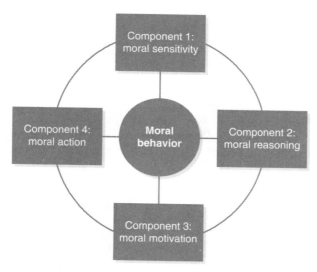

Figure 9-2 Depiction of Rest's Four-Component Model of Moral Behavior

Figure created by Lauren Petersen. Data from Rest, J.R. (1982). A psychologist looks at the teaching of ethics. *The Hastings Center Report, 12*(1), 29–36. https://www.jstor.org/stable/3560621 & Rest, J. R. (1983). Morality. In J. H. Flavell & E. M. Markman (Eds.), *Handbook of Child Psychology: Vol. 3. Cognitive Development* (4th ed., pp. 556–629), John Wiley & Sons.

1983; Robinson et al., 2014; Robichaux et al., 2022). These components are not necessarily linear nor a decision-making model; instead, they serve as a model for moral education as the components can be foci for proficiency attainment. The components are all interactive through feedback and/or feedforward loops and deficiency in any one component may result in the failure to behave morally (Rest, 1982; Rest, 1983). Robichaux et al. (2022) suggest this model for structuring an educational strategy to address moral development and the competency achievement in the *Essentials*. It will continue to be necessary to have learning content for ethical competencies presented in a variety of educational formats throughout DNP programs to support learner competency (Lee et al., 2020; Milliken & Grace, 2017; Robichaux et al., 2022).

Assume Accountability for Working to Resolve Ethical Dilemmas

As previously mentioned, Milliken and Grace (2017) suggest that all nursing practice is ethical and every action or decision is subject to ethical evaluation as outlined in the *Code of Ethics for Nurses*. Further, that *moral agency* is expected from professional nurses. Moral agency in the professional nurse "is having the intent and then acting to pursue, achieve, and maintain optimal beneficial outcomes consistent with the moral/ethical principles of one's practice" (AACN, n.d.-a., para. 2). Grace (2023a) describes moral agency as "the capacity and motivation to provide good care despite barriers and to support others in doing so" (p. 38). In this expectation for all nurses, it is important that DNP graduates are practiced in moral reasoning and ethical decision making to be accountable for engaging and leading in situations that benefit from nursing's ethical perspective. Particularly challenging will be situations where one needs to navigate the discordant intersections of personal values, beliefs, or emotions and professional moralities and principles.

Considering Rest's FCM, component 1 is the ability to recognize the presence of a dilemma or the presence of actions/contexts that may produce a dilemma and is critical for engaging in moral reasoning. Often referred to as moral or ethical sensitivity, Milliken and Grace (2017) contend that this critical antecedent to moral agency should be a more robust definition to include ethical awareness "recognizing that all of [nurses or healthcare professionals] actions are subject to ethical appraisal and the maintenance of this awareness is daily practice" (p. 519). Without ethical awareness or sensitivity, there are risks for patient safety or substandard care (Millikin & Grace, 2017). For example, nurses with insufficient ethical awareness or sensitivity are at risk for violating the principle of nonmaleficence, specifically related to negligence. Beauchamp and Childress (2019) describe negligence as "falls short of due care" (p. 160). Certainly there are times where negligence is flagrant, but it can also be unintentional and due to inattentiveness by the provider. The new-to-practice DNP graduate will buffer this risk through seeking out learning opportunities and building interprofessional care teams that strive to maintain current best practices. Likewise, seasoned APRNs, leaders, and educators who actively pursue current research and evidence-based practices resist the slide into "that's how I've always done it" attitudes that increase risk for negligence. Astute ethical awareness and sense of accountability, as part of a nursing identity, will foster safe, holistic care in all settings.

Analyze Current Policies and Practices Using an Ethical Framework

Analyzing practices or system policies with an ethical lens is supported using ethical principles and frameworks. Continuing with the use of Rest's FCM, components 2 and 3 offer structure for how one might approach an ethical dilemma or questions related to policies/practices (Rest, 1982; Rest 1983). The second component of Rest's model is moral reasoning or "formulating the morally ideal course of action" (Rest, 1982, p. 31). Robichaux et al. (2022) describes it as the process where the nurse seeks understanding to fully capture the situation for determining a moral course of action. In this step, a DNP-prepared nurse might draw on a variety of sources of knowledge including past learning and experiences, skills in empathy and compassionate care, appropriate ethical principles, and/or the stories of those involved to create a clear picture of understanding that can guide plans for an intervention. Methods for facilitating this learning in the academic environment might include coursework in ethical reasoning, case analysis, or simulation (Robichaux et al., 2022).

In the third component of Rest's FCM, moral motivation, nurses decide what course of action to take (Rest, 1982). A challenge within this phase is that ethical decision making does not occur in a vacuum. The nurse may be burdened with other pressing factors that confound or lean away from ethical actions (Liaschenko & Peter, 2016; Rest, 1983; Robichaux et al., 2022; Storaker et al., 2022). This may prompt action that is not in line with the moral action, or a movement back into moral reasoning as some of these factors may require evaluation of other ethical principles, such as justice and the equitable distribution of resources. Within this process, ethical accountability is inherent (Robichaux et al., 2022). An effective practice in self-reflection and self-evaluation of personal biases and perspectives can facilitate the nurse in developing their ethical awareness and subsequently their moral agency (Grace, 2023b; Wocial & Robinson, 2023). DNP curriculum in leadership, policy, social justice, and social determinants of health can bolster skills in moral motivation and agency (Robichaux et al., 2022).

Although DNP students may have background in ethical practice, their advancing education, skills, and roles will continue to influence their moral compass and ultimately their ethical comportment in a variety of settings. Ethical frameworks can be helpful for navigating ethical concerns and can be invaluable tools for DNP students. Codes of ethics are the most frequently used ethical framework for decision making in nursing practice and research (Mallari & Tariman, 2017). In *Nursing Ethics and Professional Responsibility in Advanced Practice* (4th ed.), Grace (2023a) offers a decision-making tool with common themes for guiding ethical evaluations. Actions in this resource include identifying and understanding the presence of an ethical concern, seeking to inform gaps in knowledge, understanding perspectives of those involved, deciding courses of action, and evaluation. It provides straightforward guidance and could be used in the DNP classroom for ethical competency development or in practice for real-time decision-making support. Astute ethical awareness and skilled knowledge in ethical evaluation prepare DNP nurses to critique ethical concerns in their work environments, including policies and practices, or to navigate ethical dilemmas.

Model Ethical Behaviors in Practice and Leadership Roles

The final concept of Rest's FCM is "executing and implementing what one intends to do," or moral action (Rest, 1982, p. 34). This is a critical step, as nurses can identify and reason through an ethical problem, but without action, all is for naught. DNP-prepared nurses taking moral action on ethical issues in practice help build moral communities which in turn fosters increased moral agency (Liaschenko & Peter, 2016). Wocial and Robinson (2023) describe four components of ethical competence in advanced practice nursing that can be applicable to all DNP practices: knowledge development, skill acquisition, ethical environments, and preventive ethics. The first two components align with the Rest's FCM of moral sensitivity and the processes through moral action. In these, DNP-prepared nurses develop a working knowledge of ethical language, theories, frameworks, and moral actions. The application of theories and decision-making frameworks can guide prompt engagement in conflict resolution from the nursing perspective. As a DNP-prepared nurse hones skills in ethical decision making and dilemma resolution, they can create a more significant impact as a leader by creating moral environments through mentorship. In this component, the focus is on relationship building that is respectful and inclusive to create systems change. The final component is movement toward preventive ethics and promoting social justice within the healthcare system (White et al., 2011). Preventive ethics refers to the policies or practices that preemptively mitigate the development of ethical issues (McCullough, 2005). In this final stage of ethical competency, the DNP-prepared nurse reflects the epitome of professionalism and ethical comportment through actions of empathy, moral agency, and mentorship that engenders an ethical environment where accountability, respect, and varied perspectives are valued.

Suggest Solutions When Unethical Behaviors Are Observed

As discussed above, honing an astute ethical awareness is imperative for DNP graduates as they are positioned as leaders in creating moral communities. Prepared with skills for building moral agency and community, DNP graduates can facilitate reduction in the occurrence and impact of *moral distress* by identifying unethical behaviors and taking action with ethical comportment. Originally defined by Andrew Jameton, *moral distress* is the emotional response to a time when an individual knows the correct moral action, but they are impeded from the action for various reasons (Jameton, 1984; Liaschenko & Peter, 2016; Rushton et al., 2016). Frequent encounters with morally distressing situations may lead to erosion in moral integrity and possibly one's overall sense of moral agency (Liaschenko & Peter 2016; Rushton et al., 2016). Further, unaddressed moral distress can introduce risks for patients and healthcare professionals (Grace 2023b; Rushton et al., 2016; Wocial & Robinson, 2023). Provisions 3 and 7 of the *Code of Ethics* directly address the responsibility of nurses to patients and the practice environment to uphold ethical care (ANA, 2015a). Active listening, concerted effort to understand perspectives, and collaborative solution development are critical for addressing ethical conflicts (Wocial & Robinson, 2023). The ultimate goal for addressing unethical behavior is to find an "integrity-preserving solution that is satisfactory to all parties" (Wocial & Robinson,

2023, p. 356). Through the development of skills to address ethical issues and interprofessional conflict, nurses can reduce their experiences with moral distress, resulting in better nursing practice and adherence to the guiding *Code of Ethics for Nurses* (Grace 2023b; Robinson et al., 2014; Rushton et al., 2016).

As outlined in the *Essentials,* moral agency and ethical competency is first nurtured in the learning environment. In the academic setting, DNP students will benefit from a variety of approaches and strategies for developing their moral compass and skills for analyzing ethical situations. Learning structures, such as the one presented by Robichaux et al. (2022), provide DNP educators a foundation to build ethics into the curriculum. DNP graduates will be prepared to identify ethical concerns and acknowledge their accountability as a professional nurse through understanding didactic concepts related to ethical principles and theories. Further, skill building with role-play and simulations prepare DNP graduates in a safe learning space to seek engagement as a leader in ethical dilemma resolution (Lee et al., 2020; Robichaux et al., 2022). As ethical care is synonymous with good care according to Grace (2023b), fostering confidence and competence in the classroom encourages future nursing clinicians, leaders, and educators to evolve their ethical practice and nurture its maturation over time and experience to fully reflect the ways a nurse thinks and acts as a member of the nursing profession.

Employ a Participatory Approach to Nursing Care

Creating a person-centered, participatory approach to care is a core value in the nursing discipline across all levels of practice. In provision of the "good" that the nursing profession offers, key aspects are a commitment to the uniqueness of individuals and preservation of autonomy. The BASE of nursing developed by Dr. Teddie Potter offers a framework to articulate nursing's unique contributions to health care. This includes *Ways of Relating* and *Ways of Knowing*, which describe the way that nurses engage with people and the ways they incorporate knowledge learned into practice (Eisler & Potter, 2014; Potter, 2013). The BASE of nursing identifies four unique domains of nursing: Being present, Active caring, Stories/narratives, and Evidence from science (Eisler & Potter, 2014). Nurses garner participatory partnerships by being present emotionally and physically as well as providing nursing care with skill, knowledge, and advocacy (Eisler & Potter, 2014). Further, respecting autonomy fosters independence and shared decision making. Beauchamp and Childress (2019) state that two conditions are required for autonomy: "*liberty* (independence from controlling influences) and *agency* (capacity for intentional action)" (p. 100). Further, they assert that "respect is shown through *action,* not merely by a respectful *attitude*" (p. 104). As such, DNP-prepared nurses can foster participatory care and learning environments through their active engagement in therapeutic and/or interprofessional relationships that respect an individual's worth and contribution as well as autonomy in pursuit of creating partnerships for best outcomes.

Foster Opportunities for Intentional Presence in Practice

To reflect the contributions and role of the professional nurse in any practice setting, a first step is ensuring that one's presence and role is articulated. In Buresh and

Gordon's (2013) *From Silence to Voice,* the importance of all nurses, in any capacity, to articulate their name, title, and include a handshake in greeting is highlighted. However, it should be acknowledged that the COVID-19 pandemic forced change around the use of handshakes; likewise, it is important to be respectful that not all individuals are comfortable or familiar with handshakes as a form of greeting. After an introduction of name and title, providing a brief description of the DNP-prepared nurse role and anticipated contributions to the setting serves to create a presence of the professional nurse as well as setting expectations. For example, a valuable practice in the clinical setting is to facilitate agenda setting for a visit. This intentional action helps the APN establish for the patient and family their practice role as well as welcoming shared decision-making to reflect the value of person-centered care. Through a practice of being present and using clear communication, DNP-prepared nurses can facilitate expectation setting and invitations for all to engage.

Identify Innovative and Evidence-Based Practices That Promote Person-Centered Care

From the practice of Active caring described in the BASE of nursing, DNP-prepared nurses are positioned to be innovators given their RN experience as problem solvers for an individual's concern or advocates in creating healthy, healing environments and interprofessional partnerships. Additionally, as reflected in Evidence in science, DNP nurses are guided by a commitment to evidence-based care. DNP graduates are experienced in moving scientific evidence to practice from their quality improvement coursework and project implementation. Competence in the AACN domains of "Knowledge for Nursing Practice" and "Person-Centered Care" fortifies the DNP-prepared nurse's professional identity and supports innovative, evidence-driven practices.

Advocate for Practices That Advance Diversity, Equity, and Inclusion and Policies/Practices That Promote Social Justice and Health Equity

In 2020, approximately 42,000 registered nurses (RN), representing a national sample, responded to the 2020 National Nursing Workforce survey (Smiley et al., 2021). The self-reported data showed that in the United States registered nurses identified 90.5% as female, 9.4% as male, and 0.1% as other. The RN workforce also self-reported on race with 81% identifying as White/Caucasian, 0.5% American Indian or Alaskan Native, 7.2% Asian, 6.7% Black/African American, 0.4% Native Hawaiian/Other Pacific Islander, 0.2% Middle Eastern or North African, 2.3% other, and 2.1% identified more than one race. Further, 5.6% self-reported as Latinx/Hispanic. Finally, of the responding RNs, 1.4% reported a DNP as their highest level of academic degree. In contrast, United States Census Bureau data (2020) reflects 50.5% of respondents identifying as female. Further, 75.8% identify as White, 1.3% American Indian or Alaskan Native, 6.1% Asian, 13.6% Black/African American, 0.3% Native Hawaiian/Other Pacific Islander, 2.9% as more than one race. Additionally, 18.9% responded as being Latinx/Hispanic. By these numbers it is clear that the nursing workforce, including the DNP-prepared nurses, have a demographic profile that is predominantly White and female, which is discordant with the public and presumably the populations served.

Given these differences in distribution of identities within the workforce compared to the public, advocacy for diversity and inclusion within the healthcare workforce to create dynamic interprofessional practices is imperative. By creating more diversity within the provider population, advances in health equity and reduction in health disparities are possible through increased *provider–patient concordance,* a term used to describe shared identities between providers and patients based on race, language, gender, age, social class, ethnicity, and values, among others (Cooper & Powe, 2004). Researchers have been trying to delineate the impact that concordance or discordance between providers and patients has on health outcomes and the potential to reduce health disparities (Cooper et al., 2003; Cooper & Powe, 2004; Johnson et al., 2011; Kurek et al., 2016; Meghani et al., 2009; Otte, 2022). As reflected in the literature review by Otte (2022), this is a complex, dynamic, multifaceted question and, in the current context of the workforce not being representative of the patient population, striving for more diversity in the workforce is critical, but cannot be the lone strategy employed. Training in cultural humility, implicit bias, communication, and patient-centered care is necessary for all health professionals to mitigate health disparities in all provider–patient relationships (Kurek et al, 2016; National Academies of Science, Engineering, and Medicine [National Academies], 2021; Otte, 2022). DNP nurses in all settings are prepared to lead and advocate for training in their learning environments and in future practices. Similarly, in the reciprocity of professional development, DNP-prepared nurses can coordinate opportunities to provide information, shadowing experiences, and/or recruitment events to inspire diverse students to enter the nursing profession at all levels.

Strategies that advance DEI in the healthcare professional sector can promote health equity through increased awareness and competence in all providers along with increased *patient–provider concordance.* However, DNP-prepared nurses can also increase their impact through engagement in health advocacy aimed at issues of social justice and health equity. The DNP-prepared nurse should consider all the aspects that impact the health of individuals and communities at local, regional, state, national, and global levels and how this intersects with social justice and health equity.

Model Professional Expectations for Therapeutic Relationships

The application of BASE of nursing clearly articulates nursing's professional expectations for therapeutic relationships as well as partnerships (Eisler & Potter, 2014). Relationship building and maintenance is present in direct patient care, in boardroom leadership, in advocating for a policy change, and/or when starting an entrepreneurial endeavor. A DNP-prepared nurse models *being present* in a clinical setting through undivided attention to the patient, in an interprofessional meeting by listening intently to the ideas and thoughts of their colleagues, and in the community hearing the needs of the members. A DNP educator demonstrates *active caring* by developing content and a classroom that is welcoming and inclusive. The DNP nurse leader uses *storytelling* when engaging a community, within a health system or the public, and listens to stories with intent for positive change and partnership. Finally, the DNP-prepared APN shares evidence-based information while inviting shared decision making and respecting autonomy, even if disagreement is present. To promote a partnership culture, a DNP-prepared nurse can set the stage for professional expectations by inviting collaboration and then clearly articulating the professional expectations agreed upon. Through professional comportment and communication, DNP-prepared nurses ensure they convey the professional expectations of nursing and create healthy, functional relationships in any practice setting.

Facilitate Communication That Promotes a Participatory Approach

Behaviors in communication that demonstrate a welcoming environment for participation includes active listening, eye contact, showing respect, honoring the words and thoughts of others, and displaying positive body language. These are not only valuable and beneficial skills, but also are focused on the actions of the DNP-prepared nurse as means for inviting participation. A more inclusive action would be to invite input to understand what is needed for an individual(s) to feel safe to participate. This prompt will invite individuals to articulate what may be necessary to create a safe, inclusive environment in which they feel valued and respected and can be applied to patients, students, teams, or organizations. For example, in a DNP classroom, faculty might ask students how they can be best supported to feel safe to engage in the content and offer anonymous modalities to share ideas. Starting with a premise of valuing each person and their perspective along their unique ways of learning or thinking creates environments that foster participation. Further, if care is taken to offer individuals time to process and generate responses, a rich and robust space for understanding and learning is supported. Presuming these differences exist within any given team, efforts to ensure that each member feels valued and their unique ways to participate identified will subsequently elicit contributions from all members. Similarly, this approach can apply to the clinical space or executive space. APNs can listen intently to their patients and families to determine what unique communication needs are present or preferred to move forward in the healthcare discussions. DNP leaders can create environments and settings in which people across the system feel safe to speak up and articulate difficult conversations. DNP-prepared nurses can lead in building collaborative and fully inclusive processes for communication and participation in any setting. This participatory approach supports nursing's mission to society to improve health and well-being in all settings.

Demonstrate Accountability to the Individual, Society, and the Profession

According to the *Code of Ethics for Nurses* (2015a), accountability means "to be answerable to oneself and others for one's own actions." However, what does accountability to oneself, others, and to the profession mean? Snowdon and Rajacich (1993) explored the meaning of nurse accountability and found varying definitions within the literature ranging from a responsibility to answer for one's actions to a moral obligation and concern over nursing care. Similarly, Krautscheid (2014) identified that there was a lack of consistent definition or language for professional accountability in nursing as well as a discrepancy in the connection between responsibility and accountability. Dohman (2009) identifies the distinction stating that responsibility is when a nurse has the authority to accomplish an activity, and authority is when the nurse has the free choice to achieve a result. Further delving into the concept of accountability, Krautscheid (2014) offered a definition of professional nursing accountability to be:

> taking responsibility for one's nursing judgements, actions, and omissions as they relate to life-long learning, maintaining competency, and upholding both quality patient care outcomes and standard of the profession while being answerable to those who are influenced by one's nursing practice. (p. 46)

To be accountable to oneself, the DNP-prepared nurse must remain vigilant of the current literature and practice recommendations for their unique settings. Further, being cognizant of what one does not know and confident in seeking help are attributes necessary to ensure due diligence. To be accountable to others, one must be responsible for providing care to patients, families, and communities and ensuring that the systems are set up appropriately for providing effective care. To be accountable to the profession, the DNP-prepared nurse should practice to the top of their license, work in partnership with interdisciplinary and transdisciplinary colleagues, and continue to advocate for autonomous nursing practice (Snowdon & Rajacich, 1993). The *Code of Ethics for Nurses* reflect these levels of accountability within the provisions as previously discussed and captures the foundation of the "Values & Ethics" in professional identity in nursing (see Figure 9-1).

Demonstrate Leadership Skills When Participating in Professional Activities/Organizations and Engage in Professional Organizations That Reflect Nursing's Values and Identity

An important aspect of professional identity is the influence of socialization and group membership within the profession. The application process and acceptance into a program is the first step into a new professional community for DNP students. Within a DNP program, their professional identity formation will undergo transformation with influences coming from the socialization in the classroom and practice environments. Crigger and Godfrey (2014) describe professional identity as two paradigms, a social one and a psychological one. In the social paradigm, nurses learn the expectations of the profession as it relates to ethics, scope and standards, and the expectations from society. Participation in a professional community is important for identity formation as these social interactions and context influence both identity development directly as well as professional competencies (Jarvis-Selinger et al., 2012). Professional socialization will occur in the classroom, in precepted clinical environments, and/or in leadership experiences. DNP graduates can seek support in professional identity development and socialization within their specialty or areas of interest by engaging in professional organizations as it is important that the process of socialization continue after program completion. As DNP-prepared nurses develop their competence and confidence in their practice setting, they may participate in leadership roles within an organization to support the contributions of nursing to health care or other professional interests. Further, the socialization process of professional identity formation relies on all nurses to "pay it forward" through mentorship and development of other nurses (AACN, 2021). **Box 9-1** provides a sample list of organizations that support professional nurses.

Box 9-1 Professional Nursing Organizations

American Academy of Nurse Practitioners (AANP)
American Nurses Association (ANA)
American Association of Colleges of Nursing (AACN)
American Association of Nurse Anesthetists (AANA)
American College of Nurse-Midwives (ACNM)
American Organization of Nursing Leadership (AONL)
American Organization of Nurse Executives (AONE)
National Coalition of Ethnic Minority Nurse Associations (NCEMA)
National Association of Clinical Nurse Specialists (NACNS)
National Association of Pediatric Nurse Practitioners (NAPNAP)
National Association of Hispanic Nurses (NAHN)
National Black Nurses Association (NBNA)
American Nursing Informatics Association (ANIA)
National Rural Health Association (NRHA)
National Organization of Nurses with Disabilities (NOND)

Lauren Petersen and Stephanie Gingerich

Address Actual or Potential Hazards and/or Errors and Foster a Practice Environment That Promotes Accountability for Care Outcomes

While errors occur within every profession, medical errors are a leading cause of death within the United States (Rodziewicz et al., 2022), and thus an important topic when considering systems changes for patient safety. Should an error occur, it is the responsibility and obligation of all professionals to speak up and identify the error. As a DNP student, understanding medical errors and pursuing ways to decrease their existence is necessary for promoting safe and effective changes. Error evaluation includes understanding the type of medical error, the basis for the error, and what barriers lead to the occurrence. To address errors in practice, The Joint Commission (2023) has developed the National Patient Safety Goals (NPSGs) yearly since 2003. The NPSGs target strategies to reduce errors across the various healthcare settings. While these strategies, if followed, may reduce the risks of errors in practice, a systems-level evaluation is vital to understand all points for patient risk mitigation. Too often, errors are viewed as shameful and an individual failure on the part of the provider. However, the processes, equipment, and systems in place may prove to be a significant factor in error risk and may instigate repeat events. Therefore, a comprehensive evaluation of both behaviors and processes that contribute to an error is necessary. Critiquing the causes holistically and seeking clarity of understanding can lead to change that prevents similar errors in the future.

While nurses have ethical responsibilities in error reporting, a culture of safety in which individuals feel secure in holding themselves and others accountable must be present. Leaders can create a culture of reporting safety by establishing anonymous reporting policies and investing resources into systems that are designed to prevent errors. "Rather than placing blame, administrators and review boards need to move toward eliminating the blame-shame-discipline structure and move toward a prevention and education structure" (Rodziewicz et, al. 2022, para. 13).

Additionally, some organizations employ strategies such as a Root Cause Analysis, a process used to identify the core issues resulting in the problematic event (Singh et al., 2022). Part of this process is to investigate the source of the error from human behaviors to systems processes. After identifying the root cause or core issue, the follow-up actions must be appropriately targeted toward the identified cause and evaluated for effectiveness. All nurses share the commitment to patient safety and advocating for practices that support best outcomes. For the DNP graduate, a new role may be in systems quality improvement and error reduction. DNP graduates leading in systems change reflect nursing's ethics and professional comportment by identifying errors, holding themselves and others accountable, and advocating for changes. Ensuring safe and effective practices for patients, colleagues, and the community reflects the professional expectations of nursing.

Lead in the Development of Opportunities for Professional and Interprofessional Activities

Working in silos with limited communication and collaboration will not adequately address the current health inequities, surging costs, and healthcare access issues in the United States. Rather, an intentional focus on gathering various disciplines together and sharing professional perspectives can provide new and innovative ideas for overdue healthcare change. In 2010, the World Health Organization developed the *Framework for Action on Interprofessional Education and Collaborative Practice* stating that interprofessional education "occurs when two or more professions (students, residents, and health workers) learn with, about, and from each other to enable effective collaboration and improve health outcomes." This statement was updated in 2016 to reaffirm the need for collaboration and intentional preparation of future healthcare professionals to work in team-based settings to address population health outcomes (Interprofessional Education Collaborative, 2016).

The Health Professions Accreditors Collaborative (2019) developed a set of recommendations for interprofessional education across academic and healthcare settings (see **Box 9-2**).

Interprofessional collaboration is key to addressing the health challenges that persist today. DNP students can promote and lead activities from the academic setting across the healthcare continuum to ensure that interprofessional collaboration occurs. DNP students engaged in interprofessional learning are prepared to be future healthcare innovators and change agents.

Comply With Relevant Laws, Policies, and Regulations

"Fight for things that you care about, but do it in a way that will lead others to join you."

— Ruth Bader Ginsburg

Nurses have an incredible opportunity to effect change in the transformation of healthcare, patient outcomes, and the nursing practice environment. The *Code of Ethics for Nurses* outlines the role and commitment of the nurse to influence health outcomes further than the individual patient in provisions 7, 8, and 9 (ANA, 2015a). Likewise, the *Nursing: Scope and Standards of Practice* outlines standards

---

Box 9-2 Recommendations for Interprofessional Education Across Academic and Healthcare Settings

---

- Strategic direction and approach, through a compelling vision to "set the tone at the top" led by academic and institutional leaders (e.g., Presidents, Chancellors, Vice-Chancellors, Provosts, Councils of Deans);
- Appropriate resources to develop, implement, evaluate, and sustain IPE plans (e.g., dedicated faculty time to IPE, staff, space, and finances) at the institutional and education and/or training program levels;
- Logistical support and management (e.g., alignment of academic calendars, scheduling, classroom and facilities planning and design, common affiliation agreements with health systems);
- Dedicated leader and/or team of leaders with sufficient protected time, responsibility and accountability for IPE at the institutional level;
- Coordinating structure to facilitate joint IPE curricular planning and oversight involving faculty and administrative leaders from participating education and/or training programs;
- Development of financing models, including tuition-attribution for IPE in concert with individual program models;
- Identification and development of solutions for institutional policies that may hinder interprofessional collaboration;
- Faculty development related to the planning, implementation, and assessment/evaluation of IPE activities in classroom, simulation, and clinical/experiential education settings; and
- Formal recognition of faculty effort toward successful implementation of IPE (e.g., job expectations, the promotion/tenure process).

related to advocacy, collaboration, and leadership (ANA, 2021). The complexity of today's healthcare environment and the increase in volume of scientific knowledge demand the involvement of nurses to be prepared to influence policy on the local, state, and national levels (Mund, 2021). Arguably, the nursing profession has expectations that members will be engaged and at the table with interprofessional colleagues to guide and influence health policy.

Most nurses can identify and/or feel passionate about policies that they believe do not serve patients or the profession well. Some nurses might be particularly passionate about health policies where their professional and personal identities intersect. Advocacy starts with being well versed in an issue by understanding the evidence and the history, but requires action for change. A challenge for most is knowing how to get involved or start to take actions. The new *Essentials* incorporate the concept of health policy in the domain of professionalism because, as pragmatically raised by Oestberg (2012), nurses must advocate for important issues, otherwise, those with little knowledge about nursing or with competing interests with nurses will lead decisions in policies that affect nurses and patients. The DNP curriculum provides foundational knowledge and skills for advocacy in health policy. Learning strategies that incorporate active participation in legislative or regulating processes will reduce the perceived barriers to getting involved.

Advocate for Nursing's Professional Responsibility for Ensuring Optimal Care Outcomes and Participate in the Implementation of Policies and Regulations to Improve the Professional Practice Environment and Healthcare Outcomes

DNP graduates are positioned to influence the content and quality of healthcare legislation. They have extensive clinical background and are able to curate well-developed analyses of issues. With a working knowledge of the language of legislation and regulation, DNP graduates can influence and lead in health policy and resources allocation consistent with the values and perspectives of nursing (Mund, 2021). The *Nursing: Scope and Standards of Practice* (ANA, 2021) articulates the need for professional nurses to advocate and lobby for issues, such as:

- evaluation and restructuring of health care and healthcare systems
- reimbursement for the value of nursing care
- funding for nursing education
- identifying the role of nurses and nursing in health and medical homes
- comparative effectiveness, transparency, and quality of care
- advances in health information technology (pp. 35–36)

Further, nurses can serve as members in legislative bodies, organizational boards, and/or scientific committees (ANA, 2021). Overall, the DNP-prepared nurse can serve as an active voice of the nursing profession to advocate for optimal care outcomes at the bedside, within organizations.

Influencing the Health Policy Agenda. Public policy is created by governmental legislation and involves laws and regulations. Public policy can be divided into social policy, which concerns communities, and health policy, which focuses on the health of the individual (Mason et al., 2021, Mund, 2021). As DNP-prepared nurses are increasingly empowered to engage in the process of transforming health care, the following sections offer ideas for both DNP students and educators to engage in health policy (Mund, 2021).

Write a Health Policy Brief. A potential avenue for influencing health policy is to author a policy brief. A policy brief serves as a written communication that summarizes an issue and offers policy options based on evidence and expertise to influence a selected course of action for addressing the issue—it is not an opinion piece or a specific call to action (Wong et al., 2017). Specifically, it is a means to inform those without a background in health care, but with political sway, about the most pressing issues affecting nurses, patients and the delivery of health care.

A policy brief can be defined as a short report that addresses the interests and needs of policy makers through application of best evidence in an effort to produce a solution to a problem (DeMarco & Tufts, 2014; Mund, 2021). See **Box 9-3** for considerations on developing a policy brief.

Policy briefs are a valuable modality for DNP graduates to get involved in health policies that impact nursing and patient outcomes. Although "brief" in words, such documents can be a challenge to write as each sentence will need to capture critical information or arguments. Demarco and Tufts (2014) and Wong et al. (2017) offer

Box 9-3 Considerations for the Development of a Policy Brief

Make it brief and understandable for a non–healthcare provider audience.
Know the audience and what problems they are interested in solving.
The brief should be no longer than four pages and as succinct as possible.
A typical format consists of four sections: an executive summary, background
    and significance, statement of the author's position, and a reputable
    reference list.
Determine the most efficacious timing for submitting the brief.
A sense of urgency is a powerful motivator in seeking solutions.
Provide a convincing argument through a systematic review of the literature.
Advocate for a desired solution based on the information.
Provide data that refute objections to the solution proposed within the brief.
Demonstrate credibility and expertise in the area of concern.
Clearly articulate the action you request of your audience.

Data from DeMarco, R., & Tufts, K. A. (2014). The mechanics of writing a policy brief. *Nursing Outlook, 62,* 219–224.

practical, accessible recommendations for brief writing in health policy. Application in a classroom serves as a space for DNP students to practice and prepare skills in persuasive writing and argument articulation.

Engage as a Nurse Expert in the Legislative Process. The legislative process is rarely the linear, rational process described in textbooks. Instead, it is a process whereby competing interests attempt to influence policy making by creating bargains, trading votes, and using rhetoric to convince legislators that their policy agenda is best. As previously mentioned, DNP-prepared nurses have the opportunity and responsibility to educate lawmakers regarding concerns for nursing and healthcare as legislation moves through the legislative bodies and government agencies (Mund, 2021). A common way for DNP-prepared nurses to influence legislation is through partnership with interested and supportive legislators in the state or federal House of Representatives or Senate. The most successful partnerships are developed over time instead of forced during times of crisis or expedience, as this creates a relationship of trust and mutual respect (Mund, 2021).

A DNP-prepared nurse may get involved by participating in the legislation drafting process. In pursuit of upholding the interests of the nursing profession, it will be beneficial at the drafting stage to allow any nursing stakeholders to review the language of proposed legislation. This is important as not all language will be viewed the same by all nursing groups, and what may be good for one group may be detrimental to another. Nurses may also serve as content experts in advocacy for the profession of nursing or topical concerns to help shape the healthcare agenda. The opportunity to share expertise in favor of or against a piece of legislation will be completed through oral or written testimony. It is imperative to know the opposition of your legislation and be able to generate a strategy for managing any counterarguments. Well-prepared testimony includes a description of who is doing the testifying (e.g., a family NP in a rural practice), the background of the issue, and why the legislation is supportive or detrimental in resolving the issue. Effective testimony must also include commentary by the expert regarding preferred actions or outcomes they'd like to see from the committee (Mund, 2021).

An important role for DNP nurses throughout the legislative process is to contact their representatives or senators and to build coalitions with other professional associations. The importance of creating these relationships prior to the introduction of any legislation will become evident as the bill moves through Congress. Nurses must not wait until the proposed legislation is being voted on—this is too late! Instead, nurses must be involved early and through all stages to develop the relationship before a request for action is warranted (Mund, 2021).

Exemplars. Safe staffing in nursing discussions is a common practice concern, but commanded more attention across the country amidst the COVID-19 pandemic given the demands for staff and resource shortages compounded by the influx of patients. In response to this pervasive issue, a new bill was introduced in Washington State in 2023 which includes discussions on safe staffing standards, staffing committees, and enforcing existing laws such as meal breaks (Washington State Nurses Association, 2023). Similarly, Colorado recently enacted legislation which stipulates that hospitals have a staffing committee of at least 60% clinical staff nurses to address safe staffing alongside ancillary staff and hospital leaders (Colorado General Assembly, n.d.). DNP-prepared nurses can provide expertise for crafting such legislative documents and serve on committees to discuss potential solutions and barriers to issues with proposed interventions. DNP-prepared nurses are able to advocate for the interests of both the nursing profession and patients as well as articulate policies and processes to support both. DNP educators support advocacy skill development by offering DNP students opportunities and examples of how to engage in political discussions at the local, state, and national legislative levels.

Advocating for optimal care outcomes may also be initiated when gaps are identified. Within the United States, Black women giving birth have higher rates of babies born premature, with low birth weight, or infant mortality as compared to White women (Burris & Hacker, 2017; CDC, 2019). One organization addressing the inequities within birthing care outcomes in minority and impoverished communities is the Nurse Family Partnership (NFP), a nursing-led home visitation program (American Academy of Nursing [AAN], 2021). This program offers in-home services for low-income, first-time parents, with services which have demonstrated reduction in preterm delivery for women who smoke and fewer hypertensive disorders of pregnancy as well as a reduction in injuries among children as demonstrated by lower incidence of emergency visits for accidents and poisonings from birth to age 2 (AAN, 2021). Regardless of the practice issue, professional nurses are positioned to advocate for environments, policies, and practices grounded in nursing's values and commitment to promoting optimal care outcomes.

Advocate for Policies That Enable Nurses to Practice to the Full Extent of Their Education

Continued concerns persist across the country regarding issues of healthcare access, staff attrition exacerbated during the pandemic, and worrisome patient outcomes as compared to other industrialized countries (The Commonwealth Fund, 2021; The Commonwealth Fund, 2023). The United States ranks last compared to other industrialized countries regarding access to and timeliness of care as well as affordability (The Commonwealth Fund, 2021). According to the American Hospital Association (2022), 136 rural hospitals closed between 2010 and 2020, limiting rural access to health care. These are just glimpses of the strain and dire need for transformation in the United States healthcare system. As part of the nursing's ethical code, nurses need to be involved at the political level to drive healthcare change and promote full scope nursing practice for the health of patients and populations (ANA, 2015a).

One integral part of addressing the complexity of health care and the current gaps is to acknowledge and promote the practice of nurses to the full extent of their education. With nurses prepared as APNs, policies should be addressed to ensure that they are able to practice at the top of their license to improve access to health care across the country. To address the topic of healthcare access and related barriers for patients in Minnesota (MN), advanced practice registered nurse (APRN) leaders from MN met in 2009 (MN APRN Coalition, n.d.). Over the course of several years, they formed the APRN Coalition to advocate and propose legislation to allow for APRN full practice authority so MN APRNs could practice to the full scope of their education and support enhanced healthcare access to residents in MN (MN APRN Coalition, n.d.). Legislation was passed in 2015 allowing MN APRNs to practice without physician oversight, due largely in part to the partnership and collaborative efforts of the MN APRN coalition, interdisciplinary team members, and healthcare leaders across the state. Work continues to ensure that outdated legislation is updated to reflect language that allows MN APRNs to practice to the top of their license (MN APRN Coalition, n.d.). For example, a MN statute now allows nurse practitioners to evaluate teachers on their disability status; previously, MN APRNs were not included in the list of acceptable providers (Teachers Retirement, 354.48 Permanent disability benefits, n.d.). Likewise, the Improving Care and Access to Nurses (I CAN) Act is proposed legislation which would allow "other health care providers besides physicians (e.g., nurses) to provide certain services under Medicare and Medicaid . . . [including] a nurse practitioner or physician assistant to fulfill documentation requirements for Medicare coverage of special shoes for diabetic individuals" (I CAN Act, H.R.8812, 117th Cong., 2022). Ensuring nurses at all levels can practice to the top of their education and license will allow for a more accessible healthcare system and create opportunities for innovation.

Assess the Interaction Between Regulatory Agency Requirements and Quality, Fiscal, and Value-Based Indicators

As healthcare leaders consider their organizations and best care delivery formats, they must also identify, measure, and evaluate the quality, fiscal, and value-based indicators as part of the overall strategic planning. They must follow the regulatory requirements set at the state and national levels. In addition, they must address the issue that healthcare outcomes in the United States have continued to rank the lowest among international industrialized countries despite spending at least double what other countries spend on health care (The Commonwealth Fund, 2023). As such, work needs to be done to address not only lower level outcomes but also costs associated with healthcare in the United States.

In 2009, Teisberg and Wallace identified three main strategies that were needed to address costs and for health care outcomes in the United States to improve:

> (1) reorganizing care delivery into clinically integrated teams defined by patient needs over the full cycle of care; (2) measuring and reporting patient outcomes by clinical teams, across the cycle of care and for identified clusters of medical circumstances; and (3) enabling reimbursement tied to value rather than to quantity of services. (p. 1)

Since their 2009 work, they have continued as thought leaders in methods to improve the value of healthcare and in 2016 created the *Value Institute for Health and Care* at the University of Texas, Austin (Value Institute for Health and Care, 2023). Their further research into health care organizations around the world (Teisberg, et al., 2020) led to development of a strategic framework for value-based healthcare implementation which includes the following concepts:

> (1) Understand shared health needs of patients; (2) Design solutions to improve health outcomes; (3) Integrate learning teams; (4) Measure health outcomes and costs; and (5) Expand partnerships. (p. 4)

As discussed, focusing only on one aspect of healthcare will likely not improve the value of healthcare. DNP-prepared nurses must be aware of the patient and family perspective, the providers involved in the care, organizational structures, quality, fiscal, and value-based indicators, as well as regulatory agencies requirements. The DNP-prepared nurse can partner with individuals, organizations, and agencies to implement such models as offered by Teisberg and Wallace. Regulatory agencies exist to monitor, inform, guide, and ensure high safety standards in health care. Agencies such as the Center for Disease Control (CDC), Environmental Protection Agency (EPA), Food and Drug Administration (FDA), and Occupational Safety and Health Administration (OSHA) maintain regulations and update recommendations to ensure safe practices across healthcare. The DNP-prepared nurse should be aware of the internal resources and metrics within an organization and of the regulations at the state and national levels that will drive practice and ensure thoughtful planning for use of resources and effective partnerships across healthcare systems.

Evaluate the Effect of Legal and Regulatory Policies on Nursing Practice and Healthcare Outcomes and Analyze Efforts to Change Legal and Regulatory Policies That Improve Nursing Practice and Health Outcomes

As a DNP student, it is necessary to be aware of legal and regulatory policies being proposed or discussed at the state, regional, and national levels and consider the potential impact on nursing practice. Some may have ramifications for how care is delivered, how documentation must be completed, and how staffing must be managed. To effectively advocate in support of or against legal and/or regulatory policies, DNP-prepared nurses should maintain awareness of proposed changes to policies of interest and be prepared to share evidence from a nursing perspective as previously described.

As an example, workplace violence is considered "any act or threat of physical violence, harassment, intimidation or other threatening, disruptive behavior from patients, patients family members, external individuals, and hospital personal . . . [including] physical, sexual, and psychological assaults" (ANA, 2023, para. 2). The World Health Organization (WHO) and the International Council of Nurses (ICN) expand this definition to also include violence related to work that occurs during work or when commuting to or from work (International Labour Organization et al., 2002). "From 2016 to 2020 there were 207 deaths due to violence in the workplace in the health care and social assistance industry within the private sector" (CDC, 2020, para. 2). Recent fatal events such as at the Methodist Dallas Medical Center, where an individual shot and killed a patient care manager and a nurse, has brought to light the ubiquity and severity of this issue (Southwick, 2022).

Nurses continue to be assaulted in the workplace and recent legislation has been proposed to address workplace violence within healthcare settings known as the Workplace Violence Prevention for Health Care and Social Service Workers Act (2022). If passed, covered facilities will need to have an identified and unique workplace violence plan (developed by employees and leaders) based on the setting and risks present, with processes, procedures, training, and responses clearly identified. As a DNP student or graduate, consider how this legislation may impact the work settings in which you are employed. What policies may need to be adjusted? How will this impact patient care? What impact would this legislation and new protocols have on the statistics of workplace violence for healthcare providers?

Demonstrate the Professional Identity of Nursing

Often, nurses will simplify their profession to *just* a nurse. In addition, the public often views nursing as a caring profession that completes the orders provided by a physician without truly understanding the skill and evidence incorporated into the practice of nursing. In Buresh and Gordon's (2013), *From Silence to Voice,* the authors depict the ways the profession of nursing is misunderstood, erroneously portrayed, and sidelined despite the critical work of nursing in health care. Cingel and Brouwer (2021) argue that long-standing stereotypes of being a task-oriented, subordinate, and female profession is obstructing the advancement of the profession and professional identity which may result in long-term impacts on health systems if active change is not pursued. In continued calls for change by experts in nursing ethics, policy, academia, research and practice, as a profession, nurses at all levels are positioned to participate in changing the narrative to accurately convey what it is to think, act, and be a nurse (Godfrey & Young, 2021).

Formation of professional identity is not a linear process; rather, it is a dynamic process that is responsive to academic experiences, clinical learning, and mentorship. In addition, it demands the intentional drive of nurses to develop their own unique professional identity. At times, the maturation may be slow and seemingly undetectable, as it evolves from the decisions and experiences of everyday work. Other times there may be distinct formative moments, such as navigating an ethical dilemma or serving as an expert in the legislative process. These developmental and maturational processes happen across all nursing practices including the new graduate registered nurse, the retiree, nurses at the bedside, or those in leadership. Nurses pursuing DNP degrees are intentionally seeking advanced clinical knowledge and scopes of practice, these endeavors will produce transformations in professional identity. For the DNP student, the development of a professional identity includes both the construction of the new identity, a doctorally prepared nurse, and the deconstruction or reconstruction of the previous identity, as a registered nurse (Jarvis-Selinger et al., 2012). Through this process, professional comportment will be necessary to continue to reflect the values and characteristics of the nursing profession.

Articulate Nursing's Unique Professional Identity to Other Interprofessional Team Members and the Public

In *The Future of Nursing 2020–2030: Charting a Path to Achieve Health Equity* by the National Academies of Sciences, Engineering, and Medicine (National Academies, 2021) there is a frank call to not only increase the nursing workforce, but for increasing nursing's contributions through full scope of practice. The unique knowledge, skills, and perspectives of nursing will facilitate equitable and innovative healthcare delivery. For too long, the dominant stereotypes and narrative of nursing being female, subordinate, and/or task-oriented have persisted and been reinforced in healthcare institutions, media, and by nurses themselves (Buresh & Gordon, 2013; Cingel & Brouwer, 2021; Godsey et al., 2020). Therefore, nursing today is at a critical nexus to doff the old stereotypes and instead articulate the discipline and the necessity of nursing practice as an independent professional entity within the healthcare setting. Further, as professional identity includes the intersection of personal and professional identities, communicating the vital role of nursing in both personal and professional arenas will help garner understanding in the populations that nurses care with and care for in practice. Through professional comportment, DNP graduates demonstrate the value of the nursing perspective and expertise in healthcare transformation (see Figure 9-1).

A particular challenge for DNP-prepared nurses to be aware of is the potential for intraprofessional discord and workplace bullying. Anderson et al. (2020) found three thematic relationships between APNs and RNs including *conciliating nursing* (positive relationship building), *vertical discounting* (dismissiveness and undermining between APNs and RNs) and *lateral othering* (APNs undermined by other APNs). Such relational interactions potentially undermine the professional identity of individuals and of nursing as a discipline by fortifying stereotypes or creating toxic environments due to bullying (Edmonson & Zelonka, 2019). Lacking a unified sense of professionalism leaves nursing stereotypes space to persist or be reinforced, instead of reflecting the contributions of the nursing profession. Edmonson and Zelonka (2019) offer strategies to address and reduce intraprofessional bullying. DNP students have an evolving identity, but it remains grounded in an RN background. By reflecting on their new role and recognizing their active role in the nursing community, DNP-prepared nurses can support and advance the profession in unity with other nurses to achieve the goals outlined in the *Future of Nursing 2020–2030* (National Academies, 2021; Grace, 2023a).

Again, in Buresh and Gordon's (2013), *From Silence to Voice,* they describe ways in which nursing is understood in the public. Examples that may be most pertinent for the DNP graduate in a clinical setting will be preparing responses that reflect the professional identity of nursing to questions such as, "Why didn't you just go to medical school?" Or for the DNP-prepared nurse leaders being asked, "Oh, so you aren't really a nurse?" Recognizing the importance of word choice, DNP-prepared nurses will need to take care to avoid perpetuating the stereotype of "just a nurse" in their responses to such questions given their new roles and perspectives. Likewise, APNs can reflect the skills and knowledge of the profession through purposeful introductions as previously discussed and actions that reflect expertise and knowledge in clinical reasoning and care planning. DNP graduates in academia or leadership positions can use their space of influence to create a systems-level understanding of the nursing profession and support future nurses in professional identity development. The classroom environment remains an ideal place for crafting statements, role-playing responses, and simulations to bolster DNP students in their confidence and competence for articulating their professional identity.

Evaluate the Practice Environment to Ensure That Nursing Core Values Are Demonstrated

In the 1980s, the American Academy of Nursing developed a task force to identify the unique characteristics of work environments that attracted and retained nurses providing quality care during a nursing shortage period (American Nurses Credentialing Center [ANCC], n.d.). The task force identified specific institutions with characteristics they defined as "forces of magnetism" to attract and retain these high-quality healthcare workers (ANCC, n.d.). Today, hospital and healthcare institutions can apply to earn Magnet designation by demonstrating a culture supportive of nursing with five model components: transformational leadership; structural empowerment; exemplary professional practice; knowledge, innovation, and improvements; and empirical quality results (ANCC, n.d.). Currently, there are over 600 facilities worldwide that have Magnet designation. Studies have shown that organizations with Magnet designation were associated with improved nursing satisfaction and retention (Kutney-Lee et al., 2015). Whether a healthcare organization chooses to pursue Magnet designation or an alternative method of evaluation, it is important that time and resources are committed to emphasizing the value of the nursing culture within the organization.

DNP graduates have expertise in patient care at both the RN and DNP practice level and have skills in system needs assessment. Therefore, DNP-prepared nurses are prepared for advocacy, making recommendations to mitigate issues and bolster the magnetic qualities that may be present. DNP-prepared nurses might facilitate workplace improvements by applying Gallup's four phases of culture change when issues arise. The four phases are: "1) Understand the current state of your culture; 2) Define the gap between aspirational and actual culture; 3) Align activities, initiatives and systems; 4) Establish accountability and ongoing evaluation" (Gallup, 2018, p. 17). While addressing these aspects of culture, it is vital that DNP-prepared nurses continually re-evaluate the culture and the value that the organization places on nursing. Questions such as: does the organization support nurses in practice with policies and process?; does the organization support nurses to advance their career?; does the organization allow nurses to practice at the top of their license?; does the organization value nurses and value nursing input throughout the healthcare experience? These questions can help the DNP nurse navigate the workplace cultural changes that may be necessary to further promote the nursing profession and its core values while supporting patient care across the healthcare continuum.

Identify Opportunities to Lead With Moral Courage to Influence Team Decision Making

Understanding the concept and the need for moral courage is imperative as a nurse in any setting. Moral courage supports ethical care and creates moral practice environments. The AACN (n.d.-b) describes moral courage as "the ability to stand up for and practice that which one considers ethical, moral behaviors when faced with a dilemma, even if it means going against countervailing pressure to do otherwise" (para. 2). The trailblazers from the past and change agents of the future have cultivated and employed moral courage in advocacy for health equity, nurse practice issues, and social justice. Through development of ethical competencies and collaborative care values, DNP-prepared nurses have garnered skills around ethical decision making and moral agency and are ready to employ moral courage as needed in team decision-making processes. Through action of moral courage, nurses convey nursing's commitment to positive health outcomes and contributions to the values of inclusivity, humanity, and social justice.

Integrate Diversity, Equity, and Inclusion as a Core to One's Professional Identity

Throughout this chapter, nursing's commitment to ethical practice and compassionate care and the call to action to articulate what it means to be a nurse, all reflect aspects of professionalism and the formation of a professional identity in nursing. Within each of these concepts, the need for addressing and advocating for DEI within the nursing profession is paramount. Nurse graduates at all levels are prepared to care and advocate for all individuals, especially those who have been historically or currently marginalized, underrepresented, and underserved. Integration of the concepts of diversity, equity, and inclusion into the core of their professional identity is necessary to truly reflect the values and mission of nursing. Building practices with a foundational commitment to disrupting and dismantling discrimination in our systems, our institutions, our classrooms, and our communities will lead to social justice and health equity. This work must be done by all of us, for all of us. The following subcompetencies are intended to offer tangible actions that DNP-prepared nurses can use to be change agents in the communities where we serve and live.

Model Respect for Diversity, Equity, and Inclusion

In a survey by the National Commission to Address Racism in Nursing, 3 out of 4 nurses reported having witnessed racism in the workplace, and not just from patients (ANA, n.d.-a). Black nurses reported experiencing racist acts from patients, peers, and leaders in almost equal measure. This survey was conducted in 2021 after the launch of the National Commission to Address Racism in Nursing, a partnership of nursing organizations with a mission to "confront and mitigate racism within the nursing profession and address the impact that racism has on nursing and nurses" (ANA, n.d.-a).

On June 11, 2022, the American Nurses Association adopted "Our Racial Reckoning statement" that includes acknowledging past actions contributing to racism within the profession, apologizing for these actions, and making a commitment to change (ANA, n.d.-b). This statement reflects the expectation for the nursing profession and its membership to commit to change related to the concepts of diversity, equity, and inclusion. As a part of this commitment and ongoing evolution of professional identity in nursing, it would be valuable for all nurses to review this statement and the resources offered for individuals to begin taking action and modeling our professional commitment to diversity, inclusivity, and equity.

Critique One's Personal and Professional Practices in the Context of Nursing's Core Values

Just as a DNP-prepared nurse should be astute to evaluate the practice environment, it is also necessary to reflect on and critique one's own actions and beliefs in the pursuit of building a moral and just practice. A focus on the critical skill of reflective practice and the application of moral courage engenders the concept of DEI in professional identity formation. Hilton and Slotnick (2005) highlight reflection and self-awareness as an important domain for professionalism development in the medicine learner, which can reasonably be applied to the DNP student. Reflective practice supports professional self-awareness regarding strengths and weaknesses, supports meaning-making from complex situations, and has the potential to create better outcomes for patients (Koshy et al., 2017; Mann et al. 2009). In their systematic review, Mann et al. (2009) explored reflection in health professions and the role educators play in helping students develop reflective practice skills. Although the literature was limited, they generally found that reflective practice is a skill to develop and is most successful with clear guidance and mentorship. Educators in academic and clinical settings are well positioned to model and actively support these formative skills in all facets of nursing practice.

The National Academies (2021) report recommends that cultural humility and implicit bias training be integrated throughout nursing curriculums. In consideration of building self-assessment and reflective practice as it relates to DEI, DNP students and educators could benefit from participating in assessments from the Implicit Project from Harvard (found at www.implicit.harvard.edu) as a means to create intention around understanding one's own biases and reflecting on how this may impact one's practice. Engaging with this process of self-assessment and reflection related to identifying personal biases, can influence professional identity development through a deeper understanding of what one brings into their professional identity and what experiences have had a positive or negative impact that might influence practice. Such engagement in personally vulnerable actions to better understand oneself can be illuminating and is a critical action that DNP-prepared nurses can take to make change for equitable health care and social justice.

Analyze the Impact of Structural and Cultural Influences on Nursing's Professional Identity

In pursuit of reducing health disparities, all academic settings should actively make changes in the structure and culture to create formative learning environments that not only have more diversity in students and faculty, but are more inclusive by valuing the perspectives and experiences of individuals in the classroom and the profession (Kurek et al., 2016; Marks & McCulloh, 2016; National Academies, 2021; Otte, 2022). Classrooms and clinical settings with diversity in races, ethnicities, genders, sexual orientations, religions, immigrant status, socioeconomic status, ages, and/or disabilities create profound learning for all from the sharing of personal, lived experiences and varied perspectives (Marks & McCulloh, 2016; National Academies, 2021; Otte, 2022). What nurses and other healthcare professionals offer as full partners and healthcare innovators will be more robust if learning and working environments are filled with unique and diverse professionals. All DNP educators, students, and leaders are equipped to innovate and pursue strategies to not only recruit more diverse student bodies, but to create learning environments that are rich in diverse experiences and inclusive of all perspectives. The classroom is a place that garners skills in critiquing the influences of structures or workplace culture and support skills for being agents of change. Learning environments committed to the DEI concept will be formative in the professional identity of students and engender the core values of nursing.

Ensure That Care Provided by Self and Others Is Reflective of Nursing's Core Values

Many nurses have experienced or know of incidences of microaggressions occurring in education or health care related, but not limited, to race, gender, sexual identity, religion, and/or disability. Sue et al. (2019) describe microaggressions as the "every day" events of implicit or explicit bias and/or discrimination experienced at the individual or interpersonal level that results in negative impact. In these events, nurses may be a target, a source, an ally, or a bystander. Often these events pass by without identification or challenge, subsequently compounding their negative impact (Sue et al., 2019). As professional nurses with a commitment to values of integrity, inclusion, and humanity, activating moral agency and moral courage in these moments can minimize how often these moments go unchecked.

Inaction in these events allows a permissiveness of exclusion and inequity to persist. Even if the moment is recognized, the involved individuals are often so unsure of how to respond that they remain inert. In their work to move toward taking action, Sue et al. (2019) offer concrete, accessible strategies for individuals "to begin the process of disarming, disrupting, and dismantling the constant onslaught of microaggressions" (p. 131). Examples of strategies shared include phrases that "disarm the microaggression" by expressions of disagreement and redirection or by "making the 'invisible' visible" by naming the microaggression or putting the stereotype in question (pp. 135–137). Although the strategies described reflect a simplicity, putting them into action can be challenging and the context of the moment needs evaluation for safety (Sue et al., 2019). In similar work that offers practical skills, Ackerman-Barger and Jacobs (2020) created the *Microaggressions Triangle Model* for health professional schools. This model offers a tangible resource for all healthcare professionals to build skills in navigating microaggressions. For each role in a microaggression triangle (recipient, source, or bystander), there is an acronym representing actions to take for responding to the microaggression. For DNP educators, this tool may be helpful for structuring role-playing scenarios for the classroom.

An important aspect of the *Microaggressions Triangle Model* (Ackerman-Barger & Jacobs, 2020) is the discussion and actions offered for those who are a source of the microaggression. In the case where one is the source of a microaggression, there are ways to navigate the event with composure, trust, and hope for relationship repair. Like bringing microaggressions to light, responding to being called out for a micro-aggression takes practice and preparation. Responding may include taking a deep breath and listening while acknowledging bias, focusing on the hurt, and seeking to educate oneself to understand the offensive action and how to improve (Ackerman-Barger & Jacobs, 2020; Knight, 2020). These resources can be used by all profes-sionals to make positive change in health care, learning, and work environments. By increasing awareness of and sensitivity to microaggressions, practicing skills for navigating incidences of microaggressions, and reflecting on one's own biases, all DNP-prepared nurses can begin to disrupt the persistence of these events and build a practice reflective of nursing's core values and code of ethics.

Structure the Practice Environment to Facilitate Care That Is Culturally and Linguistically Appropriate

As previously addressed, articulating the role of the DNP-prepared nurse in a clini-cal environment is not only important for communicating the professional practice of nursing, but also to ensure a shared understanding of the scope of practice for the APN to set expectations for care. To ensure clear, understandable, communication, the APN should advocate for appropriate time needed for adequate communication for individuals with articulation diagnoses or interpreters for patients with preferred languages that the APN is not fluent in. Juckett and Unger (2014) share useful tech-niques for successful engagement of professional medical interpreters in practice to assure clear communication and high-quality care. It is not recommended to rely on family members for interpretation as there may be unknown medical terminol-ogy to navigate or there is a risk for the family member to omit content from the perspective of caring for their loved one (Juckett & Unger, 2014). At the systems levels, DNP-prepared nurses in leadership can advocate for policies and practices that create culturally and linguistically appropriate care. Considering the increasing diversity in cultures and languages within the United States, the need for creating compassionate care and learning environments that reflect the diversity of the pop-ulation requires intentionality from DNP-prepared nurses to foster inclusive spaces for patients, students, colleagues, and professional partners.

Foster Strategies That Promote a Culture of Civility Across a Variety of Settings and Ensure Self and Others Are Accountable in Upholding Moral, Legal, and Humanistic Principles Related to Health

According to the Institute of Medicine (2000), factors impacting patient safety in-clude teamwork and communication amongst the care team. In addition to this, incivility in the workplace undermines patient safety and may be costly to an organi-zation (Black, 2019; Spiri et al., 2016; Edmonson & Zelonka, 2019). The ANA sub-mitted a position statement identifying that it is the shared responsibility of nurses and employers to "create and sustain a culture of respect, which is free of incivility, bullying, and workplace violence" (2015b, p. 1). Incivility was classified as ranging from actions taken to not taken, overt to covert, and challenged nurses, employers, educators, and leaders to acknowledge the presence of incivility and to promote a culture of civility across nursing in health care and academia (ANA, 2015b).

While some recommended strategies focus on the individual, other strategies to promote a culture of civility occur at the organizational or systems level. DNP-prepared nurse leaders maintaining a professional comportment grounded in the values and ethics of nursing exemplifies and sets the expectation for behaviors that are civil, kind, and enhance interpersonal and interprofessional relationships. Additionally, when uncivil behaviors are identified, leaders take action and hold those accountable as appropriate. Equally important, leaders create space for those affected by the incivility to safely express their concerns and provide access to appropriate resources. Systems can also incorporate training programs to enhance communication and teamwork such as TeamSTEPPS, an evidence-based training that supports healthcare workers in building effective relationships with clear communication and teamwork strategies (Agency for Healthcare Research and Quality, 2013).

Beyond role modeling, it is important that those in positions of authority and leadership, such as DNP-prepared nurses, are ready to advocate in moments of incivility. Such moments may include microaggression identification as previously discussed or supporting professional colleagues in more overt cases, such as patients' refusal of care based on prejudice. Preparing a strategy for these moments is an example of a practice level commitment to a culture of civility. Paul-Emile et al. (2016) discuss the challenges of navigating a racist patient from the provider perspective and offer an insightful algorithm to support navigating medical stability and principles of autonomy while protecting the provider, abiding by legal requirements, and maintaining a no tolerance policy. DNP students and educators might consider using this work to prepare graduates with skills and resources to respond to scenarios of prejudicial basis for care refusal. Preparation for managing prejudice supports a simultaneous upholding of a commitment to patient care and a commitment to a civil work environment that protects healthcare professionals within the system.

Addressing the concepts of DEI and the impacts of prejudice and discrimination is at the forefront in discussions on how the nursing profession can better support the future of nursing and our ethical commitment to good patient care. As stated, this is work by all of us, for all of us. DNP-prepared nurses are well positioned to lead with our interprofessional colleagues for a socially just and humanity-focused healthcare system that is committed to the health and well-being of those who are served by and work in it.

Summary

The evolution of a nurse's professional identity is not static, but a cyclical, nonlinear process that evolves with influences by personal identities, educators, family/friends, clinical experiences, the media, and policy. Although the academic process is a formative time, professional identity is not granted, nor complete, on the day of graduation. Instead, throughout a DNP program, new aspects of professional identity germinate and grow, not in exception to a previous identity as an RN, but in addition to, as all nurses engage in lifelong learning.

As described throughout this chapter, the overarching concepts outlined by the *Essentials* are core areas of knowledge for DNP-prepared nurses. They provide the underpinnings to the competencies expected of the DNP graduate by the profession and the public. Nurses practice across healthcare and academic settings in service to patients, families, students, communities, states, nations, and the world. The DNP-prepared nurse has an obligation to serve their intended population while leading healthcare change broadly. A commitment to DEI is critical to being change agents in the pursuit of nursing's fundamental commitment to improvement in the health and well-being of all. Application of the code of ethics and core values provides the basis for a practice of moral agency and courage in any setting in which a DNP-prepared nurse practices. In nursing's unique ways of knowing and relating, DNP graduates are prepared to provide compassionate care and be accountable for their practice. In synthesis of the unique knowledge and skills of nursing, DNP graduates are poised to engage in health policy and advocacy to wield the greatest impacts. All DNP graduates will need professional comportment and clear articulation of the nursing profession to dispel deeply rooted stereotypes and establish nursing as a unique discipline and professional partner in health care. In doing so, nurses will be an integral part of the change required to address the health concerns present within our communities and abroad.

As we look to the future of the nursing profession, DNP-prepared nurses are in a position to make profound changes across healthcare systems. In pursuit of these changes, DNP-prepared nurses can be role models in "rebranding" the profession and articulating to patients, interprofessional colleagues, and the public what it means to think like, act like, and be a nurse. Further, DNP-prepared nurses can follow the lead of the National Commission to Address Racism in Nursing and lean into some discomfort to begin dismantling prejudice and discrimination within one's own professional identity and the larger professional identity of nursing. Through this, real transformation in healthcare can begin. Finally, DNP-prepared nurses will need to reflect on experiences that have influenced and molded their professional identity and then pay it forward to those new or early in the profession of nursing. By committing to lifelong learning and engaging in the cycles of professional identity formation, DNP-prepared nurses are grounded with the Professional Identity in Nursing domains because they have engendered the ethics and values of nursing, have unique knowledge supported by evidence and influenced by stories, and are prepared to lead with intentionality and professional comportment.

References

Ackerman-Barger, K., & Jacobs, N. N. (2020). The microaggressions triangle model: A humanistic approach to navigating microaggressions in health professional schools. *Academic Medicine, 95*(12, suppl), s28–s32. https://doi.org/10.1097/ACM.0000000000003692

Agency for Healthcare Research and Quality. (2013). *TeamSTEPPSTM Pocket Guide-2.0: Team strategies & tools to enhance performance and patient safety*. Publication #14-0001-2. http://www.ahrq.gov/professionals/education/curriculum-tools/teamstepps/instructor/essentials/pocketguide.html.

American Academy of Nursing. (2021). *Edge-Runners: Nurse-family partnerships helping first-time parents succeed*. https://www.aannet.org/initiatives/edge-runners/profiles/edge-runners--nurse-family-partnerships

American Association of Colleges of Nursing. (n.d.-a) *Moral Agency*. https://www.aacnnursing.org/5B-Tool-Kit/Themes/Moral-Agency

American Association of Colleges of Nursing. (n.d.-b). *Moral Courage*. https://www.aacnnursing.org/5B-Tool-Kit/Themes/Moral-Courage

American Association of Colleges of Nursing. (2021). *The Essentials: Core competencies for professional nursing education*. AACN.

American Hospital Association. (2022). *Rural hospital closures threaten access: Solutions to preserve care in local communities.* https://www.aha.org/system/files/media/file/2022/09/rural-hospital-closures-threaten-access-report.pdf

American Nurses Association. (n.d.-a) *National commission to address racism in nursing.* https://www.nursingworld.org/practice-policy/workforce/racism-in-nursing/national-commission-to-address-racism-in-nursing/

American Nurses Association. (n.d.-b). *Our Racial Reckoning Statement.* https://www.nursingworld.org/practice-policy/workforce/racism-in-nursing/RacialReckoningStatement/

American Nurses Association. (2015a). *Code of ethics for nurses with interpretive statements.* Nursingbooks.org.

American Nurses Association. (2015b). *Incivility, bullying, and workplace violence.* https://www.nursingworld.org/practice-policy/nursing-excellence/official-position-statements/id/incivility-bullying-and-workplace-violence/

American Nurses Association. (2021). *Nursing: Scope and standards of practice* (4th ed.). Author.

American Nurses Association. (2023). *End nurse abuse.* https://www.nursingworld.org/practice-policy/work-environment/end-nurse-abuse/

American Nurses Credentialing Center. (n.d.) *About magnet.* https://www.nursingworld.org/organizational-programs/magnet/about-magnet/

Anderson, H., Birks, Y., & Adamson, J. (2020). Exploring the relationship between nursing identity and advanced nursing practice: An ethnographic study. *Journal of Clinical Nursing, 29*(7–8), 1195–1208. https://doi.org/10.1111/jocn.15155

Beauchamp, T. L., & Childress, J. F. (2019). *Principles of biomedical ethics* (8th ed.). Oxford University Press.

Benner, P., Sutphen, M., Leonard, V., & Day, L. (2010). *Educating nurses: A call for radical transformation.* Jossey-Bass.

Black, A. (2019). Promoting civility in healthcare settings. *International Journal of Childbirth Education, 34*(2); 64–67.

Buresh, B., & Gordon, S. (2013). *From silence to voice: What nurses must know and communicate to the public* (3rd ed.). Cornell University Press.

Burris, H. H., & Hacker, M. R. (2017). Birth outcome racial disparities: A result of intersecting social and environmental factors. *Seminars in Perinatology, 41*(16), 360–366. https://doi.org/10.1053/j.semperi.2017.07.002

Centers for Disease Control and Prevention. (2019). *Racial and ethnic disparities continue in pregnancy-related deaths.* https://www.cdc.gov/media/releases/2019/p0905-racial-ethnic-disparities-pregnancy-deaths.html

Centers for Disease Control and Prevention. (2020). *The national institute for occupational safety and health (NIOSH).* https://wwwn.cdc.gov/WPVHC/Nurses/Course/Slide/Unit1_6

Cingel, M., & Brouwer, J. (2021). What makes a nurse today? A debate on the nursing professional identity and its need for change. *Nursing Philosophy, 22,* e12343. https://doi.org/10.1111/nup.12343

Colorado General Assembly. (n.d.). HB22-1401: Hospital nurse staffing standards concerning the preparedness of health facilities to meet patients needs, and, in connection therewith, making an appropriation. https://leg.colorado.gov/bills/hb22-1401

The Commonwealth Fund. (2021). *Mirror, mirror 2021: Reflecting poorly health care in the U.S. compared to other high-income countries.* https://www.commonwealthfund.org/publications/fund-reports/2021/aug/mirror-mirror-2021-reflecting-poorly#access

The Commonwealth Fund. (2023). *U.S. health care from a global perspective, 2022: Accelerating spending, worsening outcomes.* https://www.commonwealthfund.org/publications/issue-briefs/2023/jan/us-health-care-global-perspective-2022

Cooper, L. A., & Powe, N. R. (2004). Disparities in patient experiences, health care processes, and outcomes: The role of patient-provider racial, ethnic, and language concordance. *The Commonwealth Fund.* https://www.commonwealthfund.org/publications/fund-reports/2004/jul/disparities-patient-experiences-health-care-processes-and

Cooper, L. A., Roter, D. L., Johnson, R. L., Ford, D. E., Steinwachs, D. M., & Powe, N. R. (2003). Patient-centered communication, ratings of care, and concordance of patient and physician race. *Annals of Internal Medicine, 139*(11), 907–915.

Crigger, N., & Godfrey, N. (2014). From the inside out: A new approach to teaching professional identity formation and professional ethics. *Journal of Professional Nursing, 30*(5), 376–382.

Cruess, R. L. , Cruess, S. R. , Boudreau, J. D., Snell, L., & Steinert, Y. (2014). Reframing medical education to support professional identity formation. *Academic Medicine, 89*(11), 1446–1451. https://doi.org/10.1097/ACM.0000000000000427

Cruess, S. R., Cruess, R. L., & Steinert, Y. (2019). Supporting the development of professional identity: General principles. *Medical Teacher, 41*(6), 641–649. https://doi.org/10.1080/01421 59X.2018.1536260

DeMarco, R., & Tufts, K. A. (2014). The mechanics of writing a policy brief. *Nursing Outlook, 62*, 219–224. https://www.nursingoutlook.org/article/S0029-6554(14)00057-8/pdf

Dohman, E. (2009). *Accountability in nursing: Six strategies to build and maintain a culture of commitment.* HCPro, Inc.

Edmonson, C., & Zelonka, C. (2019). Our own worst enemy: The nurse bullying epidemic. *Nurse Administration Quarterly, 43*(3), 274–279. https://doi.org/10.1097/NAQ.0000000000000353

Eisler, R., & Potter, T. (2014). *Transforming interprofessional partnerships: A new framework for nursing and partnership-based health care.* Sigma Theta Tau International.

Fitzgerald, A. (2020). Professional identity: A concept analysis. *Nursing Forum, 55*(3), 447–472. https://doi.org/10.1111/nuf.12450

Frank, J. R., Snell, L. S., Cate, O. T., Holmboe, E. S., Carraccio, C., Swing, S. R., Harris, P., Glasgow, N. J., Campbell, C., Dath, D., Harden, R. M., Iobst, W., Long, D. M., Mungroo, R., Richardson, D. L., Sherbino, J., Silver, I., Taber, S., Talbot, M., & Harris, K. A. (2010). Competency-based medical education: Theory to practice. *Medical Teacher, 32*(8), 638–645. https://doi.org/10.3109 /0142159X.2010.501190

Gallup. (2018). *Gallup's approach to culture: Building a culture that drives performance.* http://acrip .co/contenidos-acrip/gallup/2020/noviembre/gallup-perspective-building-a-culture-that-drives -performance.pdf

Giddens, J., Douglas, J. P., & Conroy, S. (2022). The revised AACN essentials: Implications for nursing regulation. *Journal of Nursing Regulation, 12*(4), 16–22.

Godfrey, N., & Young, E. (2021). Professional identity. In J. F. Giddens (Ed.), *Concepts for nursing practice* (3rd ed., pp. 363–370). Elsevier.

Godfrey, N. (2022). New language for the journey: Embracing a professional identity of nursing. *Journal of Radiology Nursing, 41*(1), 15–17. https://doi.org/10.1016/j.jradnu.2021.12.001

Godsey, J. A., Houghton, D. M., & Hayes, T. (2020). Registered nurse perceptions of factors contributing to the inconsistent brand image of the nursing profession. *Nursing Outlook, 68*(6), 808–821. https://doi.org/10.1016/j.outlook.2020.06.005

Goodolf, D. M., & Godfrey, N. (2021). A think tank in action: Building new knowledge about professional identity in nursing. *Journal of Professional Nursing, 37*(2), 493–499. https://doi .org/10.1016/j.profnurs.2020.10.007

Grace, P. (2018, January 31). Enhancing nurse moral agency: The leadership promise of Doctor of Nursing Practice preparation. *OJIN: The Online Journal of Issues in Nursing, 23*(1), Manuscript 4. https://doi.org/10.3912/OJIN.Vol23No01Man04

Grace, P. J. (2001). Professional advocacy: Widening the scope of accountability. *Nursing Philosophy, 2*, 151–162.

Grace, P. J. (2023a). Nursing ethics. In P. J. Grace & M. K. Uveges (Eds.), *Nursing ethics and professional responsibility in advanced practice* (4th ed., pp. 36–76). Jones & Bartlett Learning.

Grace, P. J. (2023b). Philosophical foundations of applied and professional ethics. In P. J. Grace & M. K. Uveges (Eds.), *Nursing ethics and professional responsibility in advanced practice* (4th ed., pp. 2–36). Jones & Bartlett Learning.

Health Professions Accreditors Collaborative. (2019). *Guidance on developing quality interprofessional education for the health professions.* https://healthprofessionsaccreditors.org/wp-content /uploads/2019/02/HPACGuidance02-01-19.pdf

Hilton, S. R., & Slotnick, H. B. (2005). Proto-professionalism: How professionalisation occurs across the continuum of medical education. *Medical Education, 39*(1), 58–65.

I CAN Act, H.R.8812, 117th Cong. (2022). https://www.congress.gov/bill/117th-congress/house -bill/8812?s=1&r=6

Institute of Medicine. (2000). *To err is human: Building a safer health system*. National Academies Press.

International Labour Organization, International Council of Nurses, Work Health Organization & Public Services International. (2002). *Framework guidelines for addressing workplace violence in the health sector.* https://www.ilo.org/wcmsp5/groups/public/---ed_dialogue/---sector/documents/normativeinstrument/wcms_160908.pdf

Interprofessional Education Collaborative. (2016). *Core competencies for interprofessional collaborative practice: 2016 update*. Interprofessional Education Collaborative.

Jameton, A. (1984). *Nursing practice: The ethical issues*. Prentice Hall.

Jarvis-Selinger, S., Pratt, D. D., & Regehr, G. (2012). Competency is not enough: Integrating identity formation into the medical education discourse. *Academic Medicine, 87*(9), 1185–1190. https://doi.org/10.1097/ACM.0b013e3182604968

Johnson Thornton, R. L., Powe, N. R., Roter, D., & Cooper, L. A. (2011). Patient-physician social concordance, medical visit communication and patients' perceptions of health care quality. *Patient Education and Counseling, 85*(3), e201–e208. https://doi.org/10.1016/j.pec.2011.07.015

The Joint Commission. (2023). *National patient safety goals*. https://www.jointcommission.org/standards/national-patient-safety-goals/

Juckett, G., & Unger, K. (2014). Appropriate use of medical interpreters. *American Family Physician, 90*(7), 476–480.

Knight, R. (2020, July 24). You've been called out for a microaggression. What do you do now? *Harvard Business Review*. https://hbr.org/2020/07/youve-been-called-out-for-a-microaggression-what-do-you-do

Koshy, K., Limb, C., Gundogan, B., Whitehurst, K., & Jafree, D. J. (2017). Reflective practice in health care and how to reflect effectively. *International Journal of Surgery Oncology, 2*(6), e20. https://doi.org/10.1097/IJ9.0000000000000020

Krautscheid, L. C. (2014). Defining professional nursing accountability: A literature review. *Journal of Professional Nursing, 30*(1), 43–47. https://doi.org/10.1016/j.profnurs.2013.06.008

Kurek, K., Teevan, B. E., Zlateva, I., & Anderson, D. R. (2016). Patient-provider social concordance and health outcomes in patients with type 2 diabetes: A retrospective study from a large federally qualified health center in Connecticut. *Journal of Racial and Ethnic Health Disparities, 3*, 217–224. https://doi.org/10.1007/s40615-015-0130-y

Kutney-Lee, A., Stimpfel, A. W., Sloane, D., Cimiotti, J., Quinn, L., & Aiken, L. (2015). Changes in patient and nurse outcomes associated with Magnet hospital recognition. *Med Care, 53*(6), 550–557. https://doi.org/10.1097/MLR.0000000000000355

Landis, T., Godfrey, N., Barbosa-Leiker, C., Clark, C., Brewington, J., Joseph, M. L., Luparell, S., Phillips, B. C., Priddy, K. D., & Weybrew, K. A. (2022). National study of nursing faculty and administrators' perceptions of professional identity in nursing. *Nurse Educator 47*(1), 13–18. https://doi.org/10.1097/NNE.0000000000001063

Lee, S., Robinson, E. M., Grace, P. J., Zollfrank, A., & Jurchak, M. (2020). Developing a moral compass: Themes from the Clinical Ethics Residency for Nurses' final essays. *Nursing Ethics, 27*(1), 28–39. https://doi.org/10.1177/0969733019833125

Liaschenko, J., & Peter, E. (2016). Fostering nurses' moral agency and moral identity: The importance of moral community. *The Hastings Center Report, 46*(5), S18–S21. https://doi.org/10.1002/hast.626

Mallari, M. G. D., & Tariman, J. D. (2017). Ethical frameworks for decision-making in nursing practice and research: A integrative literature review. *Journal of Nursing Practice Applications & Reviews of Research, 7*(1), 50–57.

Mann, K., Gordon, J., & MacLeod, A. (2009). Reflection and reflective practice in health professions education: A systematic review. *Advances in Health Sciences Education, 14*(4), 595–621. https://doi.org/10.1007/s10459-007-9090-2

Marks, B., & McCulloh, K. (2016). Success for students and nurses with disabilities: A call to action for nurse educators. *Nurse Educator, 41*(1), 9–12. https://doi.org/10.1097/NNE.0000000000000212

Mason, D. J., Perez, A., McLemore. M. R., & Dickson, E. (2021). *Policy & politics in nursing and health care* (8th ed.). Elsevier.

McCullough L. B. (2005). Practicing preventive ethics—the keys to avoiding ethical conflicts in health care. *Physician Executive, 31*(2), 18–21.

Meghani, S. H., Brooks, J. M., Gipson-Jones, T., Waite, R., Whitfield-Harris, L., & Deatrick, J. A. (2009). Patient–provider race-concordance: Does it matter in improving minority patients' health outcomes? *Ethnicity & Health, 14*(1), 107–130. https://doi.org/10.1080/13557850802227031

Merriam-Webster. (n.d.). Professionalism. In *Merriam-Webster.com dictionary*. https://www.merriam -webster.com/dictionary/professionalism

Milliken, A., & Grace, P. (2017). Nurse ethical awareness: Understanding the nature of everyday practice. *Nursing Ethics, 24*(5), 517–524. https://doi.org/10.1177/0969733015615172

Minnesota APRN Coalition. (n.d.) *History*. https://mnaprnc.enpnetwork.com/page/22301-history

Mund, A. (2021). Healthcare policy for advocacy in health care. In M. E. Zaccagnini & J. M. Pechacek, (Eds.), *The doctor of nursing practice essentials: A new model for advanced practice nursing* (4th ed., pp. 131–162). Jones & Bartlett.

National Academies of Sciences, Engineering, and Medicine. (2021). *The future of nursing 2020– 2030: Charting a path to achieve health equity*. The National Academies Press. https://doi .org/10.17226/25982

Oestberg, F. (2012). Policy and politics: Why nurses should get involved. *Nursing, 42*(12), 46–49. https://doi.org/10.1097/01.NURSE.0000422645.29125.87

Otte, S. V. (2022). Improved patient experience and outcomes: Is patient–provider concordance the key? *Journal of Patient Experience, 9*, 1–7. https://doi.org/10.1177/23743735221103033

Owens, R., & Godfrey, N. (2022). Fostering professional identity in nursing: How to wholly support nurse well-being. *American Nurse Journal, 17*(9), 12–16.

Paul-Emile, K., Smith, A. K., Lo, B., & Fernández, A. (2016). Dealing with racist patients. *The New England Journal of Medicine, 374*(8), 708–711. https://doi.org/10.1056/NEJMp1514939

Potter, T. M. (2013). *The BASE of nursing*. Unpublished manuscript, School of Nursing, University of Minnesota, United States of America.

Rest, J. R. (1982). A psychologist looks at the teaching of ethics. *The Hastings Center Report, 12*(1), 29–36. https://www.jstor.org/stable/3560621

Rest, J. R. (1983). Morality. In J. H. Flavell & E. M. Markman (Eds.), *Handbook of Child Psychology: Vol. 3. Cognitive Development* (4th ed., pp. 556–629). Wiley.

Robichaux, C., Grace, P., Bartlett, J., Stokes, F., Saulo Lewis, M., & Turner, M. (2022). Ethics education for nurses: Foundations for an integrated curriculum. *The Journal of Nursing Education, 61*(3), 123–130. https://doi.org/10.3928/01484834-20220109-02

Robinson, E. M., Lee, S. M., Zollfrank, A., Jurchak, M., Frost, D., & Grace, P. (2014). Enhancing moral agency: Clinical ethics residency for nurses. *Hastings Center Report, 44*(5), 12–20.

Rodziewicz, T. L., Houseman, B., & Hipskind, J. E. (2022). *Medical error reduction and prevention*. In: StatPearls [Internet]. StatPearls Publishing. https://www.ncbi.nlm.nih.gov/books/NBK499956/

Rushton, C. H., Caldwell, M., & Kurtz, M. (2016). Moral distress: A catalyst in building moral resilience. *The American Journal of Nursing, 116*(7), 40–49. https://doi.org/10.1097/01.NAJ .0000484933.40476.5b

Singh, G., Patel, R. H., & Boster, J. (2022). *Root cause analysis and medical error prevention*. In: StatPearls [Internet]. StatPearls Publishing. https://www.ncbi.nlm.nih.gov/books/NBK570638/

Smiley, R. A., Ruttinger, C., Oliveira, C. M., Hudson, L. R., Allgeyer, R., Reneau, K. A., Silvestre, J. H., & Alexander, M. (2021). The 2020 national nursing workforce survey. *Journal of Nursing Regulation, 12*(1), S1–S96. https://doi.org/10.1016/S2155-8256(21)00027-2

Snowdon, A. W., & Rajacich, D. (1993). The challenge of accountability in nursing. *Nursing Forum, 28*(1).

Southwick, R. (2022, October 24). Dallas hospital shooting marks latest attack on healthcare workers. *Chief Healthcare Executive*. https://www.chiefhealthcareexecutive.com/view /dallas-hospital-shooting-marks-latest-attack-of-healthcare-workers

Spiri, C., Brantley, M., & McGuire, J. (2016). Incivility in the workplace: A study of nursing staff in the military health system. *Journal of Nursing Education and Practice, 7*(3), 40–46. https://doi .org/10.5430/jnep.v7n3p40

Storaker, A., Tolo Heggestad, A. K., & Sμteren, B. (2022). Ethical challenges and lack of ethical language in nurse leadership. *Nursing Ethics, 29*(6), 1372–1385. https://doi .org/10.1177/09697330211022415

Sue, D. W., Alsaidi, S., Awad, M. N., Glaeser, E., Calle, C. Z., & Mendez, N. (2019). Disarming racial microaggressions: Microintervention strategies for targets, white allies, and bystanders. *American Psychologist, 74*(1), 128–142. http://dx.doi.org/10.1037/amp0000296

Teachers Retirement, § 354.48 (n.d.) *Permanent disability benefits*. https://www.revisor.mn.gov/statutes/2022/cite/354.48?keyword_type=all&keyword=aprn

Teisberg, E., & Wallace, S. (2009). Creating a high-value delivery system for health care. *Seminars in Thoracis and Cardiovascular Surgery, 21*(1), 35–42. https://doi.org/10.1053/j.semtcvs.2009.03.003

Teisberg, E., Wallace, S., & O'Hara, S. (2020). Defining and implementing value-based health care: A strategic framework. *Academic Medicine, 95*(5): 682–685. https://doi.org/10.1097/ACM.0000000000003122

United States Census Bureau. (2020). *Quickfacts: United States*. https://www.census.gov/quickfacts/fact/table/US/POP010220#POP010220

Value Institute for Health and Care (2023). *Transform health care*. https://valueinstitute.utexas.edu/

Washington State Nurses Association. (2023). *Safe staffing legislation*. https://cdn.wsna.org/assets/entry-assets/659637/Safe-staffing-legislation-summary-2023.pdf

White, K. W., Zaccagnini, M. E., Casey, K. H., & Britain, M. K. (2011). Ethics, In M. E. Zaccagnini & K. W. White (Eds.), *The doctor of nursing practice essentials: A new model for advanced practice nursing* (1st ed., pp. 317–345). Jones & Bartlett.

Willetts, G., & Clarke, D. (2014). Constructing nurses' professional identity through social identity theory. *International Journal of Nursing Practice, 20*(2), 164–169. https://doi.org/10.1111/ijn.12108

Wocial, L. D., & Robinson, E. M. (2023). Ethical practice. In M. F Tracy, E. T. O'Grady, & S. J. Phillips (Eds.), *Advanced practice nursing: An integrative approach* (7th ed., pp. 341–381). Elsevier.

Wong, S. L., Green, L. A., Bazemore, A. W., & Miller, B. F. (2017). How to write a health policy brief. *Families, Systems, & Health, 35*(1), 21. http://dx.doi.org/10.1037/fsh0000238

Workplace Violence Prevention for Health Care and Social Service Workers Act. (2022). https://www.baldwin.senate.gov/imo/media/doc/Baldwin%20Workplace%20Violence%20Protection%20for%20Health%20Care%20and%20Social%20Service%20Workers%20Act.pdf

World Health Organization. (2010). *Framework for action on interprofessional education and collaborative practice*. https://apps.who.int/iris/bitstream/handle/10665/70185/WHO_HRH_HPN_10.3_eng.pdf;jsessionid=F5FAFBCB64C40F5EEB0CA99F3CD6E942?sequence=1

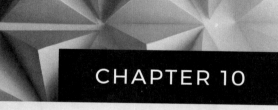

CHAPTER 10

Personal, Professional, and Leadership Development

Joy Elwell, DNP, FNP-BC, APRN, CNE, FAAN, FAANP

"Authentic service can be seen in the nurse who has nurtured herself, the healer who has been healed. It is the service we hear when the nurse can speak from her heart to the patient these simply and humble words, 'I am here. Let's heal together'"

—**Caryn Summers**

Introduction

This domain addresses the nurse's care of self. While the other domains focus externally, this domain focuses internally on the nurse. According to the 2021 *Essentials* document, this involves "Participation in activities and self-reflection that foster personal health, resilience, and well-being; contribute to lifelong learning; and support the acquisition of nursing expertise and the assertion of leadership" (AACN, p. 54).

Self-care is critical to personal, professional, and leadership development, as without self-care, the nurse risks frustration, stagnation, and burnout. There is significant literature on self-care that validates the effects of compassion fatigue and burnout on patient outcomes.

Crane and Ward (2016) identify stressors associated with nursing practice and discuss self-care techniques, including mindfulness, deep breathing exercises, meditation, relaxation exercises, yoga, tai chi, and qigong, hypnosis, and visualization. In personal interviews, nursing faculty acknowledge that self-care is not typically addressed with students at the undergraduate or graduate level. Given the ample number of nurses leaving the profession, or considering such a move, it is incumbent on faculty in prelicensure and graduate nursing programs to address this prior to graduate nurses finding themselves in difficult working situations.

Nantsupawat et al. (2016) found in their study on nurses and burnout that nurse burnout is associated with higher likelihood of negative health outcomes among patients. They recommended healthcare systems acknowledge this reality and implement interventions to reduce nurse burnout.

Ross et al. (2019), in a study examining the barriers and facilitators of health-promoting self-care among registered nurses found that the study participants revealed barriers to self-care behaviors including lack of time, lack of adequate resources/facilities, fatigue, outside commitments, and unhealthy food culture. The last, unhealthy food culture, included a lack of healthy choices in hospital cafeterias, the prevalence of calorie-dense offerings brought into work by colleagues for celebrations, and perceiving the need to reward oneself with treats, such as doughnuts or cake. Conversely, facilitators of positive self-care behaviors included sharing healthy recipes, taking walks during breaks, as well as having managers who encouraged exercise by supporting nurses to leave the unit during breaks.

While the effects of burnout on the health outcomes of patients and healthcare systems are of vital importance, no less important are the effects of burnout on nurses themselves. Filoramo (2022) identified that burnout can result in anxiety and depression, but that it is not unavoidable or unmanageable. She recommended that building resilience can help prevent burnout by facilitating the nurse's ability to cope with and recover from unexpected challenges that are intrinsic to the nursing role. Some of the approaches to building resilience include offsetting negative emotions with positive ones, finding positive meaning, mindfulness activities, developing self-awareness, and building/supporting strong interpersonal relationships.

Resilience

Self-care cannot be discussed in a vacuum. Resilience is a key component of nurses' interest in, and ability to engage in, self-care. It is defined as "the ability to adapt successfully in the face of stressful or threatening situations" (Filoramo, 2022, p. 237).

Guo et al. (2019), in a comparative cross-sectional study on burnout and resilience found that while burnout is common, and increases the risk of staffing turnover, its effects are mitigated in nurses who report resilience. Blackburn et al. (2020) implemented a program designed to develop resilience in a population of oncology nurses, which was found to be successful.

This begs the question, can resilience be taught or developed? The literature suggests that it can. Walsh et al. (2020) conducted an integrative review of the literature and their findings concluded that resilience is a valuable trait that should be included in nursing curricula.

How, then, can nursing programs incorporate resilience strategies into their curricula? One example is at the University of Connecticut. A doctoral (DNP) student developed and implemented, for their DNP Project, a mindfulness learning module, and administered it to prelicensure, graduate, and doctoral nursing students (Carini, 2023). Such programs are valuable for students and practicing nurses alike and healthcare systems should reinforce and support resiliency skills as a way to invest in the well-being of their employees.

Selected Concepts for Nursing Practice Represented in the Domain

The AACN *Essentials* concepts that can be considered as most clearly represented in this domain are communication, diversity, equity, and inclusion (DEI), and ethics. Communicating in a manner that is nonthreatening is essential to development of professional maturity and leadership capacity, as well as being crucial for mentoring and peer review (AONL, 2015; Clark, 2017; Kouzes & Posner, 2023; Voss et al., 2022). Being a champion for DEI as well as being cognizant of one's own biases is necessary to contribute to an environment that promotes well-being and an essential leadership skill (Kouzes & Posner, 2023). Also, leadership needs to be based within the concept of ethics as a foundation of nursing practice in order to advocate for social justice and address inequities present in nursing, healthcare settings, and society at large (Nardi et al., 2020). Additionally, the concept of ethics can be associated with nurses and other healthcare professionals experiencing burnout and leaving the bedside because of moral distress and moral hazards experienced in healthcare settings (DeChant, 2022). Such distress and hazards have been present for some time (Jameton, 2017) but were exacerbated by the COVID-19 pandemic. Thus, the need for an emphasis on fostering an environment that promotes self-care as an essential competency for professional nurses (AACN, 2021) as self-care is critical to supporting resilience.

Level II Competencies of the Domain

Demonstrate a Commitment to Personal Health and Well-Being

Personal health and well-being can be a challenge for many nurses, with physical and psychological stressors being often ubiquitous in healthcare work settings. Inadequate staffing in many in-patient settings contributes to a number of negative consequences. In the physical realm, nurses report not being permitted meal and bathroom breaks. Water and other drinks are typically not allowed outside the break rooms. A legitimate rationale for this is infection control, which is a real concern in the clinical setting. However, when rest breaks are limited, or nonexistent, adequate fluid intake is at risk, and the result can be inadequate hydration, and urinary tract infections (Fasugba et al., 2020). Inadequate staffing contributes to breaches in quality care for patients. It also negatively impacts the well-being of the nurse. Nurses report exhaustion, frustration, and burnout. Surveys report that up to 90% of nurses consider leaving the profession (Siwicki, 2022; Pearson, 2023). Some blame the COVID-19 pandemic, but nurses say there is more to it than the pandemic. The pandemic may have been the deciding factor for many nurses who question how well healthcare systems value their worth and their safety.

In an interview, a nurse practitioner reported that, at the beginning of the pandemic, before the advent of the vaccine, she was issued one paper surgical mask, and told not to lose it, as it was the only one she would receive. When she asked if that meant for the day, she was told that it would be for the foreseeable future. She reminded the administrator that masks were intended to be changed in between patients. She was told there were no more masks and to make do with what she had. Nurses have to question how this can be. How can it be that frontline health-care providers have their well-being disregarded by the healthcare system that so desperately needs them? How do nurses address the perceived lack of care shown to them by their employers, especially when senior administrators are earning high salaries and taking no personal risks with their health, while mandating, creat-ing, and enabling unsafe working conditions for their employees? This account is supported in the literature. Cohen and Rodgers (2020), and DeChant (2022) observed that, during the COVID-19 pandemic 87% of nurses reported having to reuse single-use masks. Beyond the risk to personal health and well-being, nurses have to question how much the healthcare system values them. Healthcare sys-tems administrators must consider the costs to the institution when nurses resign. Beyond the financial costs associated with temporarily filling staffing gaps with temporary staff, for example, agency or travel nurses, there is the cost associated with onboarding and orienting new staff. Beyond that, the human costs to morale when nurses observe their colleagues resign should be considered, as it can lead to more resignations.

Contribute to an Environment That Promotes Self-Care, Personal Health, and Well-Being

Setting and Maintaining Boundaries. Healthcare administrators consider the institution a business, with finite resources. Administrators may make decisions about staffing, salaries, and working conditions based on how effectively costs are saved, rather than the best interests of those delivering care.

To facilitate self-care, nurses must be aware of institutional philosophies and policies. Once aware of institutional policies and practice—and this should ideally occur prior to taking a position—the nurse must set boundaries and maintain them. This may be more difficult for nurses in the baby-boomer generation. One study concluded that "nurses and executives viewed generation Y as being less willing to give oneself out and as attaching less importance to work than generation X and the baby boomers" (Huber & Shubert, 2019, p. 1341). Baby boomers are considered those born 1945–1964. Generation X includes those born 1965–1980. Generation Y, or the millennials, are those born 1981–1996, and Generation Z are those born 1997–2012 (Dimock, 2019).

One has to ask, is this really true? Is it true that nurses from Generation Y are less willing to give of themselves? Do they attach less importance to work? Or are they instead, by virtue of having been raised by baby boomers and Generation X parents, more cognizant and protective of their own interests. Are those from Gen-eration Z also less willing to give of themselves? Regardless of the cause, if true, is this a problem? Is it possible that this generation of nurses can effect positive change by setting and maintaining boundaries? If so, this is a hopeful sign.

Knowing and Valuing Self-Worth. Often, particularly among newly gradu-ated nurses and advanced practice nurses, there is fear and concern that they will not be able to find a position. Some graduates are located in parts of the country where positions are not plentiful, and salaries are lower than in other areas. They may, for personal or family reasons, be reluctant to relocate. As a result, they may feel pressure to settle for sub-optimal salaries and working conditions. There is no simple answer to this quandary, particularly if the nurse holds a strong allegiance to their community.

Knowing one's value and articulating that to institutional leaders is essential. Change does not occur without some disruption. Unions can be one answer. Advocacy via the local and state legislatures can be another. Awareness of comparable compensation is important knowledge for nurses to have when discussing these matters with administrators.

Evaluate the Workplace Environment to Determine Level of Health and Well-Being

Assessing and Understanding Institutional Culture. Optimally, nurses will check on the institutional culture prior to taking a position. How does one do this? It can seem mysterious and murky. If colleagues already work there, the nurse can ask for confidential feedback. In the interview, the nurse can ask targeted questions about institutional values, what types of behaviors are encouraged, and how the institution supports its staff. Of course, platitudes can be expected. But if the nurse is specific, realistic answers can be obtained. As an example, asking about mandatory overtime, how workplace violence is handled, tuition reimbursement policies, and/or staffing ratios are all important to well-being. If vague or evasive answers are received, that should be considered a warning sign that the institution may not be a good fit. Ultimately, the nurse must value their self-worth enough to decline offers from institutions that will exploit them. They must also contribute to a culture of positivity.

Demonstrate a Spirit of Inquiry That Fosters Flexibility and Professional Maturity

All nursing programs from entry level to terminal degree are rigorous and demanding. Many new graduates of programs at all levels experience a degree of fatigue and even burnout at the point of graduation. In their integrative review, Katchaturoff et al. (2020) identified that undergraduate and graduate nursing students experience stress, and some experience burnout. It should not be surprising that new graduates of undergraduate and graduate programs may express a desire to take a hiatus from scholarly inquiry.

Awareness of the phenomenon of feeling stressed and needing a brief respite from the rigors of academic work may refresh the nurse, and inspire them to maintain the spirit of inquiry. Health care is dynamic, constantly evolving, and to be current in an area of expertise requires scholarly inquiry.

Cognitive Flexibility in Managing Change Within Complex Environments

Science is constantly evolving, undergoing change, with new technologies and treatment modalities emerging on a regular basis. It is incumbent on all practitioners to embrace change, addressing their implicit biases and fears of change, in order to prevent stagnation and obsolescence.

The seminal work, *Who Moved My Cheese?* by Spencer Johnson (1998) addresses the need for adaptability and flexibility in the face of constant change.

Although it is not a new publication, and was originally intended for a business audience, it has sold over 30 million copies, and has applicability for healthcare providers and leaders. The key message is that change is inevitable and to be successful we must embrace it. There is a temptation for nurses, faculty, and leaders to become stagnant. The attitude of "It was good enough when we were students/ new nurses" is destructive. Practitioners, both in academia and the clinical arena, need to welcome change as necessary for quality improvement. Further, support for innovation is critical for recruitment and retention. When new ideas are stifled, it encourages turnover and attrition.

Mentor Others in the Development of Their Professional Growth and Accountability

Mentoring others can contribute to a sense of self-worth. Voss et al. (2022) identify mentoring as a "powerful tool that can be leveraged in both academic programs and in the health care practice setting to foster an environment that supports the successful transition from student to novice nurse, to experienced nurse" (p. 401). The relationship between the mentor and mentee fosters positivity and resilience for both. Further, over time, the roles of mentor and mentee can reverse, in which the mentee becomes the mentor.

Foster Activities That Support a Culture of Lifelong Learning

One key strategy to foster loyalty and a culture of positivity in an institution is to show those within it that they are valued. The institution can do this by investing in continued education for their employees or students. How is this done? In the academic setting, student scholarship awards can be funded, tuition support can be provided for faculty, stipends provided for presentations, and educational sponsorships can be provided to attend conferences, for both students and faculty. Similar investments can be made for employees in the practice setting. The key is to demonstrate to the student or employee that the institution values them enough to invest in their continued learning. This should inspire in the nurse a desire to invest in themselves to continue lifelong learning. This does not necessarily mean pursing advanced or terminal degrees. It can mean pursuing certificates in an area of scholarly interest, such as dementia care, holistic nursing, innovations, interprofessional education, pain management, and others.

Expand Leadership Skills Through Professional Service

Service to the profession is one of the four domains of Boyer's Model of Scholarship (Boyer, 1990), identified within the scholarship of application. It is essential to self-governance for the profession. Engaging in professional service allows the nurse to observe leadership qualities in others and internalize and apply them to engage in problem solving. One of the challenges in encouraging nurses to engage in professional service is that it is often a volunteer activity with no compensation. This can conflict with the desire, particularly among Generation Y nurses, to protect their free time (Huber & Shubert, 2019). Other incentives can be provided, such as complementary conference registration for serving on a board.

Develop Capacity for Leadership

Leadership takes many forms and is not restricted to paid leadership positions within academia or practice. Leadership skills are valuable to the nurse in every setting and there are many ways to develop and utilize these skills and competencies. The student or new graduate may think that leadership skills are not necessary for them, but that is incorrect.

Miles and Scott (2019) posit that the time to begin leadership development is at the prelicensure level. Toward that end they developed a conceptual framework, the Nursing Leadership Development Model, providing a structure to promote leadership development for prelicensure nursing students, encouraging competence to incorporate and apply leadership skills upon entry to practice. These skills promote strength within the new graduate that can be further developed as they move through their career, regardless of their position or setting.

Provide Leadership to Advance the Nursing Profession

Leadership to advance the profession takes place in multiple arenas and offers nurses opportunities to follow their passion, utilizing leadership skills to effect positive advancement for the profession. There are opportunities in the area of health policy. Advocating for legislation that increases access to health care or improves practice conditions for nurses is one avenue. There are a few nurses in the U.S. Congress. Running for office at the local level can be a stepping stone toward higher offices. Serving on volunteer or professional association boards is also an effective way to achieve positive change.

Nurses may not think they have the expertise or time resources to engage in advocacy. Fortunately, there are numerous professional organizations representing nurses that engage in health policy advocacy, as well as providing educational opportunities, specialty certification, and networking opportunities. Examples of these include the American Nurses Association, which has a strong policy and advocacy presence, as well as a certification arm, the American Nurses Credentialing Center. An example of a specialty organization is the American Association of Nurse Practitioners (AANP). In addition to advocacy and educational offerings, AANP offers national certification for nurse practitioners through its affiliated certification body, the American Academy of Nurse Practitioners Certification Board (aanpcert. org, n.d.). State associations may be the most reasonably priced associations to join, while also providing opportunities to build relationships within the local community. State associations are also the ones that advocate for improved practice statutes that will improve practice conditions for nurses within the state. An example of this is the Nurse Practitioner Association New York State (The NPA). The NPA is solely responsible for the multitude of practice-advancing legislation and regulatory advances for nurse practitioners (NPs) in New York that have been achieved since it was formed in 1980. From the first law defining title and scope of practice for NPs in 1988 to the Nurse Practitioners Modernization Acts (2014, 2022), which afforded experienced NPs full practice authority, the NPA has led in advancing the profession in that state (https://www.thenpa.org/page/NPAHistoryRevised). In addition to advocacy, state associations typically offer continuing education opportunities and employment services.

Influence Intentional Change Guided by Leadership Principles and Theories

Leadership involves understanding its principles and theories. By intentionally learning and employing leadership principles and theories, the nurse can assess how effectively their leadership is working to effect the desired change. An example of this is seen in Lewin's Change Theory. A psychologist, Kurt Lewin (1947) developed a three-step model of change, which involves *unfreezing* (letting go of the old state), *changing* (moving toward the new state), and *refreezing* (solidifying the new state). This model is very simple and has applications to almost every type of change.

Kouzes and Posner's (2023) theory of transformational leadership can also be used as a guide to influence change. Their theory has five key components of transformational leadership:

- Model the Way
- Inspire a Shared Vision
- Challenge the Process
- Enable Others to Act
- Encourage the Heart

Kouzes and Posner's principles are similar to the *servant leader* style of leadership, as defined by Greenleaf (2012), which describes a style of leadership in which the leader serves the group, engages them in partnership, inspiring them to do their best. This can be compared against an autocratic, transactional style of leadership, in which the leader demands actions or behaviors from the group. Servant leadership is challenging as it requires obtaining buy-in from the group on decisions, and unpopular policies may still have to be implemented. However, it can result in loyalty and camaraderie that the authoritarian leader will not experience.

Evaluate the Outcomes of Intentional Change

Learning and utilizing leadership competencies allows the nurse to perform program evaluations. Change should be evaluated to see if it actually occurred, to see if the outcomes were as expected, and if it contributed to making a positive difference.

The American Organization of Nurse Leadership (AONL, 2015) identifies five core domains which can also be used to guide evaluation of outcomes of intentional change. The anchoring domain, Leader Within, supports the five core domains:

- Business Skills and Principles
- Communication and Relationship Building
- Knowledge of the Health Care Environment
- Professionalism
- Leadership

Evaluate Strategies/Methods for Peer Review

An important component of leadership is conducting peer review in a manner that is positive, fair, and equitable. Acknowledging one's own implicit bias is a key component of leadership. The ability to examine peer-review methods to ensure they are not discriminatory or result in disparities is a key leadership ability. Clark (2017) emphasizes the importance of civility in peer review. Nursing students and nurses may react with discomfort, and even dread, at the prospect of a peer evaluation.

They may fear it will be confrontational, demeaning, even cruel. This prevailing fear is disheartening, does not contribute to the mentor–mentee relationship, and can contribute to burnout. This should not be the case. Peer-to-peer evaluations should be collegial and supportive. As Clark points out, to make peer evaluations effective and productive, the evaluator must be civil, cordial, and respectful of differing points of view. The peer being evaluated must assume good will on the part of the evaluator. Both parties must listen to the other's perspectives respectfully.

Participate in the Evaluation of Other Members of the Care Team

Team-based health care is a desired model and healthcare teams are interdisciplinary, meaning that they are represented by members from all professions, including medicine, nursing, physical therapy, pharmacy, social work, psychology, and others. Utilizing an interprofessional team can improve outcomes and reduce hospital readmissions by tapping the expertise from its members.

Evaluating the various members of the healthcare team should be a collegial and peer-to-peer process. Understanding and employing leadership ability and skillsets improve this process.

Demonstrate Leadership Skills in Times of Uncertainty and Crisis

Crisis offers the opportunity for nurses to demonstrate leadership and ensure best outcomes. There are a multitude of examples of times of uncertainty and crisis during which nurses are called upon to demonstrate leadership skill, from military conflicts to natural disasters. A prime example is the COVID-19 pandemic. Wymer et al. (2021) identified three key points for nursing leadership in times of crisis:

- Nurse leaders often make decisions in an environment of conflicting data and directives.
- Nurse leaders must harness respect and goodwill while overcoming current challenges.
- Nurse leaders must develop and mature the skills necessary to quickly identify and effectively respond to crises.

Considering the conflicting theories on the genesis of the COVID-19 virus, the management of the disease, and further, managing strategies to protect healthcare professionals caring for its victims, all of which were exacerbated by conspiracy theories and misinformation, nurse leaders faced a daunting task. Utilizing leadership skills and competencies in conjunction with the consistent application of best practices of scientific evidence results in nurse leaders who are optimally equipped to lead healthcare teams during crises.

Advocate for the Promotion of Social Justice and Eradication of Structural Racism and Systematic Inequity in Nursing and Society

Structural racism and systematic inequity result in a multitude of disastrous health consequences across generations. Social justice benefits all corners of society and must be a priority. Every major nursing organization has spoken out against racism, inequities, and disparities (Nardi et al., 2020). Further, social justice addresses disparities affecting all marginalized populations including LGBTQ groups, senior citizens, the disabled, the incarcerated and post-incarcerated, people experiencing homelessness, and others. Ageism, misogyny, homophobia, transphobia, classism, and ableism all contribute to negative health outcomes.

Advocate for the Nursing Profession in a Manner That Is Consistent, Positive, Relevant, Accurate, and Distinctive

Leadership skills and competencies provide the ability to advocate in an effective manner to achieve desired outcomes. Consistency is a key element in fairness and equity. Positivity contributes to acceptance of change. Relevance is essential to authority. Accuracy is a key component of trust.

Membership in professional associations, as students are often told, is a professional responsibility. It is also an opportunity. Hann (2003) identifies that policy is about relationships, describing how forming relationships is critical to influencing policy. Policy is not solely about legislation or regulation. It is also about the policies that are set within institutions. Building relationships builds coalitions and partnerships. By joining professional associations, nurses have the opportunity to learn about innovations taking place in other institutions and can bring awareness of them to their own healthcare system. Beyond that, professional associations provide excellent opportunities for networking and relationship building.

Summary

The importance of domain 10, which addresses the personal, professional, and leadership development of the nurse, lies in its focus on the nurse, and their growth, development, and ability to achieve personal and professional excellence. It addresses the need for positivity, for maintaining well-being. The ability to develop leadership skills and competencies facilitates leading healthcare teams, as well as mentoring and supporting peers, which are essential for the sustainability of the profession.

References

American Academy of Nurse Practitioners Certification Board. (n.d.). *Welcome to the American Academy of Nurse Practitioners Certification board.* aanpcert.org.

American Association of Colleges of Nursing. (2021). *The essentials: Core competencies for professional nursing education.* https://www.aacnnursing.org/Portals/42/AcademicNursing/pdf/Essentials-2021.pdf

American Nurses Credentialing Center. (n.d.). *Our certifications.* nursingworld.org.

American Organization for Nursing Leadership and The Center for Nursing Leadership. (2015). *Dimensions of leadership.* https://www.aonl.org/system/files/media/file/2019/06/nurse-manager-competencies.pdf.

Blackburn, L. M., Thompson, K., Frankenfield, R., Harding, A., & Lindsey, A. (2020). The THRIVE© Program: Building oncology nurse resilience through self-care strategies. *Oncology Nursing Forum, 47*(1), E25–E34. https://doi.org/10.1188/20.ONF.E25-E34

Boyer, E. (1990). Scholarship reconsidered: Priorities of the professoriate. *The Carnegie Foundation for the Advancement of Teaching.*

Carini, C. (2023). *Mindfulness in nursing practice: Education to enhance caregiver wellness & task performance.* (Unpublished DNP Project). School of Nursing, University of Connecticut.

Chiu, P., Thorne, S., Schick-Makaroff, K., & Cummings, G. G. (2023). Lessons from professional nursing associations' policy advocacy responses to the COVID-19 pandemic: An interpretive description. *Journal of Advanced Nursing.* https://doi.org/10.1111/jan.15625

Clark. (2017). An evidence-based approach to integrate civility, professionalism, and ethical practice into nursing curricula. *Nurse Educator, 42*(3), 120–126. https://doi.org/10.1097/NNE.0000000000000331

Cohen J., & Rodgers, Y. V. M. (2020, December). Contributing factors to personal protective equipment shortages during the COVID-19 pandemic. *Preventive Medicine, 141*, 106263. https://doi.org/10.1016/j.ypmed.2020.106263. Epub 2020 Oct 2. PMID: 33017601; PMCID: PMC7531934.

Crane, P., & Ward, S. (2016). (Self-healing and self-care for nurses. *AORN Journal, 104* (5), 386–400. http://dx.doi.org/10.1016/j.aorn.2016.09.007

DeChant, P. (2022). *How to face the Great Resignation in healthcare.* https://insights.vitalworklife.com/the-great-resignation-post

Dimock, M. (2019, 17 January). Defining generations: Where millennials end and generation Z begins. *Pew Research Center.* https://www.pewresearch.org/fact-tank/2019/01/17/where-millennials-end-and-generation-z-begins/

Fasugba, O., Mitchell, B. G., McInnes, E., Koerner, J., Cheng, A. C., Cheng, H., & Middleton, S. (2020). Increased fluid intake for the prevention of urinary tract infection in adults and children in all settings: A systematic review. *Journal of Hospital Infection, 104*(1), 68–77.

Filoramo, M. (2022). Nurses as the patients and burnout as the condition: Self care to improve patient care. *Pain Management Nursing, 23*(2), 237–237. https://doi.org/10.1016/j.pmn.2022.02.011

Giddens, J., Douglas, J. P., & Conroy, S. (2022). The Revised AACN Essentials: Implications for nursing regulation. *Journal of Nursing Regulation, 12*(4), 16–22.

Greenleaf, R. (2012). *The servant as leader.* The Greenleaf Center for Servant Leadership.

Guo, Y., Plummer, V., Lam, L., Wang, Y., Cross, W., & Zhang, J. (2019). The effects of resilience and turnover intention on nurses' burnout: Findings from a comparative cross-sectional study. *Journal of Clinical Nursing, 28*(3–4), 499–508. https://doi.org/10.1111/jocn.14637

Hann, N. (2003, Winter). All policy is relationships. *Transformations in Public Health, 6.*

Huber, P., & Shubert, H. (2019). Attitudes about work engagement of different generations—A cross-sectional study with nurses and supervisors. *Journal of Nursing Management. 27*(7), 1341–1350. https://doi.org/10.1111/jonm.12805.

Jameton, A. (2017). What moral distress in nursing history could suggest about the future of health care. *AMA Journal of Ethics, 19*(6), 617–628.

Johnson, S. (1998). *Who moved my cheese?* Putnam.

Kachaturoff, M., Caboral-Stevens, M., Gee, M., & Lan, V. (2020). Effects of peer-mentoring on stress and anxiety levels of undergraduate nursing students: An integrative review. *Journal of Professional Nursing, 36*(4), 223–228.

Kouzes, J. M., & Posner, B. Z. (2023). *The leadership challenge: How to make extraordinary things happen in organizations* (7th ed.). Jossey-Bass.

Lewin, K. (1947). Frontiers in group dynamics: Concept, method and reality in social science; Social equilibria and social change. *Human Relations, 1*(1), 5–41. https://doi.org/10.1177/001872674700100103

Miles, J., & Scott, E. (2019). A new leadership development model for nursing education. *Journal of Professional Nursing, 35*(1), 5–11.

Nantsupawat, A., Nantsupawat, R., Kunaviktikul, W., Turale, S., & Poghosyan, L. (2016). Nurse burnout, nurse-reported quality of care, and patient outcomes in Thai hospitals. *Journal of Nursing Scholarship, 48*(1), 83–90. https://doi.org/10.1111/jnu.12187.

Nardi, D., Waite, R., Nowak, M., Hatcher, B., Martin, V., & Stacciarini, J. (2020). Achieving health equity through eradicating structural racism in the United States: A call to action for nursing leadership. *Journal of Nursing Scholarship, 52*(6), 696–703.

Nurse Practitioner Association New York State. (n.d.). *Nurse practitioner history and accomplishments.* https://www.thenpa.org/page/NPAHistoryRevised

Pearson, B. (2023, February 20). Nurses are burned out. Can hospitals change in time to keep them? *The New York Times*. https://www.nytimes.com/2023/02/20/well/nurses-burnout-pandemic-stress.html

Ross, A., Touchton-Leonard, K., Perez, A., Wehrlen, L., Kazmi, N., & Gibbons, S. (2019). Factors that influence health-promoting self-care in registered nurses: Barriers and facilitators. *Advances in Nursing Science*, 42(4), 358–373. https://doi.org/10.1097/ANS.0000000000000274

Siwicki, N. (2022, March). Report: 90% of nurses considering leaving the profession in the next year. *HealthcareITNews*. https://www.healthcareitnews.com/news/report-90-nurses-considering-leaving-profession-next-year

Stevenson, D. (2022). Academic burnout in nursing school. *Nursing 2023*, 52(3), 60–61.

Voss, J. Alfes, C., Clark, A., Lilly, K., & Moore, S. (2022). Why mentoring matters for new graduates transitioning to practice: Implications for nurse leaders. *Nurse Leader*, 20(4), 399–340.

Walsh, P., Owen, P. A., Mustafa, N., & Beech, R. (2020). Learning and teaching approaches promoting resilience in student nurses: An integrated review of the literature. *Nurse Education in Practice*, 45, 102748.

Wymer, J., Stucky, C., & De Jong, M. (2021). Nursing leadership and COVID-19: Defining the shadows and leading ahead of the data. *Nurse Leader*, 19(5), 483–488. https://doi.org/10.1016/j.mnl.2021.06.004

PART 2

The Doctor of Nursing Practice Project

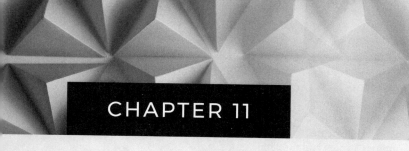

CHAPTER 11

A Template for the DNP Project

Diane M. Schadewald, DNP, MSN, RN, WHNP-BC, FNP-BC, CNE

Knowing is not enough; we must apply. Willing is not enough; we must do.

—Goethe

In his 1995 address to the AACN, Boyer proposed a reimagination of scholarship as a concept that has four interdependent aspects: the scholarship of discovery, the scholarship of integration, the scholarship of teaching, and the scholarship of application. He further proposed that each domain should be valued equally (Boyer, 1996). The DNP degree focuses on the clinical scholarship of integration and application as elucidated by Boyer in his AACN address.

While both DNP and PhD programs are doctoral degree programs, the end product of the programs differ. The DNP course of study as proposed by the AACN culminates in a scholarly product, as should any doctoral education (AACN, 2021). The nature of the product should be commensurate with the domain of scholarship of the student. For doctor of philosophy (PhD) students, the domain of discovery of new knowledge dictates an original research product, a dissertation, conducted and evaluated using traditional research methodologies, statistical analysis, and evaluation schemes. Scholarship for the DNP student is demonstrated through a practice product, the DNP project, which reflects the breadth of the student's education and is a synthesis of the knowledge gained in the course of study (AACN, 2015, 2021). The DNP project should address a complex practice, process, policy, or systems problem within the student's field of expertise or chosen specialty and include an evidence-based intervention to address that problem for a significant population as well as implementation plans. The evidence-based intervention should be implemented whenever feasible. An evaluation of the implementation process as well as the efficacy of the intervention and the outcomes of the intervention are also recommended to be included in the final product (AACN, 2021). The project may take on many forms, but the common element throughout the various DNP projects is the use of evidence to improve practice, processes, or health outcomes (AACN, 2021). That is, a review of the literature on its own or a portfolio minus a DNP project paper do not meet the level of scholarship required for a DNP program end product (AACN, 2015, 2021).

The DNP student functioning as project leader gains real-world leadership skills conducting the project. The structure and format of the final product will vary with the requirements of the degree-granting institution (AACN, 2021) in collaboration with community partners and implementation sites.

Nature of the Project

Although practice doctorate programs have grown within colleges and schools of nursing, questions remain about the nature of the DNP project. This is reflected in the many appellations previously given to this project: leadership project, scholarly project, DNP scholarly project, or capstone project. Because of this inconsistency in titling, the National Organization of Nurse Practitioner Faculties (NONPF) in a 2013 white paper proposed adopting the title, DNP Project, for the end product of DNP programs and in 2015 the AACN concurred with such titling (NONPF, 2013; AACN, 2015).

Nurses can gain insight from other disciplines that have used a project as evidence of scholarship. For example, projects are used in the fields of business and engineering to demonstrate mastery of the subject matter. The use of a project as evidence of scholarship in the engineering field is particularly interesting because of similarities between nursing and engineering. Both of these fields of study center on the application of evidence-based knowledge to practice problems, and they both integrate knowledge from other fields of scientific study as well as the base field to create interventions. In Ernest Boyer's definition of the scholarship of application, he stated that this type of scholarship moves "from theory to practice and from practice back to theory" (Boyer, 1996, pp. 1–6). Both engineering and nursing take theories and new knowledge and test them in the gritty world of real life, real people, and real institutions.

Original research, even when illuminating and well executed, may languish for lack of application in the real world. In their 2001 publication, *Crossing the Quality Chasm*, the Institute of Medicine (IOM) noted a lag time from discovery of effective treatments to the integration and application of those treatments in clinical settings was 15 to 20 years (IOM, 2001); unfortunately, this lag in time has yet to be shortened (Kirchner et al., 2020). The IOM called for development of an effective infrastructure to support more rapid application of evidence to patient care. The DNP-educated advanced practice nurse (APN) and the DNP-educated nurse in an advanced nursing practice specialty can do just that—bring evidence to patient care using the scholarship of integration, application, and implementation.

In engineering and business, capstone projects are done most frequently at the baccalaureate and master's levels. What distinguishes the DNP Project from the baccalaureate or master's capstone project is the depth of inquiry, the depth of the literature reviewed, the scope of the project, the population served by the project, and the student's use of solid scientific evidence and theory as underpinnings of the project (AACN, 2015). **Box 11-1** outlines Boyer's criteria to evaluate scholarly work in any domain.

The DNP curriculum focuses on nursing practice, leadership, collaboration, and integration of science from many fields of study. This curriculum prepares

Box 11-1 Boyer's Criteria for Evaluation of Scholarship

Are the goals of the project clearly stated?
Are the procedures well defined and appropriate for the project?
Are resources adequate for the stated goals of the project and utilized
    effectively?
Did the student communicate and collaborate effectively with others?
Are the results of the project significant?
Is there evidence of self-reflection and learning?

Data from Boyer, E.L. (1996). Clinical practice scholarship. *Holistic Nursing Practice, 10*(3); 1-6.

Table 11-1 Comparison of DNP Project and PhD Dissertation

PhD Dissertation	DNP Project
Systematic search for an answer to a research question	Systematic investigation of a practice issue
Outcome is an answer to the research question that is generalizable beyond current study; reproducible	Outcome is a solution to a practice problem that usually involves systems change; may be reproducible in other systems
Not specific to a time or place	Limited to a place and a time
Based in theory and literature	Based in theory and literature
Uses rigorous methodology that is unbiased and can be reproduced	Uses rigorous methods that are appropriate to the scope of the problem

Reproduced from Edwardson, S. (2009; January 14). *MN/DNP colloquium.* Colloquium conducted at the University of Minnesota School of Nursing, Minneapolis, Minnesota. Reprinted with permission.

APNs/DNPs to evaluate evidence for the implementation of best practices and the improvement of patient care. The PhD course of study focuses on vigorous research, generation of new knowledge, and the scholarship of discovery. Although the DNP Project is quite different from a PhD dissertation (see **Table 11-1**), it is a rigorously executed project that is clearly described and the results are documented in a paper or product of doctoral quality (AACN, 2015, 2021).

When evaluating the differences between the PhD dissertation and the DNP Project, it is useful to consider the desired outcomes for graduates of these programs. The PhD-prepared nurse will likely conduct his or her career in the academic or research setting. The DNP-prepared nurse will almost certainly conduct his or her career in practice. To that end, the emphasis of the PhD dissertation is on rigorous application of standard methodologies and meticulous evaluation of results using generally accepted scientific analysis techniques that can be reliably reproduced and are generalizable. The DNP Project focuses on a problem and the evidence-based solutions for that problem. It is specific to a place or a system and may be transferrable to other settings, but generalizability is not the goal of the project (AACN, 2015, 2021). Rather, the project focuses on the application of evidence to the problem that was identified in a specific setting. Results may be analyzed using standard statistical methods, but such analysis is not strictly necessary (Edwardson, 2009).

Some important similarities between the PhD dissertation and DNP Project emerge as well. Both approaches need to be systematic and the literature review should be in depth and rigorous. The PhD dissertation topic is narrow; the investigation is tightly controlled to eliminate extraneous influences. The DNP Project, being a real-world project, cannot control those influences. The DNP Project seeks to adapt research to real situations. Both the PhD dissertation and the DNP Project are based in theoretical concepts and literature. The PhD literature review will be focused; the DNP literature review will be broader and may have many different points at which a discussion of theory is appropriate. The final product should meet all the academic institution's requirements for scholarly work (AACN, 2021). According to the AACN (2015), graduates from both research- and practice-focused doctorates are prepared to generate new knowledge:

> Research-focused graduates are prepared to generate knowledge through rigorous research and statistical methodologies that may be broadly applicable or generalizable; practice-focused graduates are prepared to generate new knowledge through innovation of practice change, the translation of evidence, and the implementation of quality improvement processes in specific practice settings, systems, or with specific populations to improve health or health outcomes. New knowledge generated through practice innovation, for example, could be of value to other practice settings. This new knowledge is considered transferrable but is not considered generalizable. (p. 3)

The AACN white paper went on to state,

> These delineations in knowledge generation are not to be construed as a hierarchical structure of the importance of these two types of knowledge generating methods. The application and translation of evidence into practice is a vital and necessary skill that is currently lacking in the healthcare environment and the nursing profession. The DNP graduate will help to fulfill this need. As a result DNP and PhD graduates will have the opportunity to collaborate and work synergistically to improve health outcomes. (p. 3)

What does this mean for the DNP Project? It means that the project needs to be as rigorous, evidence-based, and scholarly as a dissertation. The difference is that the DNP Project is utilizing the tools of translation and implementation science to bring research findings into practice. The end result is evidence-based quality patient care outcomes or changes in practice, programs, or policy. Because this product is a synthesis of the student's work in the DNP program, it should be related to the student's advanced practice specialty (AACN, 2021). The problem to be addressed usually arises from clinical practice issues observed by the student or his or her mentors, or is proposed by the partnering institution or practice setting. The process or practice improvement project is often conducted at a clinical practice site.

1

It can also be done in partnership with an agency of the community (e.g., school, health agency, church, nonprofit organization). The leadership of the project is typically conducted by the student, along with community partner and faculty support. The project may be conducted in collaboration with another student if the educational institution permits. However, each student is accountable to meet all expectations of the DNP Project and each student is responsible for a specific portion of the project such as a separate concept and framework or intervention and outcome of the project. The project should engage a team of professionals to accomplish the change, demonstrating the student's attainment of leadership and collaboration skills (AACN, 2015, 2021).

Structure of the Project

A needs assessment and literature review should be conducted to support the need for and structure of the project. For a quality improvement project and an evidenced-based project, the improvement should benefit a significant population instead of a single patient or practitioner (AACN, 2015). Two other DNP Project types include program evaluation and policy analysis, both of which should include recommendations for change based on the evaluation or analysis as well as implementation, evaluation, and/or dissemination of the recommendations if feasible.

The review of literature for the DNP Project is not done to identify gaps in the body of knowledge, as one would do for the PhD dissertation. Rather, the DNP Project proposes to fix a gap given the available evidence. The literature review should address the efficacy of the intervention selected for the project, provide an in-depth exploration of the problem, program, or policy, and support the rationale for selection of the chosen approach for the project. It should support the validity and reliability of assessment tools, specifically surveys and data collection methodologies. Scholarly support for the project includes the use of theoretical support to describe the conceptual framework of the project. The student may need to integrate several theories from different fields of study beyond nursing to adequately describe the project framework.

The implementation of the DNP Project should meet all the ethical standards for conducting any research or quality improvement project. Consultation with an institutional review board (IRB) to determine if the project is human subjects research or not is recommended. Also, consultation with an IRB is important because many professional organizations and publishers require a determination from an IRB as a baseline requirement for consideration to present or publish project findings. A form, consisting of screening questions to determine if a project involves human subjects research and therefore need for IRB review, has been developed by some organizational and academic IRBs to assist with the review process. The expected outcomes of the project should be defined when constructing the project. Project outcomes should be measurable within the time frame of the project. The elements for implementation of the project should also be sufficiently described to allow for the project to be implemented at other clinical sites (NONPF, 2007).

Data collection during the project should be rigorous and structured. The tools and methods for data collection should meet accepted standards of practice (NONPF, 2007). Tools and methods should be defined early in the project for best-practice and best-outcomes evaluation. It is helpful to consult with a statistician early in the development of the project if advanced statistical analysis is anticipated. Data collected can be qualitative or quantitative. Statistical analysis is useful as a measure of change but may not be the only measure. The time frame of these projects often does not permit the collection of enough data points to achieve statistical significance. Other measures of change may include graphs, trends, cost analysis, narrative data, and patterns of practice.

The development, implementation, and outcomes of the project should be reviewed by an academic panel or committee per the academic policies of the degree-granting institution and disseminated to stakeholders at the project site or in a broader public forum (AACN, 2021). Modalities for dissemination are diverse and vary from project to project and degree-granting institution to degree-granting institution.

Advising the student's DNP project is different from advising the PhD dissertation and remains a highly debated topic in nursing academia. Advising is often quite intense because of the condensed time frame of the project. Instead of one or two PhD advisees, clinical and research faculty in schools of nursing that house advanced practice programs may have multiple DNP advisees, which increases faculty workload (Corey et al., 2022). Clinical faculty, who must maintain a clinical practice to maintain certification, often find their workloads unsustainable. Various strategies have been suggested to account for faculty workload, but the workload is rarely altered to allow for more advising time (Anderson et al., 2019; Corey et al., 2022). Additionally, salary disparity exists between full-time faculty and APNs in clinical practice, which is a barrier to filling academic positions. For example, the salary for nurse practitioners in clinical practice is significantly higher than in doctorally prepared academic settings (AACN, 2022).

As nursing progresses toward the goal of educating all APNs in a DNP framework, projects are evolving. A schema for the DNP Project is laid out in the remainder of this chapter. A graphic representation of the process is shown in **Figure 11-1**.

This model is one framework for the development, implementation, and evaluation of DNP projects. This section of the chapter is primarily written to assist DNP students and faculty but can be used by any practitioner who is developing a new project or program.

The Project

Getting Started

In the author's experience with baccalaureate-to-DNP students, finding a project idea is often the most difficult part of the project. This may be because students are new to the role and the clinical environment. They may not know the evidence that supports the practice. Students with a master's degree in an advanced practice nursing role or advanced nursing practice specialty don't have as much difficulty finding a project idea. A search through clinical guidelines can be utilized to discover gaps in practice that are amenable to a DNP Project. Clinical guidelines can be found in many sources. High-quality guidelines and suggested sites for locating guidelines can be found in **Box 11-2**.

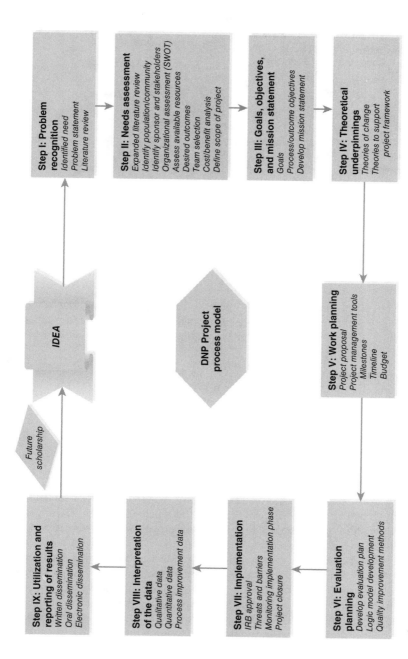

Figure 11-1 DNP Project Process Model

Box 11-2 Sources for DNP Project Ideas

Active Implementation Research Network (Heptagon Tool)
Agency for Healthcare Quality and Research
Joanna Briggs Institute
National Academy of Science
National Academy of Medicine
Institute for Healthcare Improvement
World Health Organization
Cochrane Library: Cochrane Reviews
National Quality Forum
Quality and Safety Education for Nurses (QSEN)
DynaMed
Evidence Updates
Centre for Evidence-Based Medicine (Oxford University)
Canadian Medical Association Clinical Practice Guidelines Infobase
Registered Nurses Association of Ontario Best Practices Guidelines
Clinical Key Guidelines

© Jones & Bartlett Learning

The Heptagon Tool (**Figure 11-2**) (Van Dyke, Kiser, & Blase, 2019) can be used as a planning tool to evaluate evidence-based guidelines, programs, and practices during the exploration stage of the DNP Project. Factors that can be evaluated with the Heptagon Tool include the following:

- Needs (how well the guideline meets the identified needs)
- Evidence (supporting expected outcomes)
- Fit (with initiatives already in place as well as values)
- Usability of innovation (available assistance)
- Capacity to implement (qualified staff and adequate ability to collect data)
- Resource availability (system and technology supports)
- Capacity to collaborate (communication and stakeholder support)

As the student becomes immersed in the advanced practice specialty and his or her practice area, gaps in practice will become more apparent. Perusing guidelines during the exploration phase of the DNP Project may help the student identify potential project ideas. Practice guidelines also often provide support for the project during the needs assessment phase of the project.

The second most difficult problem students often face in getting started on a DNP project is finding a community partner and site in which to implement a project. Procuring a community partner and exploring problems the community partner would like to focus on can be an ideal approach to development of a DNP project and establishes a win–win situation for the DNP student, their community partner, and the project site. A community partner ideally works with the student and the academic advisor in all phases of the DNP project. The community partner often helps the student address institutional barriers at the project site. Having a community partner that has the authority to facilitate accomplishment of the project is often vital to success of the project.

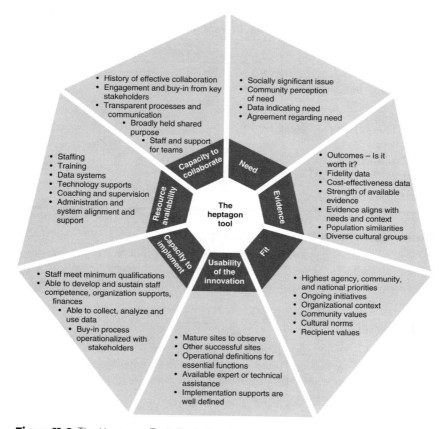

Figure 11-2 The Heptagon Tool: Exploring Context for the DNP Project

Modified with permission from Van Dyke, M., Kiser, L., & Blase, K. A. (2019). *The heptagon tool*. Chapel Hill, NC: Active Implementation Research Network.

Step I: Problem Recognition

Project ideas typically emanate from a clinical issue or opportunity identified by the nurse who is exercising critical thinking skills. In "Critical Thinking and Clinical Judgment," Facione and Facione (2008) outlined a critical thinker in part as a person who "fair-mindedly follows where evidence and reason leads." This statement continues to be reaffirmed as a model for assessment of critical thinking in health care.

The problem could be brought forth by an individual, a group, facility administration, regulatory bodies, accreditation organizations, or government agencies. Drivers for the project can be internal or external (see **Table 11-2**). The problem must be articulated clearly to the academic advisor or committee working with the student's project. The academic advisors and student must sufficiently focus the project so that it can be completed within the period defined by the academic institution. Ideally, the project should be in the student's area of practice scholarship (AACN, 2021). The project also must fit into the mission of the organization in which it will be developed and implemented as well as within the constraints of that organization. The next step is to develop a problem statement.

Table 11-2 Internal and External Drivers for Projects

Internal Drivers	External Drivers
Administration	Public policy
Healthcare professionals	Standards of practice
Budgetary issues	Evidence-based guidelines
Customer needs	Accreditation organizations
Quality improvement programs	Third-party payers
Safety issues	Government regulations
Staffing issues	Mandatory education
Educational requirements	

© Jones & Bartlett Learning

Developing the Problem Statement

A problem statement identifies a situation that requires change and puts the problem into an organized form. It answers the questions, Why this project? Why now?

Clarity is the key. The following list is a framework for developing a problem statement (Polit & Beck, 2021; Waddick, 2010):

1. Identify the deficits in the current circumstances.
2. Describe the setting of the problem.
3. Define the magnitude of the problem in measurable terms.
4. Characterize the impact of ignoring the problem on the population or organization.
5. Describe where evidence is missing in practice (identifying gaps in practice).
6. Outline evidence-based solutions.

At this juncture, one dimension of the literature review should be done to support the problem statement and should answer the questions posed earlier: Why this project? Why now? The literature review is multidimensional and iterative (see **Figure 11-3**). The purpose of the literature review for quality improvement and/or evidence-based practice projects is to identify gaps between practice and evidence, provide scientific support for the proposed intervention, support the desired goal and outcomes, and identify theoretical supports for the proposed change. The literature review for program evaluation or policy analysis projects often focuses on literature about the problem the program or policy addresses. The program evaluation or policy analysis review encompasses alternative evidence-based program or policy approaches, as well as literature about and theoretical support for the program evaluation or policy analysis process implemented for the project. The literature review may include scholarly articles, government regulations, national guidelines, clinical care models, regulatory agency policy or guidelines, professional standards and scopes of practice, organizational procedures and policies, certification requirements, reimbursement requirements, and internal institutional data.

Step II: Needs Assessment
Introduction

According to Rouda and Kusy (1995), a needs assessment is the systematic identification of the gap between the current condition and the ideal condition. It involves

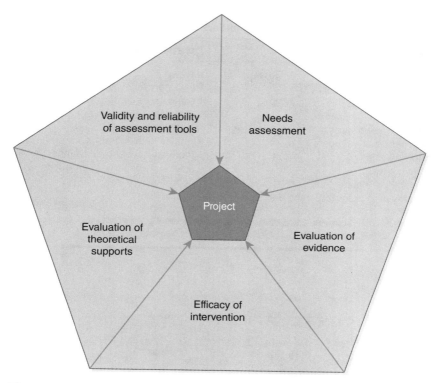

Figure 11-3 Multidimensional Literature Review for the DNP Project
© Jones & Bartlett Learning

scanning for problems, upcoming changes in regulations or clinical requirements, business opportunities, and new mandates. A good needs assessment identifies the difference between what is and what should be. A scholarly needs assessment describes the gap between the best-practice evidence and the current environment or system. Needs assessment tools and templates are readily available and can be found in multiple online sites.

Population Identification

An in-depth exploration of the population affected by the problem is often a good way to begin a needs assessment. Tools for this assessment may include demographic data from public sources, consultations, surveys, interviews, chart reviews, observations, focus groups, internal organizational data, and external data from government websites.

Identification of Project Sponsor and Key Stakeholders

The next phase of the needs assessment is identification of individuals who have a vested interest in the outcome of the project. That is, who beyond the community partner are stakeholders for the project? Stakeholders are key individuals who will be affected one way or another by the project. To identify the stakeholders, consider

Table 11-3 Identifying Key Stakeholders

Internal	External
Site administrator	Insurers
Chief financial officer	Regulatory agencies
Medical director	People in the community
Chief nursing officer	Suppliers
Department or program director	Interest groups
Project team members	Families in the community
Nurses	Health advocacy organizations
Ancillary staff	Community health organizations
Patients or residents	Support groups
Quality or process improvement officer	General public

Data from Mind Tools Content Team. (2022a). Stakeholder Analysis: Winning support for your projects. *Mind Tools.* © Emerald Works Limited 2006-2022. All rights reserved https://www.mindtools.com/aol0rms/stakeholder-analysis

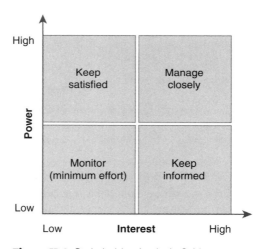

Figure 11-4 Stakeholder Analysis Grid

the individuals who not only are affected by the work but also may have an interest in its outcomes. **Table 11-3** lists examples of potential stakeholders. In addition to simply listing stakeholders, it is useful to analyze their roles, interests, and influence over your project. The example that follows (**Figure 11-4**) is a grid developed by Mind Tools for analysis of stakeholder interest and influence.

Organizational Assessment

The organizational setting and culture should be assessed. This assessment should answer these questions (W. K. Kellogg Foundation, 2004a): What are the values of the organization in which the project will be conducted? Are the values of the organization consistent with the values of the project and the project leader? To what extent is the mission of the project consistent with that of the organization in which the project will take place? The evaluation of the setting may identify challenges and stumbling blocks for the project. When such stumbling blocks are identified, plans can be made to address them, or the project can be implemented in a different setting. If the values of the project or the project leader are not consistent with those of the organization, the project is likely to fail.

Assessment of Available Resources

A thorough assessment of available resources should be conducted early in the project development and planning. These resources could include, but are not limited to, financial support, personnel, materials for the project, marketing, statistical analysis support, office space and materials, communication costs, consulting costs, grant writing support, travel expenses, survey costs, and copyright costs. The cost of the resources must be thoroughly investigated, understood, and documented before moving on to develop a cost–benefit analysis for the project proposal.

Identification of Desired Outcomes

Outcomes describe the impact of the project. Tracking outcomes involves a concerted effort to identify what impact, benefit, or change resulted from the project. Outcomes can be measured in changes in knowledge (e.g., pre-/post-program surveys), attitudes, skills, and behaviors (e.g., reduction in risk behaviors), or other improvements (e.g., decreased costs, patient satisfaction).

Early in project development, the project leader (DNP student) must develop a reasonable estimate of the desired outcomes. These can be defined through the literature review done for the problem statement; alternatively, this may be a point at which the literature review requires expansion to search for predictable outcomes based on other similar projects. In either case, some outcome statements should be developed. Outcome statements at this phase of project development are often brief and will need refinement before the implementation phase. Nevertheless, the remainder of the project plan cannot proceed without clear outcomes in mind. In health care, measurement of outcomes is the backbone of assessing the quality of the care delivered. Healthcare providers have a vast array of physiologic measures, patient self-reported functional status, and symptoms that make for rich measurements of outcomes. The difficulty is in attributing any given outcome to the care that preceded the event of physiologic change. Making the connection between any outcome measured and the care that preceded it is further complicated by the variety of care providers a patient may encounter in any one event. An example of this is a surgical patient who receives care from the surgeon, clinic staff, any number of nursing personnel with different educational backgrounds, anesthesia providers, postoperative or homecare providers, family caregivers, physical therapists, and others. Attributing outcomes to one provider or another becomes quite complex. Nevertheless, project leaders must strive to demonstrate the efficacy of interventions. Risk factors and risk stratification can be used to account for factors that impact the outcomes of care, particularly in large populations or an accountable care organization that takes responsibility for care coordination (Agency for Healthcare Research and Quality [AHRQ], 2022).

SWOT Analysis

A powerful and simple tool for needs assessment is the SWOT analysis. SWOT stands for strengths, weaknesses, opportunities, and threats. It helps the project leader discern where the strengths of the project lie, make plans to address weaknesses, know where to look for opportunities, and be aware of threats. The SWOT analysis had its origin as a business tool, but it can be adapted to the DNP project to provide a useful analysis of the project and to generate material for the project leader to consider for solutions and direction for the project. In general, strengths and weaknesses are internal to the organization or project, and opportunities and threats are external (Mind Tools, 2022b). The SWOT analysis is typically summarized in a grid that briefly touches on the important learning in each category (see **Figure 11-5**).

The first step in a SWOT analysis is to make a list for each of the categories. When the list is complete, prioritize it to a few strategic items in each category. Use verifiable data whenever possible (e.g., "The project improves compliance with Hgb A1C recommendations from the American Diabetes Association in this clinic population by 20%" rather than "We will improve Hgb A1Cs in our clinic"). Be brutally honest when assessing all categories, seek reliable opinions from outside the organization or unit, and be certain that this analysis is done at a level where it can make a difference. A SWOT analysis on a large organization may not generate enough specific data and ideas to give good direction to the organization or project (Mind Tools Content Team, 2022b). Some statements and questions to stimulate thoughts about each category include:

Strengths are just that. You can contemplate these questions: What does this organization, unit, or project do better than anyone else? What special resources do

---

SWOT Analysis

Strengths
- What do you (or your organization) do well?
- What resources do you have that others may not have available?
- What do your customers see as your strengths?

Weaknesses
- Where could you improve?
- Where do you have poor resources as compared with other similar organizations?
- What do your customers see as your weaknesses?

Opportunities
- What social, economic, regulatory, or policy changes are happening that may provide opportunities for growth?
- How can you turn strengths or weaknesses into opportunities?

Threats
- What are competitors doing that presents a threat to your core business?
- Are there impending changes in technology, regulations, policy, or organizational leadership that present threats to your business or project?

Figure 11-5 SWOT Analysis

you have access to that others might not? What advantages do you have? Why do patients choose your organization over other similar organizations?

Weaknesses are areas for improvement. What could you improve about the organizational or unit performance? What do your patients see as your weakest areas? Should you address these areas, or simply avoid them? Do you have the resources to strengthen these areas?

Opportunities often arise from an assessment of strengths and weaknesses. Do your strengths create any opportunities for additional business or a change in direction of the current project? The same is true for weaknesses. Ask yourself if elimination of weaknesses would create additional opportunities or if it would be more cost-effective to let go of a weak area. Scan the environment for changes in regulatory requirements, emerging social phenomena, new technology, new laws, and new markets to identify opportunities.

Threats include obstacles to the project, business, or organization. Identify competitors that you should be concerned about, technological threats to the project, changes in regulatory requirements, impending changes in organizational leadership, and policy changes that may negatively impact your project. At the conclusion of the SWOT analysis, the project leader should have a sense of direction for the project's best chance for success.

Team Selection and Formation

At this point, the DNP student should assemble a team of individuals with the correct skills to conduct the project. There is no defined number or recommended composition for the team. The team membership is dictated by each individual project. Special attention must be paid to the interprofessional nature of the work when engaging the members of a team. Consideration of perspectives of multiple professions, as well as the recipient of the intervention, is advisable in most project work. Members may or may not come from the list of stakeholders; however, the project leader is always the team leader.

Team formation is a process well defined in the literature. It proceeds through four phases: forming, storming, norming, and performing. These stages were first described by Tuckman (1965). In the forming stage, the people on the team get to know each other and may be hesitant to offer opinions. This is a good time to evaluate individual skills and personalities. The team leader should be directive during this phase. In the storming phase, team members may jockey for position and authority. At this point, some team members may feel overwhelmed by the scope of the project and the tasks necessary to complete the project. Some may be resistant to the project and express doubts about it. At all times, the DNP student should remember that she or he is the project and team leader and is ultimately responsible for the project and that the end product will reflect on her or his scholarship (Sipes, 2019). The project leader (DNP student) should support those team members who feel less secure, work to build positive relationships among team members, and remain positive but firm when the goals of the project or leadership are challenged.

Norming brings the team's strong commitment to the project goals, and as the team socializes more, the members are more agreeable to taking on the tasks of the project and working together as a unit. The DNP student should facilitate the development of collaboration among team members.

The last stage of team development is performing. In this stage, the team makes rapid progress toward the goals of the project. The team leader may be able to delegate much of the work but remains ultimately responsible for the outcome. The team leader must remain cognizant of the constraints of the team members. In many cases, the members are staff members with other responsibilities.

If the project is not dictated by the needs of the institution or community in which it is being conducted, there may be constraints on the time that team members can commit to the project (Sipes, 2019). Considering such constraints is important in project planning.

Cost-Benefit Analysis

A cost–benefit analysis is a powerful tool to promote the project to sponsors and others with vested interests. The development of this analysis simply adds up the real costs of the project and subtracts them from the benefits gleaned from the project. The point of the analysis is to demonstrate that the benefit of solving the problem is worth the costs (Starbird et al., 2021). For most projects, it is important that both costs and benefits be quantifiable. It is often easy to quantify costs and relatively difficult to measure benefits that are intangible and realized over a period of time. Many templates for cost–benefit analysis are available online. Use of an Excel spreadsheet is often involved. Please see **Figure 11-6** for a graphic presentation of a cost–benefit analysis.

Because outcomes can be measured in a number of ways, it is imperative to avoid double counting benefits of the project. An example of double counting benefits follows. Gaining control of Hgb A1C levels in a population will decrease the cost of care through avoidance of long-term complications of diabetes. In addition, it may decrease the number of hypo-/hyperglycemic visits to the emergency department. Counting both financial outcomes as a benefit is double counting (Ungar, 2016).

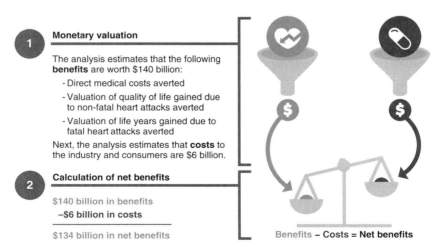

1 Monetary valuation

The analysis estimates that the following **benefits** are worth $140 billion:

- Direct medical costs averted
- Valuation of quality of life gained due to non-fatal heart attacks averted
- Valuation of life years gained due to fatal heart attacks averted

Next, the analysis estimates that **costs** to the industry and consumers are $6 billion.

2 Calculation of net benefits

$140 billion in benefits
−$6 billion in costs
―――――――――――――――
$134 billion in net benefits

Benefits − Costs = Net benefits

Figure 11-6 Cost Benefit Analysis

CDC (2021). Office of the Associate Director for Policy and Strategy, Cost Benefit Analysis. https://www.cdc.gov/policy/polaris/economics/cost-benefit/index.html

In some instances, projects are dictated by regulatory requirements, governing bodies, or organizational administration. In this case, it is still useful to do a cost–benefit analysis. If the cost–benefit analysis demonstrates more cost than benefit, the analysis will demonstrate how the costs will affect the budget. This does not imply that the project will not be done; often the institution has no choice. For example, regulatory issues may dictate the implementation of the project regardless of the cost. At times the project will proceed simply because it is the right thing to do. Examples of this might be a project that is done to benefit the community served by the organization to improve community relationships or provide service to the community.

There are four additional approaches to analyzing the financial impact of a project or intervention, and each has its own advantages and disadvantages in certain situations (Starbird et al., 2021):

- Cost minimization
- Cost utility
- Cost consequences
- Cost-effectiveness

Defining the Scope of the Project

Now the scope of the project statement can be written. A well-crafted project scope statement is essential for the project leader to make well-reasoned decisions throughout the life cycle of the project and limit potential changes in scope. Such changes are often referred to as scope creep (Sipes, 2019). The scope statement will clearly and succinctly state what the project will and will not do (Polit & Beck, 2021; Sipes, 2019). The scope will help to identify potential barriers to the project. The scope statement will bind the agreement between the project leader, the project sponsor, and the organization. A well-thought-out project scope statement will help the project leader identify changes throughout the life of the project and guide modifications to the project to adapt to the changes (Sipes, 2019).

Step III: Goals, Objectives, and Mission Statement Development

Goals

The concepts, goals, and objectives are complicated by confusing and overlapping terminology. For the purposes of this chapter, goals are defined as broad statements that identify future outcomes, provide overarching direction to the project, and point to the expected outcomes of the project. Goals should be written first. Typically, a project has several goals, and each goal will need different objectives to support its achievement. Institutional demands may dictate that the goals of the project be prioritized according to financial savings, safety, or the institutional mission. Simply stated, goals are where you want to be; objectives are how you get there.

Objectives

Objectives are clear, realistic, specific, measurable, and time-limited statements of the actions that, when completed, will move the project toward its goals. In the business literature, the commonly used template for crafting objectives is SMART, which stands for specific, measurable, attainable, realistic, and timely (Lewis, 2007). In the case of the DNP Project, *specific* means being precise. It is not enough to state that you want to improve a process or practice; you must name the who (target population), what (what the project will accomplish), where (project setting), and when (creation of a specific timeline) (Issel et al., 2022). *Measurable* implies that there are collectible data adequate for measuring change. *Attainable* and *realistic* mean that the scope of the project has been focused so that the project is feasible and meaningful with the resources at hand. Will the project really make a difference, or is it simply an exercise to attain a degree? *Timely* refers to the ability to realistically get the project accomplished in the time allotted by the academic institution. This can be an opportunity to recheck whether the scope of the project is attainable. The objectives should be rigorous but not impossible to achieve (Lewis, 2007). DNP students might find accessing the Center for Disease Control and Prevention's (CDC's) public health communities' website helpful when developing SMART objectives for their projects. A SMART objectives template is available on the CDC's website at the following: https://www.cdc.gov/publichealthgateway/phcommunities/resourcekit /evaluate/develop-smart-objectives.html.

Although many other types are found in the literature, in this conceptualization of the DNP project, there are two types of objectives: outcomes objectives and process objectives. *Outcomes objectives* simply address the outcomes of the project as they were defined earlier but state a specific time frame for accomplishment of the desired outcomes. *Process objectives* define the steps needed to accomplish the outcomes objectives. The process objectives are the actions or activities required to implement the project in the time frame stated. Process objectives should be succinct and clear. They function as a real-time check on the progress of the project so that course corrections can be made in a timely manner (Issel, et al., 2022; Burroughs & Wood, 2000). Measuring the process also helps to confirm if the outcomes achieved at the end of the project are related to the process changes implemented. Any conclusion about if the project success or failure was related to the planned intervention can't be determined without measuring that the project processes to be implemented by the project did indeed occur as planned (Issel et al., 2022).

Mission Statement

The mission statement is a succinct paragraph that accurately describes why the project is being conducted. The academic institution determines whether a mission statement will be included in the DNP Project proposal. The benefit of a mission statement is that it helps clarify the purpose of the project and the methods of getting the project accomplished. Writing a mission statement is an opportunity for the project leader to take all the information gathered thus far and focus on the problem to be solved, and the methods of solving it, in two or three sentences (Allison & Kaye, 2015). A mission statement can be used to solicit support for the project, and it can be used as an explanatory statement for "elevator conversations," well-rehearsed 30-second conversations that the project leader can turn into an opportunity to inform a person or group of people about the project. A well-crafted mission statement can help keep the project focused throughout the entirety of the project.

To draft a succinct mission statement, the project leader or project team needs to answer three questions: What is the purpose of the project? (The answer should use an infinitive verb and a statement of the problem to be addressed.) What is the population to be addressed in solving the problem? What are the methods to be used in addressing the problem?

It is often helpful to engage the project team in developing the mission statement to help clarify the mission to the team itself and cultivate buy-in from the team members and other stakeholders (Allison & Kaye, 2015).

The mission statement for this text is as follows:

"This book is intended to serve as a core text for DNP students and faculty to use to achieve mastery of the American Association of Colleges of Nursing essentials as well as a shelf reference for practicing DNPs. The AACN essentials are all covered herein; each essential is covered in adequate detail to frame the foundation of the DNP educational program. This book provides the infrastructure for students, faculty, and practicing DNPs to achieve and sustain the highest level of practice."

Step IV: Theoretical Underpinnings of the Project

Theoretical Underpinnings of Change

The DNP Project leader now has completed the work necessary to begin implementing the project plan. Each project will by definition involve change in a system or practice (AACN, 2021). Change is notoriously difficult to achieve. The change will be made easier by using a theory to support the change process and building a model of the planned change. Planning expedites change and improves the likelihood of long-term success. Theories of change come from many different fields of study: education, sociology, psychology, organizational psychology, business management, and health care. Expansion of the literature review will assist the project leader in identifying theoretical supports for the project. The DNP Project leader will use the scholarship of integration to select a theory of change that best describes the change that will occur as a result of the project.

Kurt Lewin is noted as the first change theorist. His work had a profound impact on the field of psychology and organizational psychology. His force field analysis is still used to create force field diagrams. He theorized that issues are held in balance by those forces that maintain the current state and those forces that advance change, which he called restraining forces and driving forces, respectively. Until the driving forces exceed the restraining forces, change will not occur. Lewin also created tools to map the driving forces and restraining forces. The resulting force field diagram is a powerful tool to understand the environment in which the project will take place (Lewin, 1951; Thomas, 1985) (**Figure 11-7**).

Lewin's model of the change process has three stages: unfreezing, movement, and refreezing. Most other theories of change are based in part on Lewin's theory. The first step entails an "unfreezing" of the current status or state. This can be achieved by convincing people to let go of the status quo or old way of doing something. The second step involves movement toward a new state. In this phase, people are persuaded to take a fresh look at problems from a different perspective and

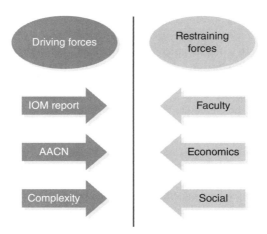

Figure 11-7 Forces for Change in Healthcare Education
© Jones & Bartlett Learning

move toward a new paradigm. Movement of the group is supported by respected leaders who understand the need for change. In the third and final step, the change becomes the new norm for the population affected by the change. One mechanism for accomplishing this is to reinforce the new behaviors and institutionalize ("refreeze") them through formal and informal mechanisms. This reinforcement is done to ensure that the change will endure past the project implementation and become incorporated into the organizational culture (Thomas, 1985). There are many other change theorists in addition to Lewin, such as Lippitt, Watson, and Westley; Wheatley; Haverlock; Rogers; Kotter; and Prochaska and DiClemente that students might consider as a fit for their project.

Theory to Support Project Framework

Domain I (Knowledge for Nursing Practice) of *The Essentials: Core Competencies for Professional Nursing Education* supports the notion of utilizing theory to create a framework for the project. Advanced-level nurses are to demonstrate competency by the following: "Apply theory and research-based knowledge from nursing, the arts, humanities, and other sciences . . . and . . . translate theories from nursing and other disciplines to practice" (AACN, 2021, pp. 27–28). The theoretical framework helps the project leader to conceptualize the project and supports it throughout the course of the project.

Theoretical frameworks can be constructed using concepts from fields of study other than nursing—for example, motivational theory in business, adult education theory, economic theory, social psychology, and theories of medicine. Often theories from different fields will need to be integrated into a theoretical framework that describes the unique project. The framework used by Felsenstein (2018) in her scholarly project incorporated the seven phases of Lippitt's change theory. This change theory provided the author with insight into the clinic staffs' "motivation and change capacity" (Felsenstein, 2018, p. 144). Furthermore, this theory was used in every stage of the project from the initial idea to the final sustainability and project closure steps. Deploying a change framework in this way provided Felsenstein with a valid and reliable structure that framed her work.

Step V: Work Planning
Project Proposal

Typically, a formal project proposal will be required by the academic institution or the organization where the project will take place. The amount of detail required varies from institution to institution. Most proposals will include a synopsis of the problem and the problem statement, a needs assessment, a description of the scope of the project, the desired outcomes, the goals and objectives, tools and procedure for implementation, and, most important for some institutions, the cost–benefit analysis. It is incumbent on the project leader to check with the organization for the details required for the project proposal.

The academic institution or organization often provides guidelines for what needs to be included in a project proposal. However, templates for project proposals can be found online. While not supporting any one software package or website, many good sources exist. One such source for templates is Google Drive (The Project Proposal Toolkit, 2018). The Project Proposal Toolkit website has many other templates (https://project-proposal.casual.pm/). Another reliable website that has templates for project proposals is Mind Tools, and their project management framework (www.mindtools.com). Many of these software packages include project management tools that will be helpful in the next phase of work planning.

Project Management Tools

Project management is a body of specialized knowledge and skills. Much of project management's body of knowledge was developed in parallel with large government projects, beginning with the transcontinental railroad and continuing through the projects of the National Aeronautics and Space Administration (NASA) that eventually landed people on the moon. The common theme is that these projects employed hundreds of thousands of people who needed to complete highly accurate work on time and within a budget. To manage these requirements, the field of project management was born.

Efficiency of work is part of project management. Around the turn of the 20th century, Frederick Taylor studied work efficiency in detail. He demonstrated that output can be improved by studying the work and breaking it down into small tasks that can be made more efficient. One of Taylor's peers, Henry Gantt, studied the order of tasks, primarily in shipyards during World War I, and crafted the familiar Gantt chart that is used by many to keep projects on task. These skills were applied to the building of the Hoover Dam, thus securing the place of project management in scientific approaches to large projects (Luecke, 2004). Any project developed today is likely to include a Gantt chart, which details the timeline for the project as well as which tasks can be done in parallel and which are sequential. An example of a Gantt chart is shown later in this chapter. Another important tool developed in the 1950s is the Critical Pathway Diagram (CPD), which adds a time and activity dimension to the scheduling of projects, and the PERT chart, which has a more detailed timeline. Activities are described as occurring in parallel or in sequence, and the relationship of activities is described before being incorporated into the timeline. Time estimates in a PERT chart are calculated using the shortest estimated time, the longest estimated time, and average time in this formula:

$$\frac{\text{Shortest time} + (4 \times \text{average time}) + \text{longest time}}{6}$$

This corrects for overly optimistic time estimates and is considered the weighted average of the time estimate. Examples of PERT charts can be found in many online resources.

Today the field of project management is a distinct field of scholarship and certifications. The DNP project leader, using Boyer's scholarship of integration (Boyer, 1990), can borrow knowledge, skills, and tools from the field of project management to use for DNP projects. The point of using project management tools is to gain benefit from careful work planning and scheduling.

Baker, Baker, and Campbell (2003) defined a project as "a sequence of tasks with a beginning and an end that is bounded by time and resources and that produces a unique product or service" (p. 404). Guided by this definition, the DNP student can discern where project management tools might aid the DNP Project and where the DNP student will need to select different tools.

Defining the scope of the project; identifying key stakeholders; assessing resources, goals, and objectives; and writing a mission statement are project management tools that have already been included in this chapter. Additional tools that can be helpful to the DNP Project leader include work breakdown, timeline tools, and project milestones. These three tools will help the project leader determine the flow of the project, predict when resources are needed, and estimate time to completion, which will in turn help the project leader estimate whether the project can be done in the allotted time.

Work Breakdowns and Milestones. Accurate planning of work requires that the work be broken down into small packages that can be easily monitored. Each task of the project is broken down into levels and sublevels or subprojects. Each subproject is then examined for milestones.

Milestones identify when an important or large part of the project is completed (Sipes, 2019). The subproject is further broken down into major activities and then into work packages (**Figure 11-8**). The purpose of this activity is to systematically identify all the work that needs to be done to execute the project. **Box 11-3** identifies the benefits of a work breakdown structure (WBS).

The WBS can be diagrammed as a simple tree diagram (Mind Tools Content Team, 2022c). Templates are available online, some at no charge to the user. The work breakdown does not have to be perfect. The amount of detail will vary from project to project. The project leader will know that the work is broken into small enough tasks when a task can be done by one individual in a defined amount of time, and that task will produce a distinct product.

Once the WBS is completed in sufficient detail, the project leader can begin to estimate the time required to complete the subprojects and tasks. At this time, it is essential to begin to identify whether tasks can be done in parallel or whether they are sequential to other tasks. This can be done by placing the activities into a simple table such as the one in **Table 11-4** (Mind Tools Content Team, 2022c). The information in the table can then be placed into a Gantt chart (**Figure 11-9**).

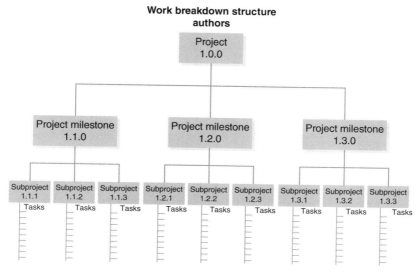

Figure 11-8 Work Breakdown Structure

© Jones & Bartlett Learning

Box 11-3 Benefits of Work Breakdown Structure

Identifies all the work needed for the project to be completed
Organizes the work in a logical sequence
Predicts when work may be completed
Identifies team members who have the best skills for the tasks
Identifies which resources are needed and when
Helps to prepare the budget
Provides a communication tool for all team members
Keeps team members attuned to the work of all team members
Organizes work tasks with milestones

© Jones & Bartlett Learning

Table 11-4 Task Length Table

Task	Estimated Start	Estimated Length to Completion	Sequential or Parallel	Dependent Upon
A	Week 1	Four weeks	Parallel	None
B	Week 2	One week	Parallel	None
C	Week 3	Two weeks	Sequential	Task B
D	Week 4	One day	Sequential	Task A
E	Week 5	One week	Sequential	Task D

© Jones & Bartlett Learning

Task	Wk 1	Wk 2	Wk 3	Wk 4	Wk 5	Wk 6
Task A *				*		
Task B						
Task C *			*			
Task D						
Task E						
*Milestone event						

Figure 11-9 Gantt Chart
© Jones & Bartlett Learning

Budget Development. Developing a budget is an important step in project management. Administrators, funding agencies, and project stakeholders will need to know the costs associated with the project to decide whether to proceed with the project. Making a detailed and accurate budget and staying within the project budget will also give the project leader credibility within the organization. Here are a few pitfalls to avoid when developing a budget (Luecke, 2004):

- *Underestimating labor costs.* Even though some of the team members may be salaried by the sponsoring institution, the project leader must include these costs in the project budget. Employee benefits, often estimated as a percentage of employee salary, must also be included in the calculations.
- *Neglecting to add in the costs of equipment in use at the institution.* Use of computers, copiers, and other business equipment should be accounted for in the budget.
- *Neglecting to add in the cost of business space.* Estimates for business space can be found from many different sources online for each city or town in the United States.
- *Underestimating the costs of external consultants and supplies.* Most professionals will provide an hourly estimate for services.
- *Forgetting about travel costs.* Mileage rates for various purposes can be found at www.IRS.gov if the institution does not have a set rate for mileage (IRS, 2022).
- *Forgetting to include all the costs for materials.* The team will need supplies such as paper, pencils, pens, printers, and folders.

Calculating Direct and Indirect Costs. The budget must account for both direct and indirect costs. Direct costs are those that are specifically attributable to the project. This includes items such as labor, materials, supplies, equipment for the project, travel, consultant fees, project training, and marketing. Indirect costs include items that are shared by many different entities in the institution, such as business space, internet access, information technology services, internal communications such as telephones and pagers, and support staff (Speilman, 2022; Luecke, 2004).

Indirect costs are often expressed as a percentage of the direct costs. A more experienced colleague or administrator at the project site may be able to assist with the development of the budget.

Templates for Budgeting. Most institutions have a template they prefer to use for developing a budget. If the institution does not have a template that it prefers, templates can be found online. Microsoft Excel, Google Docs, and Word also provide templates within the programs. Once the budget is developed and final project approval is obtained, the plan for evaluation can be created.

Step VI: Planning for Evaluation

Evaluation of project outcomes requires a broad range of data collection, often involving both quantitative and qualitative data. The focus of developing evaluation skills as a DNP student is not simply for the DNP project: These methods should become ingrained into the framework of future professional practice. Mastery of and use of these skills define clinical scholarship.

Evaluation of outcomes through data collection for DNP projects is done to measure change in a population or practice. That is, what was the impact of the DNP Project? Although some statistical methods may be useful for evaluation of the DNP Project, many of the methods for evaluation will be different from those of the research project. Evaluation provides accountability to the stakeholders, demonstrates quality improvement, demonstrates effectiveness in the population involved in the project, and provides clarity of purpose to the program (W. K. Kellogg Foundation, 2004a).

This section presents tools, methods, and resources that can be used for evaluation of the program or project. It is the responsibility of the project leader to select the correct tools and methods for evaluation of the project creating a coherent plan for evaluation. This section also presents logic models that will assist in the development of the plan. Like any other skill, development of an evaluation plan requires both tools and practice. As the DNP student uses these tools and methods, confidence and competence in project planning, implementation, and evaluation will develop.

Finding Tools to Measure Outcomes

The notion of measuring outcomes is not new and is central to demonstrating the efficacy of advanced practice nursing. Measuring outcomes provides evidence of the need for process improvements and determines whether the changes made are successful. It has been said, "If you don't know where you're going, any road will get you there" (Carroll, 1865). To develop and start a project without having clear outcomes to measure is a waste of time and talent, and it may present a hazard to the patients served. The ideal measurement tools should be valid and reliable measures that address the domain of health the project is seeking to improve. Validity refers to the degree to which an instrument measures the concept it is supposed to measure. Reliability is concerned with the accuracy of the actual measurement tool. Outcomes tools should also measure compliance with standards, evidence-based guidelines, and recommendations. That is, was the project delivered as planned? They should be useful in customizing programs to the individual and should be easily interpreted and reported to stakeholders.

Here are some questions to answer when selecting outcomes to measure for the DNP Project (Olney & Barnes, 2013):

- Does the outcome measure selected answer the question of whether the change proposed actually happened? (Appropriateness)
- Are the outcome measure data easy to collect and report? (Feasibility)
- Does the outcome measure selected produce data that are consistent? (Reliability)
- Does the outcome measure identify change over the time frame of the project? (Responsiveness)
- Is the outcome measure acceptable to the patient population? (Acceptability)

Sources for reliable tools include the AHRQ, National Guideline Clearinghouse, the IOM, and the World Health Organization.

Development of Evaluation Methods

Evaluation should be thoughtfully designed so that it measures the degree to which the outcomes were or were not met. The evaluation design should fit the unique project. The project leader must determine the appropriate methods and types of data to be collected that best demonstrate the outcomes. When choosing whether quantitative or qualitative methods are most appropriate for measurement of the project outcomes, consider the reason for collecting the data. If the outcome is to identify how much, how many, how often, or an average response, then the best method is quantitative. If the outcome is to identify what worked, what the numbers mean, how the project was useful, what it meant to the participants, or what factors influenced success or failure, then one should select qualitative methods (Olney & Barnes, 2006, 2013). Qualitative data can provide contextual meaning to the quantitative data in a project that uses both. For example, it is useful to know the number of diabetic patients in a population who develop diabetic retinopathy; it is another thing to understand the impact of blindness in a person's life. Qualitative data provide meaning to the people affected by the project, the stakeholders, the organization, and possibly outside audiences (W. K. Kellogg Foundation, 2004a). Regardless of which approach is used for evaluation, the methods should be chosen before implementation of the project.

Tools for qualitative evaluation may include observations, ethnographic interviews, structured interviews, written questions, and document review. Issues of cultural sensitivity should be kept in mind when developing survey or interview questions. Tools for quantitative data collection include surveys, health factors, laboratory test results, and chart reviews. No matter which methods the project leader selects for evaluation data collection, they should be reliable and valid (Olney & Barnes, 2006, 2013).

Logic Model Development

Basically, a logic model is a systematic and visual way to present and share your understanding of the relationships among the resources you have to operate your program, the activities you plan, and the changes or results you hope to achieve.

— **W. K. Kellogg Foundation** (2004b, p. 1)

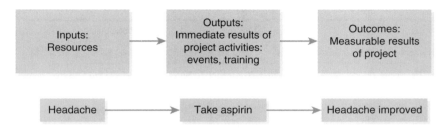

Figure 11-10 Simple Logic Model
© Jones & Bartlett Learning

The first logic models were developed in the 1970s. *Evaluation: Promise and Performance* by Joseph S. Wholey was the first text to use the term *logic model* (Taylor-Powell & Henert, 2008). Logic models have evolved since the introduction of the Government Results and Performance Act of 1993. This act was intended to improve the effectiveness of federal programs through requirements for strategic planning and program evaluation. It shifted the focus of evaluation onto results and not simply activities. The models identified in this chapter were developed in part in response to this act.

A logic model (**Figure 11-10**) is a picture of how the project developer believes the program will work. It uses a series of diagrams to indicate how parts of the program are linked together or sequenced. There is no one correct way to diagram the logic model. It depends in large part on the purpose of the model. If the diagram is used to describe the entire project plan, it should be detailed. If it is used for communication among team members, it should be less complex. The project developer may need several models for various parts of the project (Taylor-Powell & Henert, 2008). Logic models all have similar components: inputs, outputs, and outcomes (Taylor-Powell & Henert, 2008).

Only the simplest of programs will be adequately described by this model. For example, if you had a headache, it would describe the input as "headache," the output as "take an aspirin," and the outcome as "headache is better." This simple model does not identify how projects get from inputs to outputs. No activities are defined in the model. Most programs will require more detail to adequately describe the project.

The logic model template presented in this chapter is an assimilation of several models: the Kellogg Foundation Logic Model, the United Way Program Outcome Model, and the University of Wisconsin Extension Service Logic Model. Resources, templates, designs, and worksheets for development of these models are available online at no charge to the individual. **Figure 11-11** is a template created by the authors.

In the template, inputs are the resources required to implement and evaluate the project. Those resources may include personnel, facilities, equipment, time, and finances. Resources could be constrained by laws, regulations, funding, time, existing culture, and local policy. Constraints can prevent the project from advancing or limit the project in some manner. For example, financial resource allocations may be less than what was originally proposed to support the project. The project leader may either redefine the budget or reexamine the

Inputs	Constraints	Activities	Outputs	Outcomes		
				Short Term	**Long Term**	**Impact**
Personnel	Budget	Events	Number of participants	Knowledge improvement	Behavior improvement	Long-term results of the change
Financial	Physical space	Training	Amount of education delivered	Skill improvement	Motivation improvement	
Time	Law, regulations, local policy	Education	Number of hours of service	Improved level of functioning		
Materials	Time frame	Media/ technology				
Equipment	Existing culture	Meetings				
Facilities		Development of processes				

Figure 11-11 Logic Model Template

project activities that affect the budget. Activities are what the project does with the resources to achieve the intended outcomes: events, training and education, meetings, development of media and technology, and development of the processes necessary to implement the project. Outputs are the immediate results of the project. They could include the number of participants, the number of hours of instruction, the number of meetings, participation rates, and the number of hours of each service provided. Outcomes can be considered at three levels: short-term, long-term, and impact outcomes. In short-term outcomes, the project leader measures the effect of the activities on the knowledge base and skills or level of functioning. The long-term outcomes reflect a change in behavior or motivation. Impact outcomes describe the results of the change on the population served by the project.

Figure 11-12 demonstrates an application of the logic model to a more complex project completed in 2007 as part of the requirements of the DNP curriculum at the University of Minnesota School of Nursing. This model describes a DNP project completed by Mary Zaccagnini, "Development of a Computer Resourced Communication Center in a Long-Term Care Facility." This project addressed the problem of social isolation within a long-term care facility and the resultant problems caused by the isolation. The project leader developed a computer center and trained the staff and volunteers to assist the residents. It demonstrated that the residents who used the computer center experienced an increase in socialization and communication via email and a decrease in loneliness (Zaccagnini, 2007).

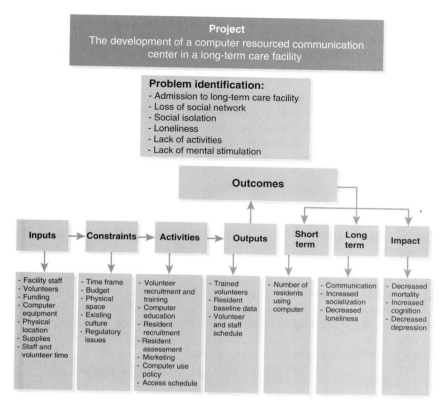

Figure 11-12 The Development of a Computer-Resourced Communication Center in a Long-Term Care Facility

Data from Zaccagnini, M. (2007). *The development of a computer resourced communication center in a long-term care facility* (Unpublished DNP project paper). University of Minnesota, Minneapolis, MN.

Quality Improvement Methods

Thinking about a program in logic model terms prompts the clarity and specificity required for success, and often demanded by funders and your community. Using a simple logic model produces (1) an inventory of what you have and what you need to operate your program; (2) a strong case for how and why your program will produce your desired results; and (3) a method for program management and assessment.

— **W. K. Kellogg Foundation** (2004b)

After a long congressional debate, the Affordable Care Act was passed and signed into law in March 2010 (Rosenbaum, 2011). One major initiative contained in this act was the directive for the Secretary of Health and Human Services to develop a national strategy for quality improvement in health care. The three aims of this national strategy were (1) to improve the delivery of healthcare services; (2) to reduce the cost of quality health care; and (3) to improve the health of the U.S. population. The strategy continues to guide the national effort to improve health care for all Americans (AHRQ, 2017). As the largest group of healthcare providers, nurses play a pivotal role in quality improvement efforts in implementing these strategies. The DNP-prepared nurse will have the skillset and an understanding of the various methodologies to develop, lead, implement, and evaluate these quality improvement efforts.

Quality improvement methods have been used in the business world for many years. The earliest quality improvement tools were developed during World War II and continue to be used in healthcare quality improvement today. W. Edwards Demming and Walter Shewhart are considered pioneers in development of quality improvement cycles. Shewhart first developed the PDCA cycle as a methodology for quality improvement. PDCA consists of the following steps (American Society for Quality [ASQ], 2022):

- Plan
  - Collect data
  - Analyze data
  - Plan the intervention
- Do
  - Develop and test potential solutions
- Check
  - Measure efficacy of solutions
  - Analyze outcomes for needed adjustments to solutions
- Act
  - Modify the plan as needed

Demming later modified the PDCA model to the PDSA model (plan, do, study, act) in order to refocus the cycle on analysis instead of inspection. Demming's PDSA model is used to this day in healthcare agencies that do *rapid cycle improvement processes* consisting of daily management and continuous development. With this model, small changes are made, evaluated in a very short time, corrected or changed, and reevaluated.

Figure 11-13 demonstrates the iterative nature of the PDSA model.

Dr. Joseph Juran broadened quality management concepts and focused on the responsibilities of management of the organization. He promoted the concept known as *managing business process quality*, which is a technique for executive cross-functional quality improvement. His model, known as the Juran trilogy (Juran, 1986), is made up of three methods—quality planning, quality control, and quality improvement—that, when complete, will lead to quality leadership. The three methods leading to quality leadership are also known as *total quality management* (TQM) (Ross, 2017). The Juran model gained popularity in business during the 1980s (Bisgaard, 2008).

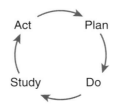

Figure 11-13 PDSA Model

Another quality improvement method, *value analysis*, also known as value engineering, was developed by Larry Miles, an engineer at General Electric during World War II. The value analysis method focuses on a very structured analysis of materials, processes, and designs by multifunctional teams to seek cost-effective alternatives. The data generated by this very structured methodology laid the groundwork for the *lean* and *six sigma* techniques for quality improvement in health care (Mandelbaum et al., 2010).

There are many quality models in use in health care. Two focus on patient care: the CARE model and the FADE model. The CARE model is used to support chronic care projects. This CARE model emphasizes the interactions between patients with chronic diseases who take an active role in the management of those diseases, and the providers who have the expertise and resources to aid the patient's self-care. The FADE model is more appropriate for acute care. The four steps of the FADE model are as follows:

- Focus (define which processes are to be improved)
- Analyze (collect and study the data)
- Develop (develop plans for improvement in processes)
- Execute (implement) and evaluate (measure outcomes for success)

The FADE model, like PDSA, is cyclic in nature. Many iterations may be needed until the desired improvement is seen and documented with data (Duke University Department of Community and Family Medicine, 2021; ASQ, 2022).

In 1986, an engineer at Motorola Corporation, Bill Smith, invented six sigma as a method to count the number of manufacturing defects in semiconductors. He noted that it takes six standard deviations from a normal curve to improve reliability of manufactured parts to compete with the Japanese manufacturers. The goal of the Six Sigma processes is to reduce errors in manufacturing. These same statistical methods are being applied to healthcare processes in an effort to improve the quality and safety of health care. Six Sigma core concepts seek to improve the quality of healthcare process outputs by identifying and removing the causes of errors (defects) and minimizing variability in healthcare practices and processes. Two of the most common methodologies used to achieve Six Sigma goals are DMAIC (design, measure, analyze, improve, and control) and DMADV (design, measure, analyze, design, and verify). DMAIC is employed when an existing process does not meet customer expectations, and DMADV is used when "developing a new product or service or when a process is optimized but still fails to meet customer expectations" ("DMAIC versus DMADV," n.d.). There are many techniques and processes available for quality improvement. This is not intended to be an exhaustive list. PDSA and Six Sigma are at the core of many healthcare quality improvement strategies. These quality improvement skills are necessary for the DNP graduate as leaders for organizational change and healthcare quality improvement strategies (AACN, 2021).

Step VII: Implementation
Institutional Review Board Process

If Steps I through VI went well, the DNP Project is ready to be implemented. Most institutions will require a review from the IRB or human subjects committee. These reviews are a mechanism to ensure that human subjects are protected and have given fully informed consent when required. It also ensures that patient privacy issues are addressed and that the data collected are secure and used correctly. Some projects may require just one review through the academic institution; other projects and settings may require an academic review and a review by the IRB of the institution where the project will be conducted. One strategy used by both academic institutions and healthcare organizations as described earlier in the chapter is an IRB determination form. This tool can be used to determine if the project is quality improvement (not requiring IRB review) or if the project meets the institutional requirement for IRB review. Whichever IRB strategy is in place, the timeline and manner in which this review is conducted will be dictated by the institutions that complete the review. Because these reviews can take some time to process, the DNP Project leader must be certain to account for this time in the project timeline. Projects cannot be implemented until the IRB determination or review is completed.

Getting the Project Implemented

The IRB review is a good opportunity to review all the project steps taken thus far. The DNP Project leader should review the goals, objectives, and work plans to be certain that they are appropriate to the problem identified in the needs assessment. The project leader should reflect on her or his own leadership style and the team she or he will be leading. In addition, this is a good time to review the evaluation plan to be certain that it will measure the correct data points to determine whether the project addressed the problem. It is a good idea to plan a formal kickoff event to reenergize the team at this time because enthusiasm can wane over the time it takes to plan the project. The team should select a firm start date for the project and avoid wavering on this date. All of this involves clear and frequent communication. This is a time when every team member should be fully informed and knowledgeable about the project plan.

Threats and Barriers to Project Success

The project leader should think very carefully about threats and barriers to the project. Threats can be divided into those that can be predicted and those that cannot. Foreseeable threats to the project are those threats that the project leader and team members can identify as potential barriers at the beginning of the planning. The threats to the project might include lack of or decreased funding, employee turnover, reduced interest over time, time-frame barriers, and technology challenges. Unforeseen threats are events that just happen and over which the project leader has no control. Events such as a change in institutional leadership, new regulations or policies that affect the project, changes in the economy, business failures, and "acts of God" such as Hurricane Katrina and the COVID-19 pandemic are examples of unforeseen threats.

Although it is impossible to predict unforeseen events, the foreseeable threats and barriers should be addressed with alternative plans for implementation. The project leader should consult with the team to develop different strategies, taking the available resources into consideration. For example, if funding is less than anticipated, the project leader will need to work with the team on a scaled-back plan. Ultimately, if the project is successful, the project can be expanded when additional funding is available (Luecke, 2004).

Monitoring the Implementation Phase

Project implementation is the exercise of leadership and control of the project. There will most certainly be unexpected events to manage. This is the time when the DNP student has to be the explicit project leader to monitor every step of implementation and measure progress against the goals and objectives, mission statement, evaluation plan, and timeline. The project leader must have a clear vision of the project and be prepared to manage threats and barriers to implementation that may arise. Barriers associated with workflow and/or providers are common. Strategies developed when planning the project to address workflow and provider barriers will be important both at the onset of implementation as well as while the project is ongoing (Fischer et al., 2016). The project leader shouldn't vacillate about the goals and objectives or the direction of the project while maintaining flexibility, acknowledging that change is dynamic and often difficult. The DNP student will need all of the leadership skills developed during their DNP program of study to successfully lead and manage their project team. Consultation with the faculty advisor and/or the community partner/mentor is often needed during implementation. Competencies gained in interprofessional teamwork and professionalism will also be important skills used during the implementation phase of the DNP project. That is, implementation is the time to showcase all the previous work of the DNP program and to turn ideas into reality.

Implementation Science. Eccles & Mittman (2006) define implementation science as "the scientific study of methods to promote the systematic uptake of research findings and other evidence-based practices into routine practice, and hence, to improve the quality and effectiveness of health services and care" (p. 1). Fixsen et al. (2015) describe implementation science as a blend of three elements of knowledge development around an innovation: (1) diffusion theory, (2) dissemination theories, and (3) implementation theory.

The field of implementation science consists of implementation research and implementation practice. Implementation research discovers an evidence base for strategies and approaches to use for successful implementation in specific settings whereas implementation practice tailors these strategies and approaches for the setting. Some of the early research on implementation to guide getting evidence and innovations into practice was done through the Knowledge Transfer Study Group at McMaster University in Ottawa, Canada (Lavis et al., 2003) and the National Implementation Research Network in the United States (Fixsen et al., 2005). This research is ongoing.

As implementation science has evolved, a role for implementation support practitioners has emerged. Such practitioners will need to be competent in domains of co-creation and engagement, ongoing improvement, and sustaining change. The implementation support practitioner needs to be empathetic, be curious, be committed, advance equity, use critical thinking, and embrace cross-disciplinary approaches (Metz et al., 2020). The principles and competencies identified for implementation support practitioners are closely related to many of the competencies of the DNP-prepared nurse. Keeping the principles and competencies of an implementation support practitioner in mind will be useful for the DNP-prepared nurse during the implementation phase of a project. See **Figure 11-14**.

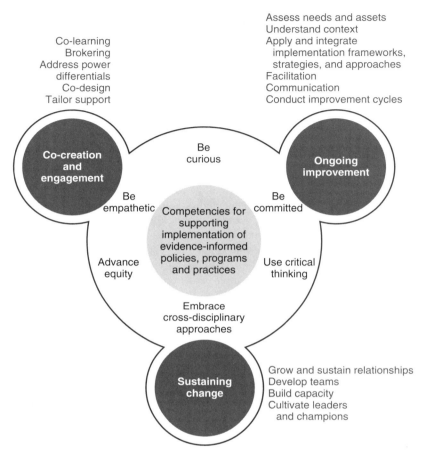

Figure 11-14 Principles and Core Competencies of Implementation Support Practitioners.

Reproduced from Metz, et al. (2020). A practice guide to supporting implementation: What competencies do we need? National Research Implementation Network, ED61057, p. 9

Project Closure

Every project should have a beginning and an end. A good project leader plans for project closure (Daneshgari & Parvin, 2022; Sipes, 2019). Not planning for closure can result in projects lingering and wasting resources (Anthony et al., 2015). Final details and loose ends must be identified and addressed. Project closure checklists and templates are available online to help the project leader develop the report that will be presented to leadership. There are also closure checklists and other tools available in print (Sipes, 2019). According to project management experts (Anthony et al., 2015; Aziz, 2015; Daneshgari & Parvin, 2022; Sipes, 2019), project closure should include the following:

- A mechanism, such as a checklist, or other audit process to assure that all aspects of the project have been completed. That is, a determination that all project objectives have been met or acknowledged to be unachievable needs to occur.

- Agreement from project personnel, leadership (management) and all stakeholders that the project is completed and the project's work approved.
- Review of lessons learned from the project and how these lessons could be applied in managing future projects. The review should include evaluation to determine if governance of the organization or project management processes need any modification.
- Formal closure of the project. Formal closure includes creation of a final project report, final payment of any project expenses, and reallocation of resources used for the project.
- Transition of the project. Transition includes delivering a final project report, sharing all project modifications, files, and other documents used in the project, as well as recommendations for how to sustain the project if pertinent.
- Hold a final project event to formalize the end of the project.

In summary, closure should include a meeting with stakeholders and an acknowledgment that the project is completed, a brief report of the results, plans for sustaining the changes due to the project, and plans for transfer of leadership to the institution. The project leader should meet with team members, thank them for their contributions, and celebrate the accomplishments of the project team. This is a time for team members to reflect on what went well and what did not go well during the project. Closure promotes sustainability of the project after implementation.

Step VIII: Interpretation of the Data
Quantitative Data

Quantitative data collected in the DNP Project serve a different purpose from those collected for the PhD dissertation. They serve to demonstrate the efficacy of the project and are not intended to meet rigorous statistical tests for significance. Nevertheless, stakeholders will be interested in the project's results, and the correct data must be collected in sufficient amounts to demonstrate the outcomes of the project. Data that describe the outcomes of the project must be collected, organized, and presented to peers, the academic community, and other parties of interest. These data will also help other clinicians with similar issues select an intervention that is likely to address the problems they are experiencing in a similar setting.

Descriptive statistical analysis is the traditional method for bringing meaning to data. This type of statistical analysis describes the population in which data were collected and what was observed in the population. The author of this chapter recommends engaging a statistician early in project planning if the plan for evaluation includes statistical analysis.

Even if the project design and sample size do not permit the application of inferential statistical analysis, there are other ways in which the project leader can bring meaning to the data. The project leader can present the findings with other visual tools and techniques, such as charts, graphs, and diagrams. Examples of these visual tools could be run charts that display a change in response over time, pie charts that show relative proportions in relationship to the whole, or flowcharts that diagram processes (Polit & Beck, 2021).

Qualitative Data

The analysis of qualitative data can be daunting because of the sheer volume of records, narratives, and interviews. An organized and logical approach is needed to gain meaning from these kinds of data. The process for analysis of qualitative data includes revisiting the data, placing the data into focus areas, coding the data while looking for themes and patterns, identifying common themes and patterns across data sets, and interpreting the results.

- Step 1 is to review all documents, tapes, videos, surveys, and field notes to get an overall sense of the data. This step will also help the project leader eliminate unnecessary or extraneous information. As this review is under way, the themes or focus areas can be identified.
- Step 2 is sorting the information into the categories and themes identified in Step 1.
- Step 3 is to code the information, naming the themes identified in a systematic manner.
- Step 4 is to look for common threads of meaning or patterns within and across the coded data sets.
- Step 5 is to interpret the data by returning to the outcomes for the project and evaluating whether the qualitative data collected and organized reflect the desired outcomes.

Programs exist to help project leaders assess and interpret qualitative data and can be found readily online. Some examples of online programs for qualitative data analysis and the websites for the applications are listed in **Table 11-5**. The cost for use of these qualitative analysis platform applications varies.

Analyzing Quality Outcomes Data

Analyzing quality outcomes data is considerably different from analysis of carefully controlled research data. Although the data collected certainly may achieve statistical significance, often they do not, and the data cannot be subjected to rigorous statistical methods. Instead, change is demonstrated through the use of pie charts, bar graphs, scattergrams, and other visual methods that show trends and patterns that have clinical significance even if the data are not statistically significant. An adequate selection of these graphic methods of showing trends and clinical change can be found on many internet sites.

Table 11-5 Online Qualitative Analysis Apps

Name of App	Website
Dedoose	https://www.dedoose.com/
Atlas.ti	https://atlasti.com/?x-clickref=1101lwBh84JW
Nvivo	https://lumivero.com/products/nvivo/
MAXQDA	https://www.maxqda.com/

Diane M. Schadewald

Step IX: Utilization and Reporting of Results
Why Disseminate Your DNP Project Outcomes?

There are two purposes for dissemination of the project results: reporting the results of the project to stakeholders and the academic community, and dissemination to other professionals in similar settings. The information and results of the successful DNP Project will have application beyond the immediate practice environment. It is very likely that the problem you identified at the beginning of the project is experienced by others as well. Therefore, it is important to share the findings of the project regardless of whether the project produced the results you expected or different results. There are many venues for dissemination of the project results. The AHRQ dissemination tool can assist authors in deciding where to publish and when they have attained successful dissemination (**Figure 11-15**).

Written Dissemination

Written dissemination is a time-honored method of sharing information. Considerations for selection of the best place to disseminate the information include

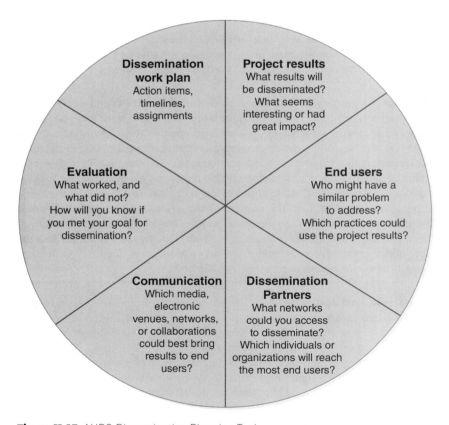

Figure 11-15 AHRQ Dissemination Planning Tool

Data from Agency for Healthcare Research and Quality (AHRQ). (2022). *Dissemination planning tool: Exhibit A from Volume 4.* Rockville, MD: Author. Retrieved from https://www.ahrq.gov/patient-safety/reports/advances/planning.html

the targeted audience, the environment in which the project is most likely to be helpful, and the forum in which the project should be published. SQUIRE 2.0 (Standards for Quality Improvement Reporting Excellence) is routinely used as the manuscript format in quality improvement journals (Ogrinc et al., 2015). The guidelines were developed in an effort to "reduce uncertainty about the information deemed to be important in scholarly reports of health care improvement and to increase the completeness, precision, and transparency of those reports" (Ogrinc et al., 2015, p. 986). If the project leader simply wants to communicate the outcomes of the project, an executive summary is a good mechanism for this purpose.

Executive Summary. An executive summary is a document that summarizes the results of the project. It should not exceed 10% of the length of the main report. It typically has a problem statement, a short description of the background, and a summary of results and recommendations. The executive summary is used quite differently from an abstract. The executive summary provides the project leader with a chance to present important information to a group that may be able to fully fund a project or continue it past the immediate project. The executive summary must be well written, succinct, smooth, and polished. When creating an executive summary, reread the project paper. Identify and extract the main themes. Create a rough draft from the ideas you have identified as the major points in each category or heading. Reread the summary until you are certain that every word in it is important and clearly communicates the outcomes of the project.

Abstract. An abstract is a very short description of the project and significant results. The purpose of the abstract is to give readers a glimpse of the main published work so they can decide whether it contains information they would find interesting or informative. Most journals are very prescriptive about the number of words and characters that may be included in an abstract. Look in the "Information for Authors" section of the journal. Some journals require as few as 200 words, making it difficult to discern which main concepts should go into this type of abstract. The author should keep in mind the purpose of the abstract: What would colleagues find interesting or informative about the project? Focusing on that will help you create a succinct and engaging abstract. Typically, the abstract should contain the introduction, method, results, and discussion (Ogrinc et al., 2015). Examples of abstracts from colleagues can be found in Chapter 12.

Peer-Reviewed Journals. If the audience for dissemination of the results of the project is a group of professionals in a similar practice setting, a peer-reviewed journal is an appropriate medium. Thousands of journals are on the market. The project leader must select the most appropriate.

For a more general project, select a journal that targets a broad base of professionals, such as the *American Journal of Nursing* or *Advanced Practice Nursing*. A more focused project should be submitted to the appropriate specialty journals. Look at several recent issues of the journal you believe may be the best for publication. Find articles that have similar subject matter to the topic you are presenting and read them to discern the style, format, and themes. Authors can also contact the editor-in-chief with the topic idea to see whether she or he believes it will be appropriate for the audience targeted by the journal. The journal will also note the publication manual used for their journal. That might be American Psychological Association, American Medical Association, Chicago, or Squire Guidelines.

The author of this chapter suggests the following methodology for writing for publication. You may find some of these tips to be helpful:

- Set a goal for publication that includes the desired journal, the target publication date, and how you will manage your time for writing.
- Good writing takes time. Set aside regular time when you can write quietly. The most difficult task will be to convey the most important findings in a four- to five-page article. Go through the major sections of your project and select the key highlights of each section to create an outline.
- Keep a folder of articles that you have cited. Make the citations in the text as you write. This is far easier than trying to go back and remember which articles support what sentences.
- Keep the material engaging. This is your chance to share important material with other professionals so they can learn about a project that improved a practice or some outcomes.
- Manuscript preparation is crucial to getting the article published. Most journals have information for authors that details how the manuscript must be prepared for that journal's editors to review it. Carefully follow those guidelines when preparing the manuscript. If questions arise, contact the journal's editorial assistant.
- Journals also have specific requirements for the abstract and keywords. Carefully follow the journal's requirements.
- Be meticulous about grammar and style. The editors will not accept an article with multiple grammar or style errors, and such errors diminish the scholarly quality of the work.
- After submission, expect feedback from expert reviewers. The feedback to the author is not intended to make the author feel good; it is intended to make the article stronger and more meaningful to the audience. In general, editors know their business well, and if you incorporate reviewer suggestions into the manuscript, it will be a better article.
- Be patient. This is a process that will take some time.
- Enjoy the results.

Other Professional Publications. Many other types of publications are not peer reviewed but may have a far larger audience. These include nonsubscription journals that come in the mail to practitioners, local publications, public media, and newspapers. All of these will be appropriate vehicles for dissemination of your outcomes if the audience is identified correctly. In general, the suggestions for peer-reviewed journals also apply to these types of publications. Reflect the scholarly nature of the project in all forms of communication.

Oral Dissemination

Nurses disseminate much information orally, and clear communication is imperative. Oral dissemination to professional audiences can be effective and oral communication gives the author the chance to express passion for the topic through voice tones and gestures. Oral dissemination opportunities include poster sessions, presentations, or lectures for professional meetings at the local, state, or national level, and presentations to population-based groups.

Preparing for oral presentations is a bit different from preparing written materials. Nevertheless, the successful presenter must identify the audience before beginning preparation, just as if the materials were being submitted to a peer-reviewed journal. Here are some tips from the chapter author on preparing oral presentations:

- Understand the setting for your presentation. If you are not familiar with the organization that requested the presentation, learn about the organization by visiting its website or reading the materials published by that organization.
- Contact an organizational officer or member of the board of directors for questions. Know why you were asked to present, what issues may underlie the presentation, the knowledge level of the audience on the topic, the organizational context, the topics of other speakers before or after the presentation, the timing of the presentation, and what is happening before or after the presentation (for example, if there is a business meeting preceding or following the presentation, the audience may be anxious about the impending meeting) (Guffey & Loewy, 2015).
- Review your project for main points and create an outline. Remember that the criteria for citations in oral presentations are the same as for written work. All the points in the presentation will need the same kind of strong support from the relevant literature. Do not use figures or tables unless you get permission from the authors. Cartoons also need permission from the author of the cartoon.
- Recognize that listening is different from reading and that it is difficult for most people to sit and listen for long periods. Thus, it is useful to change the style of presentation by interspersing scientific content with stories or case reports that break up the presentation but still present useful information in a different manner.
- Fill in the outline with the most important findings and results of the project. Be succinct. The rule of thumb is that every presentation should have three parts (Guffey & Loewy, 2015):
  - Tell the audience what you are going to say in the introduction.
  - Tell the audience the information most relevant to the project in the body of the presentation.
  - Recap your presentation in the conclusion.

Presentation Software Packages. Many presentation software packages are on the market. They will assist you in creating slides for your presentation, but the point of the slides is to enhance the oral presentation with a visual component, not to replace the oral materials. The slides should be simple and easy to read to avoid distracting the listeners from the oral materials. Each slide should cover one major point and have no more than seven lines with seven words on a line (Guffey & Loewy, 2015). Remember that many figures and tables are difficult to read when projected, so keep the tables simple and readable, or consider using bar graphs or pie charts instead of tables. Avoid using all caps—IT LOOKS AGGRESSIVE. The font size should be 24 points or larger for best readability (Guffey & Loewy, 2015). The slides should be free of grammatical errors, just as if the presentation were being published (often the presentation slides will be published for the attendees). Plan on no more than one slide per minute of presentation (Guffey & Loewy, 2015).

Tips for presenting to professional audiences include the following (adapted from Guffey & Loewy, 2015):

- Time your presentation carefully and rehearse it meticulously.
- Preparation is the key to a successful presentation. You cannot possibly rehearse too much.
- Learn to speak to the audience, not the slides.
- Check to ensure that all the embedded links work with the equipment at the site before the presentation begins.
- Bring a backup disc with the presentation materials on it.
- Get instruction on how to use the audiovisual equipment prior to the presentation.
- Establish a routine of self-care for the evening before the presentation to get a good night's rest and appear enthusiastic about the materials.
- Avoid drinking caffeinated beverages immediately before the presentation.
- Dress professionally but comfortably.

Electronic Venues for Dissemination

Electronic venues for dissemination are an exciting phenomena with options for virtual presentations expanding during the COVID-19 pandemic. Our society has quickly incorporated these forms of communication into our culture and language. One astounding example is social networking sites. SixDegrees.com was the first identifiable social network, established in 1997 (Boyd & Ellison, 2007). Since that time, the use of social networks has exploded and taken off in many different directions from the original intent of connecting friends electronically. As of this writing, there are literally hundreds of social networking sites with different purposes. Many professional organizations maintain a Facebook site, and there are thousands of informal social networking groups of professionals. Social networks are just one example of an electronic dissemination venue. Many more are available to the DNP student or practitioner who wants to disseminate project results to a specific audience. **Table 11-6** lists some of the available venues.

Table 11-6 Electronic Dissemination Venues

Formal	Informal
Peer-reviewed electronic journals	Blogs
Voice over network (VON) programs	Professional networks
Virtual/online conferences	Social networks
Podcasts	
Organizational/professional websites	
Patient education websites	
Websites with evidence-based guidelines (National Institute of Health, Agency for Healthcare Research and Quality)	

Use caution when publishing to social networks and other electronic media. There is little quality control over content, and most of these types of electronic tools are not peer reviewed. Once an article is published to many of these sites, the author has no control over where it goes or how it is used. Therefore, be cautious in publishing articles to a website or other electronic medium.

Summary

The DNP Project is not simply a requirement for a degree. At its finest, it should reflect a synthesis of all the knowledge and skills gained by the DNP student during their studies (AACN, 2021). It should also establish the basis for the student's future scholarly work—the scholarship of integration and application. The state of American health care will benefit enormously from a cadre of expert clinicians who can utilize evidence-based projects and tools to improve the outcomes of care delivered by APNs/DNPs.

Nevertheless, issues remain with the development and implementation of the project. NONPF (2013) outlined some significant issues and recommended beginning a national dialogue with advanced practice registered nurse stakeholders to accomplish the following:

- Delineate and clearly communicate the essence of the DNP project.
- Delineate and clearly communicate acceptable forms of the DNP project.
- Clarify and unify standards for DNP projects.

Since the initial publication of *The Essentials of Doctoral Education for Advanced Nursing Practice* (AACN, 2006), continued variation regarding DNP education has been noted. In 2015, an AACN task force was commissioned that offered further clarification regarding the doctorate of nursing practice, more specifically the DNP scholarly project. In 2021 the AACN, in *The Essentials: Core Competencies for Professional Nursing Education,* describes the DNP Project as (AACN, 2021):

> A scholarly work that aims to improve clinical practice . . . scholarly work should not be a separate disaggregated part of the plan of study. Instead, faculty should consider how the development of the scholarly work is integrated throughout the curriculum, allowing for dissemination of the results prior to program completion. (p. 25)

Ideally, this work provides the foundation for future scholarship in the student's chosen role as a doctorally prepared nurse. As elucidated by both the AACN (2015; 2021) and NONPF (2013), the expectations of the DNP Project have evolved over the past decade. What has remained constant is the unwavering expectation of practice scholarship at the doctoral level. The DNP-prepared nurse is well positioned to apply best practice from the bedside to the boardroom to the larger community. The AACN *Essentials* provide the competencies and curricular foundation for nurses prepared at the advanced practice nursing level of education. The final synthesis and application of these learnings in a unique practice setting, using QI tools and techniques, implementation science, policy analysis, or program evaluation methods will ensure that the DNP student is practicing at the highest level possible and is contributing to tangible improvements in health care.

References

Agency for Healthcare Research and Quality (AHRQ). (2017). *About the National Quality Strategy.* Author. https://www.ahrq.gov/workingforquality/about/index.html

Agency for Healthcare Research and Quality (AHRQ). (2022). *National healthcare quality and disparities reports.* Author. https://www.ahrq.gov/research/findings/nhqrdr/index.html

Allison, M., & Kaye, J. (2015). *Strategic planning for nonprofit organizations: A practical guide for dynamic times* (3rd ed.). Wiley.

American Association of Colleges of Nursing (AACN). (2015). *The doctor of nursing practice: Current issues and clarifying recommendations.* Author.

American Association of Colleges of Nursing (AACN). (2021). *The essentials: Core competencies for professional nursing education.* Author.

American Association of Colleges of Nursing (AACN). (2022). *Fact sheet: Nursing faculty shortage.* www.aacnnursing.org/News-Information/Fact-Sheets/Nursing-Faculty-Shortage

American Society for Quality (ASQ). (2022). *Learn about quality.* https://asq.org/quality-resources/pdca-cycle

Anderson, K. M., McLaughlin, M. K., Crowell, N. A., Fall-Dickson, J. M., White, K. A., Heitsler, E. T., Kesten, K. S., & Yearwood, E. L. (2019). Mentoring students engaging in scholarly projects and dissertation in doctoral nursing programs. *Nursing Outlook, 67,* 776-788.

Anthony, S., Duncan, D. S., & Siren, P. (2015). Zombie projects: How to find them and kill them. *Harvard Business Review.* https://hbr.org/2015/03/zombie-projects-how-to-find-them-and-kill-them

Aziz, E. E. (2015). *Project closing: The small process group with big impact.* Paper presented at PMI® Global Congress 2015—EMEA, London, England. Newtown Square, PA: Project Management Institute. https://www.pmi.org/learning/library/importance-of-closing-process-group-9949

Baker, S., Baker, K., & Campbell, G. (2003). *The complete idiot's guide to project management.* Alpha.

Bisgaard, S. (2008). Quality management and Juran's legacy. *Quality Engineering, 20,* 390–401.

Boyd, D. M., & Ellison, N. B. (2007). Social network sites: Definition, history, and scholarship. *Journal of Computer-Mediated Communication, 13*(1), article 11.

Boyer, E. (1990). *Scholarship reconsidered: Priorities of the professoriate.* Jossey-Bass.

Boyer, E. L. (1996). Clinical practice as scholarship. *Holistic Nursing Practice, 10*(3), 1–6.

Burroughs, C., & Wood, F. (2000). *Measuring the difference: Guide to planning and evaluation of health information outreach.* National Network of Libraries of Medicine.

Carroll, L. (1865). *Alice in wonderland.* MacMillan.

Corey, J. S, Roussel, L., Zellefrow, C., & Guthrie, S. (2022). National practices regarding doctor of nursing practice projects. *The Journal of Doctoral Nursing Practice, 15*(3), 131–136.

Daneshgari, P., & Parvin, S. (2022, June). The secret to better project control. *EC&M.* https://www.ecmweb.com/construction/article/21242584/project-management-best-practices-on-electrical-job-sites

DMAIC versus DMADV. (n.d.). *iSixSigma.* https://www.isixsigma.com/new-to-six-sigma/design-for-six-sigma-dfss/dmaic-versus-dmadv/

Duke University Department of Community and Family Medicine. (2021). *Methods of quality improvement?* https://josieking.org/patientsafety/module_a/methods/methods.html

Eccles, M. P., & Mittman, B. S. (2006). Welcome to implementation science. *Implementation Science, 1*(1), 1–3.

Edwardson, S. (2009, January 14). *MN/DNP colloquium.* Colloquium conducted at the University of Minnesota School of Nursing, Minneapolis, Minnesota.

Facione, P., & Facione, N. (2008). "Critical thinking and clinical judgment," from *Critical Thinking and Clinical Reasoning in the Health Sciences: A Teaching Anthology*, 2008. pp. 1–13. Published by Insight Assessment/The California Academic Press.

Felsenstein, D. R. (2018). Enhancing lesbian, gay, bisexual, and transgender cultural competence in a Midwestern primary care clinic setting. *Journal for Nurses in Professional Development, 34*(3), 142.

Fischer, F., Lange, K., Klose, K., Greiner, W., & Kraemer, A., (2016). Barriers and strategies in guideline implementation – A scoping review. *Healthcare, 4,*(36). doi: 10.3390/healthcare4030036

Fixsen, D. L., Naoom, S. R., Blase, K. A., Friedman, R. M., & Wallace F. (2005). *Implementation research: A synthesis of the literature.* University of South Florida, Louis de la Parte Florida

Mental Health Institute, National Implementation Research Network (FMHI Publication No 231), Tampa, FL.

Fixsen, D., Blase, K., Metz, A., & Van Dyke, M. (2015). Implementation science. In D. Fixsen (Ed)., *International encyclopedia of the social & behavioral sciences* (2nd ed., Volume 11, pp. 695–702). Elsevier.

Guffey, M., & Loewy, D. (2015). *Business communication: Process and product* (8th ed.). South-Western.

Institute of Medicine (IOM). (2001). *Crossing the quality chasm: A new health system for the 21st century*. National Academies Press.

Internal Revenue Service (IRS). (2022). *Publication 463: Travel, entertainment, gifts, and car expenses.* https://www.irs.gov/forms-pubs-search?search=463

Issel, L., Wells, R., & Williams, M. (2022). *Health program planning and evaluation: A practical, systematic approach for community health* (5th ed.). Jones and Bartlett.

Juran, J. M. (1986, May 20). *The quality trilogy: A universal approach for managing for quality* [Paper presentation]. ASQC 40th Annual Quality Congress, Anaheim, CA, United States.

Kirchner, J. E., Smith, J. L., Powell, B. J., Waltz, T. J., & Proctor, E. K. (2020). Getting a clinical innovation into practice: An introduction to implementation strategies. *Psychiatry Research, 283*, 112467.

Lavis, J., Robertson, D., Woodside, J., McLeod, C., & Abelson, J. (2003). How can research organizations more effectively transfer research knowledge to decision makers? *The Milbank Quarterly, 18*(2), 221–248.

Lewin, K. (1951). *Field theory in social science*. Harper Row.

Lewis, J. (2007). *Fundamentals of project management* (3rd ed.). American Management Association.

Luecke, R. (2004). *Managing projects large and small*. Harvard Business School Press.

Mandelbaum, J., Williams, H. W., & Hermes, A. C. (2010). *Value engineering synergies with lean six sigma*. Institute for Defense Analyses (IDA), IDA Paper P4586.

Metz, A., Burke, K., Albers, B., Louison, L., & Bartley, L. (2020). *A practice guide to supporting implementation: What competencies do we need?* National Research Implementation Network, ED610571.

Mind Tools Content Team. (2022a). Stakeholder analysis: Winning support for your projects. *Mind Tools*. https://www.mindtools.com/aol0rms/stakeholder-analysis

Mind Tools Content Team. (2022b). SWOT analysis: Discover new opportunities, manage and eliminate threats. *Mind Tools*. http://www.mindtools.com/pages/article/newTMC_05.htm

Mind Tools Content Team. (2022c). Work breakdown structures: Mapping out the work within a project. *Mind Tools*. www.mindtools.com/pages/article/newPPM_91.htm

National Organization of Nurse Practitioner Faculties (NONPF). (2007). *NONPF recommended criteria for NP scholarly projects in the practice doctorate program*. www.nonpf.org/associations/10789 /files/ScholarlyProjectCriteria.pdf

National Organization of Nurse Practitioner Faculties (NONPF). (2013). *Titling of the doctor of nursing practice project*. https://cdn.ymaws.com/www.nonpf.org/resource/resmgr/dnp/dnpprojects titlingpaperjune2.pdf

Ogrinc, G., Davies, L., Goodman, D., Batalden, P., Davidoff, F., & Stevens, D. (2015). SQUIRE 2.0 (Standards for QUality Improvement Reporting Excellence): Revised publication guidelines from a detailed consensus process. *BMJ Quality & Safety, 25*(12). https://doi.org/10.1136/bmjqs -2015-004411

Olney, C., & Barnes, S. (2006). *Including evaluation in outreach project planning*. National Network of Libraries of Medicine.

Olney, C., & Barnes, S. (2013). *Collecting and analyzing evaluation data* (2nd ed., Booklet 3). Seattle, WA: National Network of Libraries of Medicine.

Polit, D., & Beck, C. (2021). *Nursing research: Generating and assessing evidence for nursing practice* (11th ed.). Wolters Kluwer.

The Project Proposal Toolkit. (2018). Homepage. http://project-proposal.casual.pm/

Rosenbaum, S. (2011). The patient protection and affordable care act: Implications for public health policy and practice. *Law and the Public's Health, 126*, 130–135.

Ross, J. (2017). *Total quality management: Text, cases, and readings* (3rd ed.). eBook. Routledge.

Rouda, R., & Kusy, M. (1995). *Development of human resources part 2: Needs assessment, the first step*. Technical Association of the Pulp and Paper Industry.

Sipes, C. (2019). *Project management for the advanced practice nurse* (2nd ed.). Springer.

Spielman, E. (2022). *Direct costs versus indirect costs: What are they, and how are they different?* https://www.businessnewsdaily.com/5498-direct-costs-indirect-costs.html

Starbird, L. E., Frick, K., Cohen, C., & Stone, P. (2021). Analyzing economic outcomes in advanced practice nursing. In R. Kleinpell (Ed.), *Outcome assessment in advanced practice nursing* (5th ed., pp. 20–44). Springer.

Taylor-Powell, E., & Henert, E. (2008). *Developing a logic model: Teaching and training guide*. University of Wisconsin-Extension Cooperative Extension www.betterevaluation.org/en/resources/guide/develop_a_logic_model

Thomas, J. (1985). Force field analysis: A new way to evaluate your strategy. *Long Range Planning, 18*(6), 54–59.

Tuckman, B. W. (1965). Developmental sequence in small groups. *Psychological Bulletin. 63*(6), 384–399. https://doi.org/10.1037/h0022100. PMID 14314073

Ungar, W. J. (2016). A further examination of the problem of double-counting in incremental cost-utility analysis. *Expert Review of Pharmacoenconomics & Outcomes Research, 16*(3), 333–335.

Van Dyke, M., Kiser, L., & Blase, K. (2019). *The heptagon tool: Exploring context*. Active Implementation Research Network.

Waddick, P. (2010). *Six sigma DMAIC quick reference: Define phase*. https://www.isixsigma.com/new-to-six-sigma/dmaic/six-sigma-dmaic-quick-reference/

W. K. Kellogg Foundation. (2004a). *Evaluation handbook*. Author.

W. K. Kellogg Foundation. (2004b). *Logic model development guide*. Battle Creek, MI: Author.

Zaccagnini, M. (2007). *The development of a computer-resourced communication center in a long-term care facility* (Unpublished DNP scholarly project paper). University of Minnesota, Minneapolis, MN.

CHAPTER 12

DNP Project Types and Abstracts

Diane M. Schadewald, DNP, MSN, RN, WHNP-BC, FNP-BC, CNE

It's a bad plan that admits of no modification.

—Publilius Syrus

This chapter contains additional information about doctor of nursing practice (DNP) project types and some abstract examples of DNP Projects. The vast majority of DNP projects have followed a quality improvement (QI) or evidence-based project (EBP) format with these formats being the only acceptable formats for some academic institutions. However, for those pursuing a DNP in public health, a program evaluation format may be more pertinent for the degree and for those pursuing a DNP in health policy, a policy analysis format would perhaps fit best for the student's DNP project. The American Association of Colleges of Nursing (AACN) has provided key elements for a DNP project as listed in **Box 12-1** and acknowledges that DNP projects can take on different forms as long as the key elements are met by the project (AACN, 2021). Various format frameworks for EBP and QI projects, such as the Iowa model (Titler 2002), the PARiHS framework (Rycroft-Malone, et al., 2013) and Plan, Do, Study, Act, to name a few, are widely known as well as being described in other chapters of this text. Because information about the QI and EBP frameworks has already been covered in this text, no further guidance or description about these format approaches for DNP projects will be included in this chapter. Moran et al. (2024) have proposed a few other DNP project formats such as healthcare delivery innovation, clinical or practice-based inquiry, and demonstration project; however, these DNP project types will also not be elaborated on here. This chapter will include information about developing program evaluation and policy analysis type DNP projects as well as sharing an abstract example of a combination program evaluation/QI project and an abstract example of a policy analysis project. Three QI abstracts examples are also shared at the end of the chapter.

Box 12-1 AACN Key Elements for DNP Projects

Problem identification
Search, analysis, synthesis of literature and evidence
Translating evidence to create a strategy or method to address the problem
    identified
Design of plan for implementation
Implementation of plan if possible to implement
Evaluation of outcomes, process, and/or experience

Data from AACN (2021) *The Essentials: Core Competencies for Professional Nursing Education,* (p. 25), Author.

Program Evaluation

One format approach that may be used for guidance of a DNP project based on a program evaluation is the CDC's *Framework for Program Evaluation in Public Health.* The framework is available at the web address: https://www.cdc.gov/eval/guide /introduction/index.htm. The evaluation consists of six steps: (1) engage stakeholders, (2) describe the program, (3) focus the evaluation design, (4) gather credible evidence, (5) justify conclusions, and (6) ensure use and share lessons learned. Four standards—utility (ability to share the results in a timely manner), feasibility (degree realistic given available resources), propriety (protection of rights of participants), and accuracy (yield of reliable and valid results)—are also to be considered at each step of the evaluation (CDC, 1999). The steps and standards of the CDC program evaluation framework are similar to those used in development of QI and EBP DNP projects and appear to meet the AACN's key elements for a DNP project. Other methods considered appropriate for program evaluation include surveys, interviews, and focus groups (Moran et al., 2024).

A past DNP advisee of this author adapted the CDC's *Framework for Program Evaluation in Public Health* to evaluate a collaborative care model that had been newly instituted in a clinic setting. As part of the project the student implemented the recommendations that were drawn from the evaluation of the model and analyzed the impact that implementation of the recommendations had on the clinic setting (Jorgensen, 2020). Another past DNP advisee of this author, whose project abstract is included as the first abstract in this chapter, used an initial program evaluation approach through a survey to inform development of the intervention for a QI project (Grochowski, 2018). So, the completed DNP projects described in this paragraph were a combination of program evaluation and QI. However, these two examples of inclusion of a program evaluation as an initial component for a QI DNP project aren't meant to imply that a rigorous program evaluation on its own could not be considered sufficient for a DNP project.

Policy Analysis

Two frameworks for policy analysis that could be considered for DNP project format guidance include Bardach and Patashnik's (2020) eightfold path and McLaughlin and McLaughlin's (2019) interdisciplinary approach. Both of these policy analysis approaches start with defining the problem, similar to what is recommended as the

Table 12-1 Comparison of Policy Analysis Approaches

Bardach & Patashnik	McLaughlin & McLaughlin
Define the problem	Identification and definition
Assemble evidence	Process definition
Construct the alternatives	Process analysis
Select the criteria for analysis	Qualitative analysis
Project the outcomes	Evaluation and choice
Confront the trade-offs	Implementation strategy
Stop, focus, narrow, deepen, decide	Implementation planning
Tell your story	Feedback on policy processes

Data from Bardach, E. & Patashnik, E. M. (2020). *A practical guide for policy analysis: The eightfold path to more effective problem solving*, 6th ed, Sage CQ Press; McLaughlin, C. P. & McLaughlin, C. D. (2019). *Health policy analysis: An interdisciplinary approach*, 3rd ed., Jones & Bartlett Learning

required first key element identified by the AACN (2021) (see Box 12-1). **Table 12-1** includes a list of the steps of these two policy analysis processes for comparison. The policy analysis approaches include a literature search to find evidence and alternatives (Bardach & Patashnik, 2020) or to provide definition and analysis of the identified problem's process (McLaughlin & McLaughlin, 2019), both of which match the AACN's second key element for a DNP project. The analysis steps meet the third key AACN DNP project element by involving translation of the evidence and projection of outcomes. Bardach and Patashnik's confronting the trade-offs and McLaughlin and McLaughlin's implementation planning address the fourth and fifth AACN key elements for a project. Both of the policy analysis approaches end with sharing the outcome of the analysis and being receptive to feedback. Sharing the outcome of the analysis and receiving feedback may be considered as meeting the final AACN key element. Therefore, either of these frameworks could work for DNP project guidance.

Kingdon's model of policy change might also be useful as a guide or conceptual framework for development of a policy analysis DNP project. Kingdon describes three streams—the problem stream, the policy stream, and the political stream—and posits that these streams must converge to provide a window of opportunity for policy change (Cairney & Jones, 2016; Giese, 2020). Policy change starts with identification of a problem (the problem stream) and clearly describing it to those who can effect a change. Development of solutions to the problem involves the policy stream, with such solutions being stronger when evidence exists to support the proposed solution. Timing of the proposed change involves the political stream which can be influenced by opinion or response to a current event. Giese (2020) describes how the COVID-19 pandemic provided a window of opportunity for expansion of telehealth services. There was existing evidence that telehealth could work for delivery of health care (policy stream), lack of ability to provide outpatient services (problem stream), and the political will to address the problem (political stream). Please see **Figure 12-1** for how Kingdon's model may be applied to the AACN's key elements for a DNP project.

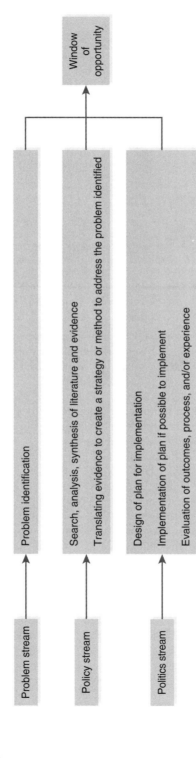

Figure 12-1 Kingdon's Three Streams Applied to AACN's Key Elements for a DNP Project

Data from AACN (2021) The Essentials: Core Competencies for Professional Nursing Education. (p. 25) Author & Cairney, P. & Jones, M.D. (2016). Kingdon's multiple streams approach: What is the empirical impact of this universal theory. *Policy Studies Journal, 44*(1), 37–58

Abstracts

Identifying Barriers to Self-Care Management in Hispanic Diabetic Patients

Provided by Suelhem A. Grochowski, DNP, RN, FNP-BC, APNP

Background

Uncontrolled diabetes mellitus type 2 (DM2) can have detrimental effects on quality of life. Self-care management (SCM) plays a pivotal role in managing DM2. Minority populations such as Hispanic adults (HA) tend to have a higher prevalence of DM2 and experience greater burden in attaining metabolic control. DM2 relies on an individual's mastering self-efficacy for management of their disease and a long-term commitment to avoid health complications. Clinic A was experiencing a high number of uncontrolled DM2 patients even with abundant DM2 resources available.

Methods

A program evaluation of Clinic A's approach to diabetic care was performed to identify barriers to SCM. A QI project was implemented focused on overcoming barriers to SCM in DM2 HA identified by the program evaluation.

Intervention

An SCM questionnaire based on the Pender's Health Belief Model was given to the HA DM2 patients to identify barriers. The healthcare staff also completed a questionnaire to assess their beliefs regarding contributing factors in poor glycemic control. Based on the results of the questionnaires, structured clinical vignettes were implemented. Effectiveness of the vignettes was measured to determine if overall glycemic control improved.

Results

There was a statistically significant difference between controlled and uncontrolled DM2 patients in regard to medication adherence ($p < .041$) and disease management at home ($p < .033$). The common themes identified between patients and providers were the need for increased education, resources, and lifestyle changes options. Unfortunately, the clinical vignettes did not have a positive impact on A1C levels.

Conclusion

The QI project identified several SCM barriers that the clinic has encountered, suggesting the important role SCM plays in managing a chronic disease such as DM2. SCM of DM2 is complex and multifactorial; therefore it is crucial to have resources to assist patients in overcoming such barriers.

Road Map to Reduce Barriers to Medical Aid in Dying for Rural Coloradans: A Health Policy Analysis and Advocacy Campaign

Provided by Ashley D. Fry, DNP, AGACNP-BC, ACHPN

Background

Medical aid in dying (MAID) is a process by which a terminally ill adult with a prognosis of six months or less can request prescription medication to end their life. Colorado's End-of-Life Options Act requires that two physicians participate in the process to certify terminal illness and prescribe medications. Nearly all rural and frontier counties face shortages of medical professionals. These conditions challenge rural residents who want to access MAID. Advanced practice registered nurses and physician assistants can address gaps in rural and frontier counties; on average, they outnumber physicians in these communities.

Aims

The aims of this health policy project were to increase awareness among state legislators of challenges rural Coloradans encounter when accessing MAID, educate legislators on useful measures for reducing barriers to access, and provide suitable language for amending Colorado's End-of-Life Option Act.

Methods

The design of this project was a governmental policy analysis and a campaign to build legislative awareness. The project employed interactions with stakeholders through in-person and virtual meetings, email, and phone calls.

Results

A total of 50 legislators from both major political parties were provided information on the barriers to patient access. They included rural and frontier legislators, members of the House Health & Insurance Committee, the Senate Health & Insurance Committee, among others. A total of 83 contacts with these legislators occurred over four months, escalating once the legislature was in session. Several legislators volunteered to support the bill if prime sponsorship could be obtained. Two legislators expressed interest in potentially serving as prime sponsors.

Conclusion

Numerous legislators were not familiar with the details of Colorado's End-of-Life Options Act, nor were they aware of access challenges. These legislators shared an appreciation for constituents' feedback and engagement. Building a statewide coalition will drive ongoing efforts to amend the Colorado End-of-Life Options Act.

Improving Compliance with Delirium Interventions Through APRN Consultation

Provided by Amy Heidenreich, DNP, RN, AGCNS-BC, PMHNP-BC, APNP

Background

Delirium is the most common psychiatric condition in hospitals leading to a longer length of stay (LOS), increased costs, and patient acuities. Patients with delirium have an average LOS of 11.6 days. Decreasing delirium incidence by 10% would save about 3,676 patient days per year. The National Institute for Health and Care Excellence (NICE) Guideline delirium bundle was a new initiative at the project site and uptake was slow. Staff were challenged with implementing the interventions for patients. Evidence supported use of APRN consultation to enhance outcomes with delirium.

Methods

This QI project utilized the APRN Project Leader as a consultant to increase knowledge of delirium and interventions, increase bundle compliance, and impact LOS, number of delirious days, and rates of delirium.

Intervention

An educational session and a pre–post knowledge survey was administered to staff on one medical unit. For 6 weeks, the APRN Project Leader performed consultations, providing recommendations from the NICE delirium bundle interventions for patients with positive delirium screening. Staff implemented the recommendations and documented per standards of care.

Results

Consultations were performed on 18 patients with average of 2.9 consultations/visits lasting an average of 43 minutes. Patients with delirium experienced a significant decrease in duration of delirium from 26.5% to 16.9% of their stay, $z=8.0$, $p < .001$. There was a clinically significant decrease in LOS of 2.7 days per patient by decreasing the duration of delirium. Compliance with delirium interventions was mixed. Nurses' confidence with delirium and the interventions significantly improved $p < .001$ and nurses on the medical unit saw value in APRN consultation.

Conclusion

An APRN consultant for delirium could be a cost-saving model of care to decrease LOS and increase the quality of care provided. Nurses struggle with implementing delirium interventions and an APRN consultation can help decrease barriers.

Implementation of Asynchronous Electronic Nurse Handoff From ED to OR

Provided by Emily Bartel, DNP, FNP-BC, APNP

Background

At the project site, handoff between ED and OR RNs often lacked all pertinent information, causing case delays, discontent among nurses, and threats to patient safety. Also, the ED RN was often uninformed of a patient's upcoming procedure. Hospitals have been implementing asynchronous electronic handoff from the ED to inpatient floors with shown benefits, and standardization of the RN handoff is recommended in literature.

Methods

A QI project using the plan-do-study-act framework and PRECEED-PROCEED theory was implemented. Data on RN satisfaction, process failure, and verification that the ED RN was notified was collected. Project implementation tools included a pre- and post-implementation RN survey, an ED2OR Handoff SmartText within Epic, and a process failure tracking tool.

Intervention

Before implementing the new handoff process, the ED and OR RNs were educated on the new handoff process. A paper bulletin was also posted when the project was implemented to inform the ED RNs of the SmartText name in Epic and to start using the new handoff note in practice. After implementation, the ED2OR Handoff Committee members were available for questions, problems, and concerns as they arose. Process failure was defined as a missing/incomplete ED2OR Handoff note.

Results

The ED2OR Handoff note, especially when properly used, was shown to have the ability to increase RN satisfaction ($p < 0.05$). However, the ED2OR Handoff Note did not show a significant increase in completeness over the course of implementation. Similarly, there was not a significant increase in timely completion of the note nor ED RN notification of the upcoming procedure.

Conclusion

While no significant increase in completeness of the ED2OR Handoff Note resulted, the percent of completed ED2OR Handoff Notes in a week was trending upward. The organization plans on future efforts to focus on strategies to increase compliance with the new handoff process.

Implementation of an Educational Booklet for Patients With Liver Cirrhosis

Provided by Megan Galske, DNP, RN, AGPCNP-BC, APNP

Background

Self-management of cirrhosis is difficult due to its complexity and systemic symptoms. Patients with liver cirrhosis are often confused about symptoms, medications, and treatment recommendations. The confusion leads to frequent phone calls and lack of compliance with treatment recommendations. The project's aim was to decrease phone calls to the hepatology care manager (HCM) and improve patient compliance with hepatocellular carcinoma (HCC) screening by increasing disease state knowledge and self-management of cirrhosis.

Methods

This quality improvement project was guided by the plan-do-study-act (PDSA) model. Over the 2 months of intervention the number of phone calls to the HCM and patient compliance with HCC screening were tracked.

Intervention

An educational booklet adapted from Dr. Michael Volk's "Liver Cirrhosis Toolkit" was reviewed with and provided to every patient seen in clinic with a diagnosis of liver cirrhosis over the course of 2 months. The booklet was also put into a folder for patients to take home for future reference. The booklet was adapted for those with compensated cirrhosis and decompensated cirrhosis. The booklet was also evaluated for readability using the Simple Measure of Gobbledygook (SMOG) and revised to a sixth-grade reading level.

Results

Phone call volumes decreased; however, this finding was not statistically significant. HCC screening rates improved but also not significantly. However, 100% of providers who participated in the project felt that the booklet decreased unnecessary phone calls from patients with cirrhosis and helped to streamline disease state education with these patients.

Conclusion

The targeted educational intervention in this project was considered useful to improve disease state knowledge and decrease unnecessary phone calls. Despite results not achieving statistical significance, findings trended in a positive direction with phone call volumes decreasing and HCC screening compliance increasing throughout the implementation phase.

Summary

This chapter has described some frameworks for students and faculty to use for developing and guiding a DNP project that is not QI or EBP-based and is meant to serve as supplementary and complementary guidance to the template provided in Chapter 11. Faculty advising students should have experience that is appropriate for the project type; however, mentors outside of the academic setting can be sought to provide support as or if needed (AACN, 2021).

References

American Association of Colleges of Nursing. (2021). *The Essentials: Core competencies for professional nursing education.* Author.

Bardach, E., & Patashnik, E. M. (2020). *A practical guide for policy analysis: The eightfold path to more effective problem solving* (6th ed.). Sage CQ Press.

Cairney, P., & Jones, M. D. (2016). Kingdon's multiple streams approach: What is the empirical impact of this universal theory? *Policy Studies Journal, 44*(1), 37–58.

Centers for Disease Control and Prevention [CDC]. (1999). *Office of policy, performance, and evaluation.* https://www.cdc.gov/eval/guide/introduction/index.htm

Giese, K. (2020) Coronavirus disease 2019's shake-up of telehealth policy: Application of Kindgon's multiple streams framework. *The Journal for Nurse Practitioners, 16,* 768–770.

Grochowski, S. (2018). *Identifying Barriers to Self-Care Management in Hispanic Diabetic Patients.* (Unpublished DNP Project Paper), University of Wisconsin-Milwaukee, Milwaukee, WI.

Jorgensen, A. (2020). *Evaluation of a collaborative care like-model and Versus technology* (Unpublished DNP Project Paper). University of Wisconsin-Milwaukee, Milwaukee, WI.

McLaughlin, C. P., & McLaughlin, C. D. (2019). *Health policy analysis: An interdisciplinary approach* (3rd ed.). Jones & Bartlett Learning

Moran, K., Burson, R., & Conrad, D. (2024). *The doctor of nursing practice project: A framework for success* (4th ed.). Jones & Bartlett Learning.

Rycroft-Malone, J., Sears, K., Chandler, J., Hawkes, C. A., Crichton, N., Allen, C., . . . Strunin, L. (2013). The role of evidence context and facilitation in an implementation trial: Implications for the development of the PARIHS framework. *Implementation Science, 8,* (28). https://doi.org/10.1186/1748-5908-8-28

Titler, M. G. (2002). Use of research in practice. In G. LoBiondo & J. Haber (Eds.), *Nursing research methods: Critical appraisal and utilization* (5th ed., pp. 410–431). Mosby.

Index

Note: Page numbers followed by "*b*," "*f*," and "*t*" indicate boxes, figures, and tables, respectively.